Improving Adolescent Dietary Behaviour

Improving Adolescent Dietary Behaviour

Special Issue Editor
Charlotte E.L. Evans

MDPI • Basel • Beijing • Wuhan • Barcelona • Belgrade • Manchester • Tokyo • Cluj • Tianjin

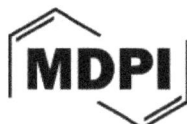

Special Issue Editor
Charlotte E.L. Evans
University of Leeds
UK

Editorial Office
MDPI
St. Alban-Anlage 66
4052 Basel, Switzerland

This is a reprint of articles from the Special Issue published online in the open access journal *Nutrients* (ISSN 2072-6643) (available at: https://www.mdpi.com/journal/nutrients/special_issues/adolescent_diet).

For citation purposes, cite each article independently as indicated on the article page online and as indicated below:

LastName, A.A.; LastName, B.B.; LastName, C.C. Article Title. *Journal Name* **Year**, *Article Number*, Page Range.

ISBN 978-3-03928-336-1 (Hbk)
ISBN 978-3-03928-337-8 (PDF)

© 2020 by the authors. Articles in this book are Open Access and distributed under the Creative Commons Attribution (CC BY) license, which allows users to download, copy and build upon published articles, as long as the author and publisher are properly credited, which ensures maximum dissemination and a wider impact of our publications.

The book as a whole is distributed by MDPI under the terms and conditions of the Creative Commons license CC BY-NC-ND.

Contents

About the Special Issue Editor vii

Charlotte E. L. Evans
Next Steps for Interventions Targeting Adolescent Dietary Behaviour
Reprinted from: *Nutrients* **2019**, *12*, 190, doi:10.3390/nu12010190 1

Stephanie Scott, Wafa Elamin, Emma L. Giles, Frances Hillier-Brown, Kate Byrnes, Natalie Connor, Dorothy Newbury-Birch and Louisa Ells
Socio-Ecological Influences on Adolescent (Aged 10–17) Alcohol Use and Unhealthy Eating Behaviours: A Systematic Review and Synthesis of Qualitative Studies
Reprinted from: *Nutrients* **2019**, *11*, 1914, doi:10.3390/nu11081914 5

Lorraine McSweeney, Jen Bradley, Ashley J. Adamson and Suzanne Spence
The 'Voice' of Key Stakeholders in a School Food and Drink Intervention in Two Secondary Schools in NE England: Findings from a Feasibility Study
Reprinted from: *Nutrients* **2019**, *11*, 2746, doi:10.3390/nu11112746 23

Maya Kamar, Charlotte Evans and Siobhan Hugh-Jones
Factors Influencing British Adolescents' Intake of Whole Grains: A Pilot Feasibility Study Using SenseCam Assisted Interviews
Reprinted from: *Nutrients* **2019**, *11*, 2620, doi:10.3390/nu11112620 35

Lucille Desbouys, Karin De Ridder, Manon Rouche and Katia Castetbon
Food Consumption in Adolescents and Young Adults: Age-Specific Socio-Economic and Cultural Disparities (Belgian Food Consumption Survey 2014)
Reprinted from: *Nutrients* **2019**, *11*, 1520, doi:10.3390/nu11071520 51

Shaojing Sun, Jinbo He and Xitao Fan
Mapping and Predicting Patterns of Chinese Adolescents' Food Preferences
Reprinted from: *Nutrients* **2019**, *11*, 2124, doi:10.3390/nu11092124 67

Guri Skeie, Vårin Sandvær and Guri Grimnes
Intake of Sugar-Sweetened Beverages in Adolescents from Troms, Norway—The Tromsø Study: *Fit Futures*
Reprinted from: *Nutrients* **2019**, *11*, 211, doi:10.3390/nu11020211 81

Joanna Myszkowska-Ryciak, Anna Harton, Ewa Lange, Wacław Laskowski and Danuta Gajewska
Nutritional Behaviors of Polish Adolescents: Results of the Wise Nutrition—Healthy Generation Project
Reprinted from: *Nutrients* **2019**, *11*, 1592, doi:10.3390/nu11071592 97

Heidi T. Lai, Jayne Hutchinson and Charlotte E.L. Evans
Non-Milk Extrinsic Sugars Intake and Food and Nutrient Consumption Patterns among Adolescents in the UK National Diet and Nutrition Survey, Years 2008–16
Reprinted from: *Nutrients* **2019**, *11*, 1621, doi:10.3390/nu11071621 113

María Isabel Santaló, Sandra Gibbons and Patti-Jean Naylor
Using Food Models to Enhance Sugar Literacy among Older Adolescents: Evaluation of a Brief Experiential Nutrition Education Intervention
Reprinted from: *Nutrients* **2019**, *11*, 1763, doi:10.3390/nu11081763 131

Matheus Mistura, Nicole Fetterly, Ryan E. Rhodes, Dona Tomlin and Patti-Jean Naylor
Examining the Efficacy of a 'Feasible' Nudge Intervention to Increase the Purchase of Vegetables by First Year University Students (17–19 Years of Age) in British Columbia: A Pilot Study
Reprinted from: *Nutrients* **2019**, *11*, 1786, doi:10.3390/nu11081786 . . . . **147**

Melissa Pflugh Prescott, Xanna Burg, Jessica Jarick Metcalfe, Alexander E. Lipka, Cameron Herritt and Leslie Cunningham-Sabo
Healthy Planet, Healthy Youth: A Food Systems Education and Promotion Intervention to Improve Adolescent Diet Quality and Reduce Food Waste
Reprinted from: *Nutrients* **2019**, *11*, 1869, doi:10.3390/nu11081869 . . . . **159**

About the Special Issue Editor

Charlotte E.L. Evans, Ph.D., (Associate Professor in Nutritional Epidemiology and Public Health Nutrition) has more than 20 years' experience in research exploring child and adolescent diet and health. She has a particular interest in improving dietary quality for optimum health in children and young people with the poorest diets. The main aims of her research are to improve the food environment, particularly in and around schools, and to make the healthier choice the easy choice. Another key area of her research is the evaluation of programs and policies to improve diet quality, such as increasing fruit and vegetable consumption and decreasing free sugars. She has more than 100 publications including papers, book chapters, and conference abstracts. She has spoken at international conferences and has presented at the UK All Party Parliamentary Group on School Food. In 2016, she was awarded the Elsie Widdowson Medal for contributions to Public Health Nutrition by the UK Nutrition Society. She regularly features on national and international television, radio, and in newspaper articles as a nutritional expert including the BBC, Sky, Channel 4, and Channel 5 news.

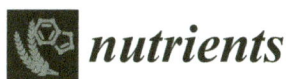

Editorial

Next Steps for Interventions Targeting Adolescent Dietary Behaviour

Charlotte E. L. Evans

School of Food Science and Nutrition, University of Leeds, Leeds LS2 9JT, UK; c.e.l.evans@leeds.ac.uk

Received: 10 December 2019; Accepted: 5 January 2020; Published: 9 January 2020

Abstract: Adolescents in many countries consume poor quality diets that include high intakes of sugary drinks and fast food and low intakes of vegetables. The aims of this Special Issue on adolescent dietary behaviour were to identify methods and approaches for successful interventions to improve diet quality in this age group and identify at risk subgroups that need particular attention. In total, 11 manuscripts were published in this Special Issue—three qualitative studies which included a systematic review, five cross-sectional studies and three quantitative evaluations of interventions. This Editorial discusses the contribution of the studies and provides suggestions to improve the success of future interventions in adolescents. It is important that adolescents are involved in the design of interventions to improve social and cultural acceptability and relevance. Interventions targeting schools or communities framed within a larger food system such as issues around climate change and the carbon footprint of food may improve engagement. Furthermore, targeting adolescents in areas of lower deprivation is a priority where diet quality is particularly poor. Potentially successful interventions also include environmental policies that impact on the cost and marketing of food and drinks, although evaluations of these were not included in this issue.

Keywords: intervention; adolescent; dietary behaviour; education; environment; nutrition policy; sugary drinks; vegetables

---

Next Steps for Interventions Targeting Adolescent Dietary Behaviour

Diets of adolescents in many countries are of poor quality when compared to those of younger and older age groups; higher in fats and sugars and lower in vegetables [1]. Intakes of fast food outside the home are often higher [2]; members of this age group are more likely to start engaging in risky behaviour including drinking alcohol and they are usually concerned with the views and opinions of their peers as well as their family [3]. This is an important age group to target as poor diet habits may persist into adulthood and increase the risk in the future of non-communicable diseases such as type 2 diabetes, cardiovascular disease and cancers [4]. These adolescents are also future parents and, therefore, good dietary habits can potentially be passed on to the next generation. This Special Issue focuses on evidence to help target and improve adolescent diet either through individual intervention or through environment-based policies. The issue includes three types of manuscripts which provide a wealth of information to inform future intervention programmes and policies targeting this age group. These are discussed below in turn, followed by a synthesis of the learnings from the body of evidence presented. First, the qualitative research from three papers based on alcohol (a systematic review), wholegrain foods (individual interviews) and school food (stakeholder focus groups) is reviewed. Second, five cross-sectional studies that include information on diet quality and dietary patterns in adolescents from five different countries are discussed. Third, three interventions based in the US and Canada targeting adolescents are examined.

Qualitative research is an important, although under-utilised, part of the process of designing successful interventions and can ensure that evaluation trials are more effective and efficient [5].

The review of qualitative research on adolescent behaviour and opinions related to alcohol in this issue was enlightening. It highlighted the difficulties and complexities inherent in influencing adolescent behaviour which includes dietary behaviour [3]. The tensions between restraint and fun, which may be due to acting on family values and beliefs versus those held by groups of peers, are high in this age group. Conflicting behaviour and views are common, leaving adolescents in challenging positions where they are expected to join in and drink and eat fast food but still maintain a healthy lifestyle and not get drunk or be overweight [3]. The review also highlighted the high rate of personal problems at this age, which may well mean that immediate mental health issues are far more of a priority than long-term physical health. Further and much-needed qualitative work from secondary schools highlighted the fact that most adolescents would choose unhealthier foods if available but primarily wanted food that was easy to purchase and carry around [6]. The challenge is to design one-pot portable meals that, unlike fast food, are not deep fried and do contain useful amounts of vegetables. Innovative methodology using a SenseCam camera to collect data reported on barriers and facilitators to improve wholegrain intake revealed that knowledge is often patchy but poor availability of healthy products aimed at this age group made it particularly difficult to make quick healthy choices [7]. Taste was mentioned as an important factor in all the qualitative studies when referring to food but not for alcohol, highlighting the importance of peers and the differences between drinking and dietary behaviours.

Cross-sectional research is useful for identifying specific foods and nutrients that are far from optimal, particularly poor or good dietary patterns and disparities in diet between specific subgroups of the adolescent population. We included a range of populations in this Special Issue, namely adolescents from Belgium [8], China [9], Norway [10], Poland [11] and the UK [12]. Different types of foods rather than nutrients were more likely to be reported, and the top dietary behaviours reported by all of the five cross-sectional studies were sugary drinks or foods and vegetables. Wholegrain foods, fruit, fast food or school food and skipping breakfast were also mentioned by at least two studies. A number of factors had an impact on sugary foods and drinks; consumption of sugary drinks was reported to rise with age [11], was more common in adolescent boys [10] and more common in less educated or lower social class households [8,10]. For example, in Belgium, authors also reported that amounts of sugary drinks were around 50% higher and wholegrain foods were 50% lower in households where education was lower [8]. Some of the studies also reported that unhealthy behaviours clustered together, pointing to the fact that interventions targeting more than one behaviour might be more effective [9–11]. Dietary data from the UK indicated that high intakes of extrinsic or added sugars are driven mainly by high intakes of sugary drinks in this age group as well as cakes, biscuits and confectionery. Furthermore, higher intakes of pasta and rice, wholemeal bread and fish were associated with lower sugar consumption. The very low proportion of adolescents meeting the recommendation (4%) and the findings that the most nutritious diets in the UK are for categories of 10–15% extrinsic sugars indicate that dietary patterns need to change dramatically in many countries in order to meet current guidelines. Although sugary drinks are a key driver of high free sugar intake, it is unlikely that solely targeting this food group will be sufficient to improve overall diet quality.

Three papers in this Special Issue reported on interventions aimed at adolescents to improve diet. One looked at how a small number of education classes on sugar literacy increased adolescents' intention to limit sugar intake and their confidence to read food labels [13]. A second study tested a nudge-based intervention to increase vegetables that had a small impact on vegetable intake [14]. A third study was a two-part intervention based on education followed by an adolescent-designed promotional activity focussed on food choices and food waste [15]. This study was successful in reducing vegetable waste in adolescents. The intervention studies published here support the need for interventions to provide high quality information, the skills to interpret complex dietary information and the framing of nutritional problems in a wider food system. Improving dietary behaviour in this age group, such as reducing portion sizes of energy dense food and encouraging higher intakes of plant-based diets, may be more likely to engage adolescents if linked to larger issues such as climate change. This could include interventions to reduce portion size to reduce food waste and increase high-fibre nutritious plant foods to reduce food's carbon footprint. Co-designed and adolescent-led interventions are likely to be more attuned to adolescent needs and values and therefore are potentially more effective.

It is worth mentioning what is missing from this Special Issue. No manuscripts were submitted evaluating interventions targeting the wider environment, including marketing and offering incentives or disincentives such as a subsidy (on vegetables) or a tax or levy (on sugary drinks or foods). In the UK, Public Health England have reported that as a result of the recent levy, half of sugary drinks have been reformulated to contain lower levels of sugars and this is likely to have a disproportionate impact on behaviour in adolescents as they are the largest consumers of sugary drinks. Furthermore, a reduction in marketing of foods high in fats, sugars and salt is identified by the WHO as a priority area, which is also likely to impact this age group more than others [16] and has already been implemented in some countries in Europe but was not featured here.

In conclusion, this Special Issue provides insights into designs of interventions and policies that have the potential to improve adolescent dietary behaviour. Policies that frame the issues within a larger food system and that target multiple eating behaviours may be more likely to be successful at changing overall diet quality and, consequently, health in this age group. Education is still needed despite nutrition education being part of the curriculum in schools. Furthermore, it is important that interventions take into account aspects of young people's emotional, social and cultural lives if they are to be successful. Interventions targeting adolescents in more deprived regions are particularly needed due to the inequalities in diet. Digital and online platforms are important sources of information in this age group, sources that have been implemented to improve dietary behaviour albeit with limited success so far [17]. This approach could have potential but is fraught with ethical issues due to problems with fake news and misinformation that particularly target this age group. It is essential that adolescents are at the heart of co-designing these complex interventions as it will be difficult for others to truly understand the social and cultural issues involved.

Funding: This Editorial received no external funding.

Conflicts of Interest: The author declares no conflict of interest.

References

1. Llaurado, E.; Albar, S.A.; Giralt, M.; Sola, R.; Evans, C.E. The effect of snacking and eating frequency on dietary quality in british adolescents. *Eur. J. Nutr.* **2015**, *55*, 1789–1797. [CrossRef] [PubMed]
2. Taher, A.K.; Evans, N.; Evans, C.E. The cross-sectional relationships between consumption of takeaway food, eating meals outside the home and diet quality in british adolescents. *Public Health Nutr.* **2019**, *22*, 63–73. [CrossRef] [PubMed]
3. Scott, S.; Elamin, W.; Giles, E.L.; Hillier-Brown, F.; Byrnes, K.; Connor, N.; Newbury-Birch, D.; Ells, L. Socio-ecological influences on adolescent (aged 10–17) alcohol use and unhealthy eating behaviours: A systematic review and synthesis of qualitative studies. *Nutrients* **2019**, *11*, 1914. [CrossRef] [PubMed]
4. Craigie, A.M.; Lake, A.A.; Kelly, S.A.; Adamson, A.J.; Mathers, J.C. Tracking of obesity-related behaviours from childhood to adulthood: A systematic review. *Maturitas* **2011**, *70*, 266–284. [CrossRef] [PubMed]
5. O'Cathain, A.; Thomas, K.J.; Drabble, S.J.; Rudolph, A.; Hewison, J. What can qualitative research do for randomised controlled trials? A systematic mapping review. *BMJ Open* **2013**, *3*. [CrossRef]
6. McSweeney, L.; Bradley, J.; Adamson, A.J.; Spence, S. The 'voice' of key stakeholders in a school food and drink intervention in two secondary schools in ne england: Findings from a feasibility study. *Nutrients* **2019**, *11*, 2746. [CrossRef] [PubMed]
7. Kamar, M.; Evans, C.; Hugh-Jones, S. Factors influencing british adolescents' intake of whole grains: A pilot feasibility study using sensecam assisted interviews. *Nutrients* **2019**, *11*, 2620. [CrossRef] [PubMed]
8. Desbouys, L.; De Ridder, K.; Rouche, M.; Castetbon, K. Food consumption in adolescents and young adults: Age-specific socio-economic and cultural disparities (belgian food consumption survey 2014). *Nutrients* **2019**, *11*, 1520. [CrossRef] [PubMed]

9. Sun, S.; He, J.; Fan, X. Mapping and predicting patterns of chinese adolescents' food preferences. *Nutrients* **2019**, *11*, 2124. [CrossRef] [PubMed]
10. Skeie, G.; Sandvaer, V.; Grimnes, G. Intake of sugar-sweetened beverages in adolescents from troms, norway-the tromso study: Fit futures. *Nutrients* **2019**, *11*, 211. [CrossRef] [PubMed]
11. Myszkowska-Ryciak, J.; Harton, A.; Lange, E.; Laskowski, W.; Gajewska, D. Nutritional behaviors of polish adolescents: Results of the wise nutrition-healthy generation project. *Nutrients* **2019**, *11*, 1592. [CrossRef] [PubMed]
12. Lai, H.T.; Hutchinson, J.; Evans, C.E.L. Non-milk extrinsic sugars intake and food and nutrient consumption patterns among adolescents in the uk national diet and nutrition survey, years 2008–16. *Nutrients* **2019**, *11*, 1621. [CrossRef] [PubMed]
13. Santalo, M.I.; Gibbons, S.; Naylor, P.J. Using food models to enhance sugar literacy among older adolescents: Evaluation of a brief experiential nutrition education intervention. *Nutrients* **2019**, *11*, 1763. [CrossRef] [PubMed]
14. Mistura, M.; Fetterly, N.; Rhodes, R.E.; Tomlin, D.; Naylor, P.J. Examining the efficacy of a 'feasible' nudge intervention to increase the purchase of vegetables by first year university students (17–19 years of age) in british columbia: A pilot study. *Nutrients* **2019**, *11*, 1786. [CrossRef] [PubMed]
15. Prescott, M.P.; Burg, X.; Metcalfe, J.J.; Lipka, A.E.; Herritt, C.; Cunningham-Sabo, L. Healthy planet, healthy youth: A food systems education and promotion intervention to improve adolescent diet quality and reduce food waste. *Nutrients* **2019**, *11*, 1869. [CrossRef] [PubMed]
16. World Health Organization. *Reducing the Impact of Marketing of Foods and Non-Alcoholic Beverages on Children*; World Health Organization: Geneva, Switzerland, 2019.
17. Sharps, M.A.; Hetherington, M.M.; Blundell-Birtill, P.; Rolls, B.J.; Evans, C.E. The effectiveness of a social media intervention for reducing portion sizes in young adults and adolescents. *Digit Health* **2019**, *5*. [CrossRef] [PubMed]

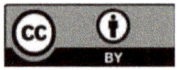

© 2020 by the author. Licensee MDPI, Basel, Switzerland. This article is an open access article distributed under the terms and conditions of the Creative Commons Attribution (CC BY) license (http://creativecommons.org/licenses/by/4.0/).

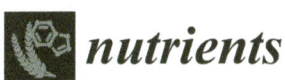

Review

Socio-Ecological Influences on Adolescent (Aged 10–17) Alcohol Use and Unhealthy Eating Behaviours: A Systematic Review and Synthesis of Qualitative Studies

Stephanie Scott [1,2,*], Wafa Elamin [1], Emma L. Giles [3], Frances Hillier-Brown [4], Kate Byrnes [3], Natalie Connor [1], Dorothy Newbury-Birch [1] and Louisa Ells [3]

1. School of Humanities and Social Sciences, Teesside University, Middlesbrough TS1 3BA, UK
2. Institute of Health and Society, Newcastle University, Newcastle upon Tyne NE1 4AX, UK
3. School of Health and Social Care, Teesside University, Middlesbrough TS1 3BA, UK
4. Department of Sport and Exercise Sciences, Durham University, Durham DH1 3HN, UK
* Correspondence: s.j.scott@tees.ac.uk or steph.scott@ncl.ac.uk

Received: 1 July 2019; Accepted: 12 August 2019; Published: 15 August 2019

Abstract: Excess body weight and risky alcohol consumption are two of the greatest contributors to global disease. Alcohol use contributes directly and indirectly to weight gain. Health behaviours cluster in adolescence and track to adulthood. This review identified and synthesised qualitative research to provide insight into common underlying factors influencing alcohol use and unhealthy eating behaviours amongst young people aged 10–17. Sixty two studies met inclusion criteria. Twenty eight studies focused on alcohol; 34 focused on eating behaviours. Informed by principles of thematic analysis and meta-ethnography, analysis yielded five themes: (1) use of alcohol and unhealthy food to overcome personal problems; (2) unhealthy eating and alcohol use as fun experiences; (3) food, but not alcohol, choices are based on taste; (4) control and restraint; and (5) demonstrating identity through alcohol and food choices. Young people faced pressure, reinforced by industry, to eat and drink in very specific ways, with clear social consequences if their attitudes or behaviour were deemed unacceptable. No qualitative studies were identified with an explicit and concurrent focus on adolescent eating behaviours and alcohol consumption. Further exploratory work is needed to examine the links between food and alcohol in young people's emotional, social and cultural lives.

Keywords: adolescent; eating; alcohol use; qualitative research; systematic review

1. Introduction

Excess body weight and heavy alcohol consumption are two of the greatest contributors to global disease burden in high-income countries [1,2]. Despite reductions in the overall prevalence of youth drinking in recent years, risky or heavy alcohol use remains the leading cause of death and disability-adjusted life years in both 15–19-year-olds and 20–24-year-olds globally [3]. Meanwhile, the number of children and adolescents (aged 2–19 years) overweight or obese in developed countries is estimated to be 24% of boys and 23% of girls [4]. Weight status and consumption of alcohol are both associated with a number of negative social, emotional and cultural outcomes during adolescence and early adulthood such as risky sexual behaviour, poor quality of life, negative effects on mental and physical health, poor educational outcomes, youth offending, and the development of alcohol-use disorders [5–12]. Further, weight gain during adolescence may to lead to disordered patterns of eating and overeating, reported to be triggered by social and emotional factors, and in particular, bullying [13,14]. Body mass index (BMI) and alcohol consumption interact, with a steeply elevated risk of liver disease observed for those with both high BMI and alcohol consumption [15]. Heavy drinking is also associated with greater waist-hip-ratio in mid-life even when taking other lifetime influences into account [16]. Adverse health behaviours such as risky drinking and unhealthy eating begin to cluster during adolescence [17], and both have been demonstrated to track into and throughout adulthood [18–20].

A growing body of quantitative, epidemiological data has identified that energy intake from alcohol, type of beverage, and drinking pattern (i.e., high volume, high frequency) can contribute substantially to total energy intake, and are associated with excess body weight and weight gain amongst adults [21–23]. Current results from the National Diet and Nutrition Survey Rolling Programme (NDNS RP, Years 1–9, 2008/9 to 2016/17) demonstrate a downward trend in the percentage of people consuming alcohol for all age groups surveyed [24]. This was statistically significant for adults aged 19–64 years (−2% per year) and for girls aged 11–18 years (−1% per year). However, for those who consumed alcohol, there was little change over time in alcohol intake as a percentage of total energy. The exception was the 11–18 years population group, where there was an average yearly decrease of 0.3 percentage points. For young people specifically (children aged 11–18), data from 2014/15 and 2015/16 of the NDNS programme highlights a mean average of 0.5% total energy intake from alcohol per day [25]. A recent systematic review and meta-analysis demonstrated that, across 22 identified studies, with 701 participants, alcoholic beverage consumption significantly increased food energy intake and total energy intake compared with a non-alcoholic comparator, suggesting that adults do not compensate appropriately for alcohol energy by eating less, and that a relatively modest alcohol dose may lead to an increase in food consumption [26]. Further, focusing specifically on young adulthood, and using pooled cross-sections of the 2008–2014 Health Survey for England and the Scottish Health Survey, Albani et al. (2018) found young adults aged 18–25 drinking the highest levels of alcohol on a single occasion were more likely to be obese than those with the lowest intake [27]; whilst Giles and Brennan (2014) highlighted that young adults make 'trade offs' between alcohol consumption, physical activity and eating patterns, by seeking to compensate 'unhealthy' behaviours with healthier ones [28]. More recently, Scott et al. (2019) identified that cultural, physical and emotional links between food and alcohol consumption were an unquestioned norm among 18–25 year-olds in the UK, with young adults calculating risks to weight, appearance and social status rather than to long-term health (in press). The latter study remains the only study to date to utilise qualitative data to examine the deeply interconnected nature of eating and drinking behaviour.

A number of influences on diet and drinking behaviours in young people (those under the age of 18) have been identified, and appear to cut across both behaviours. These include food and alcohol environments (including commercial factors such as urban space, price, promotion, and access), sometimes described as the 'foodscape' or 'obesogenic' and 'intoxigenic' environments, peers, family, and socio-economic status [29–39]. Further, there are emotional, social and symbolic benefits for young people to participating in both unhealthy eating and alcohol consumption practices for young people such as perceptions of pleasure, distinction and identity, or social status [40–43]. For example, a recent UK longitudinal study of young adults found that, contrasting with a recalled lack of concern in mid-adolescence, body-consciousness and weight-related concern generally increased around the time of school-leaving (traditionally aged 16) [44]. The authors suggest that this change resulted at least in part from increased autonomy and control over their own diet and the acknowledgement of health as personal responsibility.

Nevertheless, whilst extensive bodies of qualitative literature explore the influences on young people's eating practices and alcohol consumption, respectively, to our knowledge, no qualitative studies explicitly focus on how young people's eating and drinking behaviours interact and intertwine. This systematic review and qualitative synthesis aimed to address this evidence gap by bringing together two separate bodies of qualitative research evidence to examine young people's (aged 10–17) perspectives on socio-cultural, interpersonal and structural influences upon unhealthy eating behaviours or alcohol use. Most existing reviews focusing on health behaviours answer a very specific question, such as alcohol industry efforts to influence alcohol marketing policy [45] or barriers and enablers of healthy eating in young adulthood [46]. Therefore, it was not deemed appropriate to synthesise from these reviews as a 'review of reviews'. Instead, our intention was to capitalise on what is known from independent streams of research, enabling analysis and comparison across two associated fields of study. Thus, our primary review question is to derive socio-cultural, inter-personal and structural factors from a systematic review and synthesis of qualitative literature that might influence young people aged 10–17 among whom risky drinking and unhealthy eating co-occur, and subsequently, utilise review findings to develop a model structure of common underlying influences which cut across both behaviours in this population group.

2. Materials and Methods

The study protocol was pre-registered (Ref: CRD42017060624) [47] in compliance with the 'Preferred Reporting Items for Systematic Reviews and Meta-Analyses' (PRISMA) statement [48]. Whilst the Joanna Briggs Institute (JBI) approach was not adopted, and this review was not registered as a JBI review, it was carried out using data extraction and quality appraisal tools designed by JBI.

2.1. Eligibility Criteria

The following studies were eligible for inclusion: studies that reported primary data of any qualitative design and which explored the views of young people (aged 10–17 inclusive) on factors which shape their eating behaviours or alcohol consumption. Mixed method studies were considered eligible if findings from qualitative study components were reported in full and were distinguishable from other findings. We included studies published in English, from 2006 onwards. This date limit reflected limited time/resources for the review. Age criteria was determined using the age range cited in the study or mean age at interview. For longitudinal studies, this was the age at recruitment and/or first interview. If results were analysed separately for groups of different ages, and studies included younger children or participants aged 18 or more, only data relating to those aged 10–17 were extracted. If these data were not easily distinguished from other findings, the study was excluded. Unpublished data, abstracts, conference proceedings and studies that did not include primary evaluation data (e.g., protocols, reviews, editorials) were excluded from the review. Studies were excluded if they: (a) sought and reported the views of others (e.g., parents) rather than young people themselves; (b) analysed texts alone (e.g., discourse analysis); (c) used self-report or researcher-administered surveys, including those analysing data from open-ended questions. We also placed restrictions upon the study population, and studies were excluded if participants: (1) required specialist treatment for alcohol dependency or weight loss and gain; and (2) were pregnant or breastfeeding adolescent women whose current eating pattern was time-limited and not reflective of usual diet behaviours.

2.2. Search Strategy

In accordance with the SPIDER tool [49], the search strategy was split into five core concepts. This search strategy is documented in Supplementary Table S1. Nine electronic databases (MEDLINE, Scopus, PsychINFO, Sociological Abstracts (via ProQuest social science premium collection), CINAHL, ERIC, IBSS (via ProQuest social science premium collection), and Web of Science Core Collection) were searched from January 2006 to October 2017, using appropriate thesaurus headings and title or abstract keywords. Studies retrieved included Online First articles. Electronic database searches were supplemented by searches of Google Scholar, checking reference lists cited by included studies and checking reference lists already held by the study team.

2.3. Study Selection and Data Extraction

Figure 1 provides a visual representation of the methodological process, according to the PRISMA framework [48]. The title and abstract of all records retrieved were downloaded to Endnote X7 and independently screened by five reviewers (SS, ELG, DNB, KB, NC), with full-text copies of potentially relevant papers retrieved for in-depth review against the inclusion criteria. The JBI Qualitative

Assessment and Review Instrument (QARI) was adapted to an Excel spreadsheet to facilitate data extraction, with JBI SUMARI (JBI, Adelaide, SA, Australia) used to code and store thematic data. Data were extracted on: the phenomena of interest, methodological approach, conceptual or theoretical basis underlying the study, participant characteristics, and findings of significance to the review. Full-text screening and data extraction were carried out primarily by one researcher (WE) and checked by another (SS). Discrepancies were resolved by discussion and referral to an additional member of the review team.

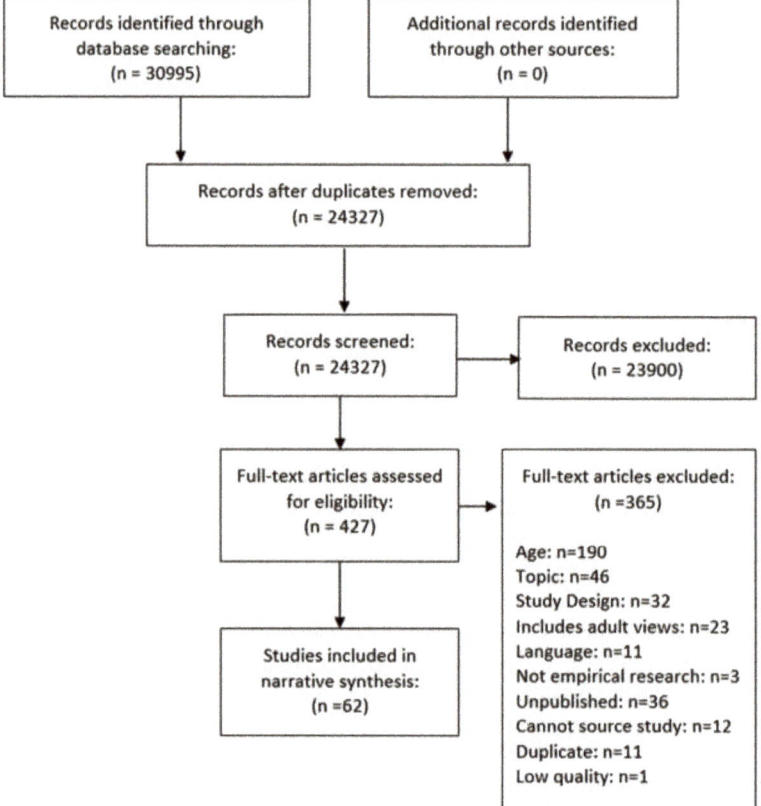

Figure 1. Flow chart showing study selection process.

2.4. Data Synthesis

Participant quotations and text under the headings "findings" or "results" were extracted from identified papers and entered verbatim into the JBI SUMARI software, where data was stored and coded. As our review involved bringing together two fields of literature (alcohol consumption and eating behaviour), we first coded papers which focused on alcohol use, followed by papers which focused on eating behaviours. Finally, we compared all themes recorded in order to identify those common only to both consumption behaviours. Based on Thomas and Harden's thematic method [50] and informed by the principles of meta-ethnography [51,52], qualitative synthesis involved three core phases: line-by-line coding of findings, development of descriptive themes, and development of analytical themes. Themes and concepts identified were explored for convergent or divergent cases, using a process referred to as reciprocol translation, similar to the constant comparative techniques used in primary qualitative research. In this way, the synthesis presented here is intended to move beyond the identification of second-order constructs (interpretations offered by the original researchers) and towards the development of third-order constructs (new interpretations beyond those offered in individual studies). Key concepts and contextual details were recorded to help understand the interpretations of every paper; regular meetings were held to discuss disagreements at all stages of assessment, but most notably, to discuss the themes and subthemes that arose from the data synthesis stage.

2.5. Quality Assessment

Included studies were assessed for quality by two independent reviewers using the 10-item JBI Qualitative Research Checklist, available via JBI SUMARI software (SS, WE). This checklist evaluated different domains of each study including appropriateness of study design, data collection techniques and analysis methods employed. Analysed together, these 10 questions determined the quality of each paper. Although no quantifiable scoring system exists for this checklist, the researchers created one to aid the process of quality assessment. Every question was allocated a score of 1 and each paper was scored out of a maximum of 10. Studies scoring 8 or above were deemed high-quality papers; studies that scored 6 or 7 were categorised medium quality. All studies that scored 5 or less were deemed low-quality papers and subsequently, excluded from the review. There were no disagreements in the assessment of methodological quality between the two reviewers.

3. Results

3.1. Description of Included Studies

The search provided 24,327 studies for screening, of which 23,900 were excluded during title and abstract screening. A further 364 studies were excluded during full-text screening ($n = 427$, completed by WE). Ten percent of studies assessed at full-text stage ($n = 43$) were double-screened (by SS). Of these, 63 studies matched full inclusion criteria. One further study was deemed low quality and later removed after quality appraisal, leaving 62 included studies (see Figure 1). The characteristics of included studies can be found in Supplementary Table S2. Of the 62 studies included in the review, 45% ($n = 28$) of studies focused on alcohol, whereas 55% ($n = 34$) focused on eating behaviours. No identified studies focused on the interaction between alcohol consumption and eating behaviours. Fourteen papers (23%) were categorised to be medium quality, while 48 (77%) were deemed high quality. The 62 studies represented over 4188 participants aged between 11 and 17 years old. European studies dominated our review findings ($n = 39$; 63%). A further nine studies (15%) were carried out in North America; four in South America (6%); four in Australia (6%); five in Asia (8%). Only one study was carried out in Africa (2%). The study settings varied among the papers but the majority recruited adolescents from schools. The findings presented below focus only on overlapping and divergent factors which influence alcohol-use behaviour and eating behaviour for young people aged 10–17, and which might be particularly pertinent for further study amongst those for whom these behaviours co-occur. Analysis yielded five themes: (1) alcohol and unhealthy food can be used by young people to overcome personal problems; (2) young people felt that unhealthy eating and alcohol use are fun experiences; (3) young people chose food based on taste—this is not the case for alcohol; (4) exercising control and restraint over eating and drinking behaviours; and (5) alcohol and food choices can be used by young people to demonstrate identity. Themes are illustrated narratively below with representative quotes from the original studies.

3.2. Alcohol and Unhealthy Food Can Be Used by Young People to Overcome Personal Problems

Study participants reflected on emotional and personal issues that they wanted to overcome through drinking or eating. Young people explained how they used alcohol to forget their problems [53–55] or to overcome sadness and *"drown their sorrows"* [56]. One participant reflected on her drinking experience and the reasons she drank (*"Once I was drunk because I was depressed; parents* were in conflict, the brother ran away from home, and I quarreled with my boyfriend..."*) [55]. Personal issues play a key role and one participant mentioned how (*"Life can go wrong and they begin to drink or to regret something. also, to forget. I think that's the reason"*) [53]. In this way, alcohol was a cushion that can be used for comfort in tough situations as (*" ... it's a way like any other to forget or to let off steam, it depends on the person"*) [54]. Similarly, young people also used food as a way to relieve stress [57,58] and to push away negative feelings or emotions: (*"If something has happened to you, and you really want it to go away. I eat, I comfort eat, and I listen to music"*) [57]. Participants were aware of their actions and the use of food to overcome depression. Interestingly, one participant mentioned how comfort food can be used if (*" ... you are depressed. It feels like the food is there for you when no one else is around"*) [57]. For this participant, these foods were replacing the human interaction he needed. Participants did not specify which type of food they ate in these circumstances, but they were concerned that (*"comfort food is probably not the healthiest stuff right, but it's what you want to eat"*) [58].

3.3. Young People Felt That Eating Unhealthy Food and Drinking Alcohol Are Fun Experiences

In a number of studies, young people highlighted the joy they experienced when eating unhealthy food [59,60] and drinking alcohol [55,61–64]. Certain foods and snacks were most enjoyable (*"For each night five days in a row you probably would get Snickers, Twix, bag a chips, and a soda, and probably a night for every day that week. Or switch up on the candy, and the soda ... "*) [65]. When asked which food type excited them most, participants were more excited about eating unhealthy options, such as junk food, than eating healthy food. The taste of food was an important motivating factor underlying this choice (*"Yeah. If you see a basket of fruit, you're like "Oh. Fruit" [Spoken in monotone]. You know, we've had fruit forever. And then you see Cheetos® and you're like, "Wow! Food! Like, real food" [Spoken enthusiastically]. For some reason, junk food is better"*) [60]. The word "fun" was used to describe the experience of eating foods such as crisps and this was particularly the case when young people got together with friends at events such as sleepovers or parties. At these events, there was a focus on enjoyment and relaxation and unhealthy options were more appealing (*"Because [if my friends are] at a place, like at a sleepover, they don't want to have healthy food. They want to have junk food because they just think that it's funner [sic] to have junk food than healthy food"*) [59].

Similarly, drinking was also described as a fun experience, to have a *"good time"* [61] and to *"relax and loosen up"* [43]. A gathering or party was expected to be much more enjoyable when not sober and so some started drinking early on in the night [63]. Alcohol also allowed young people to talk with no boundaries and to be carefree around their friends [66]. Thus, they appreciated the change in behaviour that drinking offered (*"I'm not saying it's a habit, but when you go to a party, yeah you just go there to have fun and enjoy the atmosphere. You're free not to be yourself and to let yourself go"*) [67]. On the other hand, if alcohol was unavailable at a party, this negatively impacted young people's attitude towards that event. Without the alcohol, the party was not the same (*"Often, many kids associate fun with alcohol in the sense that if a party is alcohol-free it's usually a party no one attends, because if there's no alcohol then there's no fun. I don't think it's true though"*) [62]. Across studies, participants dismissed the negative consequences of drinking alcohol that might follow a heavy session of drinking. Instead, young people focused on having a good time and convinced themselves that the negative consequences would only happen to other people. One participant highlighted that when things did go wrong, young people would *"trick themselves into thinking it's brilliant ... "* [61]. For this reason, participants continued drinking anyway and described themselves as *"courageous"* for doing so [55].

3.4. Young People Choose Food Based on Taste—This Is Not the Case for Alcohol

Fifteen studies discussed the importance of taste when it comes to eating food [60,68–80]. For many young people, healthy food has an unpleasant taste (*"Healthy foods all taste awful. The manufacturers want to sell more unhealthy foods. Therefore, they add a lot of additive to make the food tasty. These foods make us feel good. The taste is exactly what we want"*) [70] with some arguing explicitly that food *"gotta taste good"* if they are to continue to eat it [71]. One participant highlighted that *" ... Once I begin to eat* [unhealthy food], I cannot stop" [70] and craving 'addictive' foods was a regular occurrence ("*I crave the taste of soda in my mouth, especially when I see someone else drinking it*") [60]. Further, young people acknowledged that this does not always signal hunger ("*Like the other day at lunch we were walking past Annie and she had a burrito. I wasn't even hungry, but she had it so I was like, 'Can I have a bite?'*") [60], and the calorie count of unhealthy food was of secondary importance where taste was concerned ("*I don't really care how high the calories are as long as it tastes good*") [74]. The taste of alcohol, on the other hand, was described as bad ("*I thought that it should taste great but after I drank it, wow, it tasted horrible. I have no idea why people drink. I will not drink again*") [66]. Across several studies, participants questioned why young people drank when the taste is so undesirable [66,81]. However, unlike the consumption of unhealthy food, where taste could be described as pleasurable, alcohol was predominantly consumed for social purposes and with the primary objective of intoxication ("*Most people drinking like that in ninth grade don't drink because it's good, they drink to get drunk*") [81].

3.5. Exercising Control and Restraint over Alcohol and Unhealthy Food Consumption

For most participants drinking alcohol at social events was expected. Although they did it to experience fun and enjoyment, drinking alcohol was not always a good experience for them, and experienced negative consequences, which they reflected on ("*The worst feeling is being sick like and then trying to be sick and then bringing up all the beer n all or whatever you're drinking. It's terrible*") [82]. Such negative events and consequences left some young people questioning why they drank and whether it was a truly enjoyable behavior ("*I think drinking's good and then it gets worse. Like if you get completely paralytic then where's the fun in that?*") [82]. Many participants mentioned the desire to control their drinking habits [54,55,62,63,66]. Thus, self-control and having a "*good head*" [54] were important factors that young people considered when drinking alcohol ("*You've got to restrict yourself, you've got to have a certain amount of self-control to go to these parties. Like at a party you go to you don't have to necessarily get drunk, you've just got to drink the right amount, so you have fun with your friends, you don't throw up and you're ok*") [62]. Becoming uncontrollably drunk at parties was criticized as " ... *stupid and just trying to show off and it's not rational*" [62]. Nevertheless, to stop or not initiate drinking alcohol was a social challenge and very difficult to achieve. Thus, one young person highlighted that "*when I try to quit drinking, the alcohol always wins*" [55]. Therefore, to prevent alcohol from winning over their habits, narratives from young people centered on 'knowing your limits', achieved through experimentation and practice, almost akin to 'learning' how to drink alcohol ("*You know your own limitations when you drink alcohol, and my friends know their limitations too. When you are aware of your own boundaries, you know when you need to stop*") [66]. The concept of self-control was predominantly associated with studies focusing on alcohol consumption. Just one of 34 studies focusing on eating behaviours mentioned self-control [73]. In this study, one participant spoke of the hunger associated with excess intake of sugary foods ("*I see it is that when I eat something sweet, I'll be hungry for more so it is difficult to manage, so I try to stop*"). Another participant vowed to take action and stated that "*from now on I'd like to eat fruit instead of a cake in the evening*".

Other people also appeared to exercise control over young people's drinking and eating behaviours. Some young people encouraged each other to drink within their limits ("*We do tend to emphasise to each other that you should know your limitations so if someone doesn't know his limits then we would be he's not really that cool to hang out with...I guess there is a borderline between funny and embarrassing...like the new people who come in sometimes they go over the top of it and then they know that that's not really the way to go, so they kind of buckle down next time*") [63]. However, peers can also be a negative influence upon behavior and some young people described being 'coerced' by friends to drink and gave in so as to avoid looking 'bad' [83]. In this particular study, much was attributed to the dynamics of the social group as drinking habits developed at a time "*when all the groups are forming...so then you want to fit in...so then you feel the pressure to do what everyone else is doing so you're like them*" and participants feared that " ... *if I didn't drink they wouldn't want to hang out with me anymore*". Wanting to be accepted as part of a social group was also addressed in other studies [81,84] and participants explained that "*It's kind of* what you have to do to be a part of the group. There are lots of people experiencing such pressure. If you want to be one of the cool people, then you need to just start doing it—to try alcohol and do stuff you don't want to then"* [81]. Young people were not always happy to consume alcohol but saying "no" to their friends was difficult to do [85]. Commonly used phrases such as " ... 'ah, go on, give it a try' ... '" [62] or " ... try it, try it" [84] were employed by their friends to push them into trying a drink. Participants discussed being initially hesitant to try alcohol, especially if they did not intend on drinking it at a certain event. Choosing not to drink came with its own stigma and resulted in teasing and bullying (" ... people will start to tease you and all stuff like that, people are a lot meaner now, and if you don't do the same what they do, they'll start to pick on you ... ") [61]. Name-calling was another tactic used such as " ... oh you're a chicken ... " [83] and some young people ended up drinking to please friends and avoid ridicule [86]. Some attempted to use excuses such as having to participate in sporting activities the next day and the need to remain sober, although this rarely worked to their favour ("like if you say [to your peers] I'm not going out [and drinking] because of netball, you'll like cop a bit of flack for that...because they [peers] don't understand the pressure to perform...and your performance would be like totally affected [if you drank]...there's been a few times where we've gone out not intending to drink and have ended up drinking") [86].

Pressure relating to eating habits was discussed in several studies [40,60,70,71,87,88]. One participant highlighted how *"My friends are all around me eating good [unhealthy] food and I'll be like, "Oh I'm gonna buy that. I wanna go get one too." Either you won't eat or you'll have the junk food"* [60]. Eating food that was deemed undesirable by the social group also had negative social consequences for young people including gossiping or teasing (*"If you don't eat it while others are eating, you appear to be different from others. Others may say something [bad] behind your back"*) [70]. Eating healthy food or home-made packed food resulted in ridicule (*"[Some teenagers] just don't eat [healthy food] in front of other people. They're probably afraid they might get teased"*) [59]. Therefore, to avoid this, young people opted to buy food from the canteens at school, just as their friends did (*"I do not know. I believe that they might think that people will assume that their mums are preparing sandwiches for them. People feel more comfortable buying food from the canteen like everyone else, rather than having home-made food, even if it is healthier. If someone is eating a home-made sandwich, he might think that the others are going to make fun of him"*) [87]. Not only was there pressure to eat unhealthy food, but young people also felt pressured to buy expensive foods as eating cheaper foods might mean *"[peers] give you dirty looks and talk about you to your friends"* [40]. As such, participants suggested that eating cheaper brands may indicate that they are " ... *poor or something. Not exactly poor but not a lot of money"* [40]. Yet, peer influence appeared to work both ways, albeit heavily dependent on the choice of friends young people kept. In other words, peers who ate more healthy food, in turn, influenced their friends to eat healthy (*"I was eating heaps of unhealthy food then and I'd see people, like, bring in heaps of fruit and then I noticed that I was eating unhealthy, so I changed to their foods"*) [88].

Perversely, overeating and drinking to excess were also frowned upon, leading to a social 'tightrope' that had to be navigated in order to fit in. Several studies addressed young people's attitude to overeating [40,68,77,89,90]. Some participants sympathised with overweight and obese peers (*"I think that if you're overweight, you still belong. I mean, you're the same as other kids, just a little heavier"*) [68]. They argued that overweight young people may be suffering from a chronic disease and should not be discriminated against [68]. However, others had very negative attitudes towards overweight peers (*"Being overweight is not healthy. You just become so ugly. You are bullied"*) [77]. Some young people were shamed for being overweight (*"Yes, if you're fat in school they call you 'fatty' and stuff like that"*) [40] and excluded from team activities at school *"so they won't get picked on ... girls think that if they're fat, they'll get picked on a lot more"* [90]. Further, not only were overweight young people teased for being overweight, they were also teased when they tried to adopt more healthy food choices to reduce weight, adding to the complexity of their social situation (*"I usually don't eat at school. I mean, er'body be eatin' stuff at lunch that ain't really healthy, but they ain't alot a choices. If I eat a salad or somein' then they gonna crack on me. They say stuff like "What's up biggie, you tryin' to lose some pounds' and stuff. I dunno"*) [89]. Young people were also criticized for intoxication and drunken behavior [54,64,85,91–93].

Excess drinking was defined by one young person as " ... *about you getting high, about you getting drunk, about you not being able to control yourself, about you not knowing, about you not being able to decide on your own. About you doing stupid things and being different from how you really are, also about you feeling bad the day after*" [91]. Acting out and becoming sick was not appreciated by peers, especially when at house parties ("*you don't want them inside while they become sick*") [64]. Young people even chose to exclude peers from events if they continued to drink excessively and were disruptive ("*We won't invite you again if you can't control it. You shouldn't drink any more now*") [93]. Some participants found drunken behaviour both "*disgusting*" while still being "*hilarious*" to watch [92]. Nevertheless, negative attitudes remained ("*Above all, in my opinion, a twelve year old girl who drinks many glasses of vodka only makes herself look ridiculous, because no one could hold that*") [54]. Females, in particular, were criticized for being promiscuous when drunk and were looked down upon. They became a topic of conversation among their peers ("*She went skinny-dipping with another man*") [92]. Further, it was female peers who were particularly vocal about this behavior ("*I'm not a fan of girls who get really drunk and then do things [of a sexual nature] with guys and then blame it on the fact that they were drinking...I really don't like that because I kinda go, well I'd never get to that point*") [86].

Such pressure on eating behavior and alcohol use often led to young people conforming to fit in with others ("*I simply go with the flow of my era and I do not confine myself to eating beans, for instance. That is a 'no-no' for our times. I am a follower of today's fashions. Young people today believe in eating in Pizza Hut, hamburgers,* etc. *[pause] this shows that I am 'in' and not cut off from the rest*") [87]. In relation to alcohol, they tended to drink in the same ways in order to reach the same consumption level ("*It is so much more fun when all of us are on the same level—when there isn't anyone higher or lower than the rest of us*") [94]. This was not something they always wanted to partake in, however, they choose to do it regardless of whether they liked the experience or not ("*It happened to me as well, we were at the beach, we ate there, I don't like beer, but everyone drank and then I took the beer and drank it all and bleah*") [54]. Those who did not drink were excluded from social events with their peers and were described as "*weakling*" or "*a loser*" [55], placing immense social pressure on adolescents to participate in drinking sessions as they did not want to " ... *just stand there looking*" while everyone else drank alcohol [84]. For many this was " ... *a bit embarrassing*" [66]. Instead, the social norm for adolescents was to drink and be " ... *caught up in the spur of the moment. You see all your pals drinking and* ... *then you end up just joining in with them*" [61].

3.6. Alcohol and Food Choices Can Be Used by Young People to Demonstrate Identity

Drinking alcohol allowed young people to demonstrate a sense of identity, be perceived as cool, and to be praised for it (" ... *your friends think you're great, and they're good if you drink* ... ") [55]. Part of maintaining a "*cool*" image was to show off in front of friends and "*brag*" about drinking while being underage [95]. This helped them appear tough in front of their friends ("*They want to make themselves look hard, like oh yeah I drink*") [83]. Young people tended to exaggerate their drinking experience and this in itself was perceived negatively by their peers ("*They're loads of people who come in the next day, they exaggerate so much and they'd be like, 'Oh I drank two bottles of Buckfast and two wee bottles of vodka' and all this shit like you would be dead*") [95]. Coolness, popularity and being trendy were interlinked ("*It's because it's the fashion. It's the fashion that we get drunk every weekend (laughter)!*") [84]. Not everyone shared this sentiment and one participant had a different view ("*Young people only drink because it's supposed to be cool. They are trying to act tough in front of groups of guys or girls. That they kind of "yes, we are drinking and we are really cool". That was how it was earlier but now, at least in our grade and maybe ninth grade as well, they have started to think that it is really childish to stand there trying to be tough by drinking*") [81]. Nevertheless, the majority of young people who drank remained popular and influential among their peers ("*If one starts who may be popular and others, like, fancy him and think that he's cool. And if he starts, like, to drink, then he might influence a lot of other people. Because they want to be in his group*") [91].

Being 'cool' and demonstrating a sense of identity was also an important factor when choosing which foods to eat around their peers [40,69,87]. Certain foods such as sweets or fast food (for example, hamburgers or pizzas) were viewed as trendy (*"YES, YES the Mac style is more modern. It is more in, modern for young people"*) [87]. Young people felt pressure to *"be cool and be like everybody else—It is just a chain reaction"* [69]. Subsequently, those who chose other food options such as home-made and healthy options were ostracized (*"The one who eats healthy food will be more of a dumb person ... [He] cannot be modern or cool"*) [87]. This extended beyond simply eating certain foods and included how food products looked or were branded, and how they could be eaten (*"You wouldn't have a yoghurt I don't think because then you'd have to have a spoon!" "Yes." "That is not cool." Moderator: "Spoons are not cool?" "Not." Moderator: "Really?" (All laughing) "You look stupid getting a big metal spoon out of your bag."*) [40]. One participant highlighted that part of the appeal of eating certain unhealthy food products was the ability and ease of sharing it with friends. This built social bonds and cemented popularity among peers (*"But people are more excited when somebody brings sweets—you are more popular. It is easier to say do you want to have a piece of chocolate than do you want a bite of my apple"*) [69]. Media and advertisements played an influential role in choices of food and alcohol brands. Young people highlighted the role of advertising and social media in promoting certain alcohol brands [63,79,86,96]. Alcohol promotion lingered in the memories of participants (*"Ad[vertisement]s for Smirnoff are really classy and you really want to drink them 'cause they look awesome. Because everyone's doing it [drinking Smirnoff] you want to do it too"*) [86]. Participants were curious to discover the taste of the drinks that were promoted in advertisements and certain brands conjured up a persona that young people wished to imitate (*"I seen one of the adverts off Jack Daniels...I was like 'oh I wonder if I'd do that if I'm on Jackie D's' and I just had to get a bottle of Jackie D's and nowt happened...I liked the taste of it and that. Same with Southern Comfort. I've seen the advert for that and I was like 'oh' and decided to have a drink of it"*) [63]. While advertisements promoted both healthy and unhealthy food, those that focused on unhealthy food were perceived as more exciting and fun (*"The advertising promotion of unhealthy food is very good. For example, a candy is able to change the color of your tongue. There are always some new foods coming up. Young people will find them playful"*) [70]. Like the alcohol industry, the food industry also focused on the fun aspects of eating unhealthy foods. The lifestyle associated with this was more appealing to young people (*"Well, they advertise it a lot more than fruit. Like have you seen the swirly commercial? The kid comes home and his hair's all crazy because he goes on a roller coaster. And he is the guy that makes it all fun. You know, it's like we're gonna go on a trip and eat these Cheetos®"*) [60].

In many studies, young people wanted to be viewed as mature individuals (*"We started to party in the seventh grade and I have always felt, how should I put it, a bit ahead of the others ... a bit older ... Some of the others have only just started to party now"*) [97]. They wanted to drink alcohol to mimic adults and be viewed as more mature individuals by their peers (*"Drinking is associated with being an adult, like you know, smoking, doing all those things which like adults do, if you are younger and you do the things adults do then it makes you seem older and I think that's what they want"*) [83]. This helped young people to *"feel superior to others. You feel great!"* [84]. Boasting about drinking experiences helped elevate this feeling and participants used phrases such as *"I got totally smashed"* [84] to help them feel older amongst their peers. Part of appearing older was choosing different types of alcohol beverages (*"when I get older I'll start drinking beer and wine...I think they're classy drinks like they're drinks you'll have at a restaurant rather than the one that like you drink at a party"*) [86]. On the other hand, unhealthy eating habits were associated with being young and modern; such young people were viewed as attractive and independent (*"When you have delivery food you show a different character, more outgoing and attractive than having home-made food prepared by your mum or grandmother. You come over as a person with a degree of independence who does not depend that much on his family; you look cooler"*) [87]. Healthy foods were eaten by more 'mature' young people and, unlike alcohol use, this was an undesirable trait to have (*"I think, it's more mature to say that you want a piece of fruit—and then if somebody asks if you want to go downtown for a bag of crisps, that's what you'll do"*) [69].

Ultimately, young people wanted to *"feel like being grown up and to be the coolest person in school"* [91]. Achieving this balance was complex, and participants believed that they would change their drinking and eating habits as they grew older (*"When I'm older, I'll probably still drink, but not to get drunk, just to *enjoy it, whereas at the moment I'm probably just drinking to get drunk*") [83]. Thus, despite knowing the negative health risks of excessive alcohol intake or unhealthy eating behaviours, participants did not appear concerned. For alcohol, young people were concerned about more immediate consequences such as having a hangover or being caught by the police for a misdemeanor (" ... *young people think about the short term more than the long term because they think about what they're going to look like right now, than think about what will happen when they're older.*") [61]. The role alcohol played in bodily harm or long-term diseases were of secondary importance to young people, with these findings mirrored in studies looking at unhealthy eating habits [87,98]. Instead, body image was a greater and more immediate concern than future health risks ("*We probably should be thinking about our health, but personally I think more about my body ... If I eat something that's unhealthy I think, Oh no! That will make "me fatter". I don't think about my future health*") [98]. Peer influence also appeared to have a role to play. One participant described that her peers may dismiss health concerns related to unhealthy eating habits. They would even tease more health-conscious young people who choose to eat more nutritious foods (" ... *you are afraid that something will happen to you, so they might make fun of you that you are afraid and you worry about your health. They might say that: 'We are young and we do not care about all these things'*") [87]. Further, young people expected to change their eating and drinking habits as they got older. For example, they differentiated between teenage drinking and adult drinking. While they assumed that young people drank to get drunk, they did not expect this behaviour from adults as ' ... *adults are more in control than young people*' [81]. Adult drinking was associated with meals and family gatherings and participants believed that, unlike their own behaviours, the "*[adults are] done running around partying and drinking*" [81]. One participant argued that this was because " ... *when you grow up you become smarter ...* " [62].

4. Discussion

This review and qualitative synthesis demonstrated that there are a number of socio-cultural, interpersonal and structural influences upon young people's (aged 10–17) unhealthy eating behaviours or alcohol use which cut across *both* behaviours. Studies included in this review suggest that young people regularly feel pressure to drink alcohol and eat unhealthy food, particularly when around their peers. There appear to be clear social consequences and image concerns when it comes to the restriction of either of these behaviours, leading to navigation of what could be described as a social 'tightrope'. In other words, young people must fit in but not go overboard. In relation to alcohol use, those who do not drink as well as those who drink too much can lose favour with peers. This paradox has previously been described among young adults as 'calculated hedonism' [99]. Similarly, those who eat too healthily, as well as those who over-indulge, and become overweight, can be subject to ridicule, suggesting that young people must consume in very specific, rigid ways in order to be accepted. For many, this may be an impossible feat, with clear impacts on young people's physical and mental health demonstrated in wider literature [100,101]. Such pressure to behave according to narrow, pre-defined categories appears to be reinforced by wider structural mechanisms, including but not restricted to, social media use [102] and commercial drivers, such as product marketing [36,103]. Previous work suggests that marketers ('big alcohol' and 'big food') reinforce aspects of the social ecology by encouraging links between alcohol, food and aspects of identity, culture and personal reward [63,104]. Indeed, this relationship is well underway in some young people by mid-adolescence [105]. However, this is an iterative rather than linear relationship. In other words, industry feeds off young people's concerns, as well as leading them, meaning that it may be difficult to disentangle the 'real' concerns of young people ('knowing your limits') from those seeded by industry through marketing and 'educational' programmes, including alcohol programmes which are run in UK schools, and affiliated with industry (such as 'Drinkaware for Education'). Further, commercial determinants have seen expansion in recent years into new directions such as energy drinks and gambling [106–108], and warrant further exploration in future research. Such exploration should examine the holistic impact of commercial determinants upon young people's social, emotional and cultural worlds, rather than investigating these drivers in isolation.

The volume of studies identified by this review means that we have reported only what we concluded to be major themes. We also reported only themes which cut across both eating behaviours and alcohol use. This is not to say that there were no other influences on young people's alcohol use and eating behaviours. For example, parents and extended family members appeared to exert an influence on both behaviours within a smaller number of papers. Young people discussed the importance of a trusting relationship with their parents, the ability to have open discussions about both alcohol use and nutrition and the role of both parental disapproval and initiation when it comes to their child's alcohol use. As anticipated, we found no literature focusing on how young people consume food and alcohol simultaneously. Yet, one way in which to tackle a growth in obesogenic and alcohol-related harm may be to examine the overlapping influences in these behaviours at the point in which they initiate and accelerate (late childhood/early adulthood) and use this knowledge in the design of interventions which link rather than separate out food and alcohol consumption. Emergent research with young adults suggests eating patterns linked to alcohol use are not tied only to hunger but to sociability, traditions and aspects of identity. Further, young adults conceptualized and calculated risks to their weight, appearance and social status rather than to their long-term health (Scott et al., 2019, in press); whilst a raft of quantitative studies have identified that energy intake from alcohol, type of beverage and drinking pattern are associated with excess body weight and weight gain amongst young adults [21,26]. However, these attitudes and behaviours may well be established in earlier years, suggesting the need to conduct work examining the detailed links between alcohol use and eating behaviour with younger age groups. Finally, young people felt that their alcohol use and food choices would change as they got older, and tended to 'discount' potential negative consequences. Again, this argument is well supported in both fields of literature [109]. Narratives of delay discounting do not appear to be restricted to adolescence and have been demonstrated to track into young adulthood [28]. For example, young people in this review acknowledged that the taste of food was important, whereas the taste of alcohol was not. However, young people suggested that the taste of alcohol would be more meaningful to them when they were older.

There are several limitations of our review which should be acknowledged. First, we defined 'young people' to be aged 10–17. We thought very carefully about this definition. Whilst in some developed countries the legal drinking age can be higher (aged 21 in USA), we were informed by the UK legal drinking age of 18. Further, turning 18 has further connotations in young people's lives. For example, turning 18 can signal transition from children to adult health services, transitions from further education to higher education and can mark major life transitions, meaning that the environments of 16 and 17 year-olds can be experientially different to that of those aged 18 and over. Second, papers focusing on both addiction and weight control behaviours and syndromes (such as bulimia and anorexia) were deliberately excluded from our review. We felt that papers in this field focused on targeted, psychological disorders, whereas our review synthesized literature on wider cultural, inter-personal and social perspectives on eating and drinking behaviours in adolescence. Third, many of the papers in this review did not explicitly reflect upon differences between socio-economic groups. Yet, recent work suggests that socio-spatial patterning of outlets selling potentially health-damaging products such as fast food, alcohol and tobacco tend to cluster in deprived areas [110]. Further, obesity and alcohol-related mortality and morbidity are high in socioeconomically disadvantaged populations compared with individuals from advantaged areas, characterized in terms of occupation, income or educational attainment [111]. Fourth, due to time and resource restrictions, we did not double-screen all identified studies at full-text stage. Rather than employ single screening, we took the decision to double-screen 10% of full-text studies identified in order to add rigour to our review findings. Further, whilst not all results were formally double screened, the author with responsibility for full-text screening (WE) discussed any uncertainties and discrepancies across all 427 full-text papers assessed with the second reviewer (and lead author, SS) at all times. Fifth, we attempted to contact authors whose papers we were unable to obtain during database searches, with very little success. Finally, we did not analyse the data according to country of origin and, therefore, cannot make assumptions based on geographical or cultural traditions or differences.

Findings from this study have important implications for intervention development, as well as UK public health policy and practice. Themes identified in this review, and in recent parallel work conducted by the lead author with young adults, will be used to inform a qualitative exploration of young people's (aged 10–17) views regarding their eating behaviours and alcohol use. Combined, review and interview data will be used to develop a model structure, or logic model, of the influences upon both unhealthy eating behaviours and alcohol use amongst young people. It is anticipated that this model structure will be used in future participatory design work with young people, which aims to generate ideas for a dual-focused intervention to reduce alcohol consumption and excess body weight among young people, and to promote a positive approach to body image, physical and mental health.

Supplementary Materials: The following are available online at http://www.mdpi.com/2072-6643/11/8/1914/s1, Table S1: Review Concepts and Associated Search Terms, Table S2: Characteristics of Included Studies.

Author Contributions: S.S. conceived the study idea and devised the study methodology. S.S., W.E., E.L.G., L.E. and F.H.-B. participated in the design and coordination of the study. S.S. was primarily responsible for protocol writing. S.S., E.L.G., D.N.-B., K.B. and N.C. screened identified literature. W.E. and S.S. conducted data extraction and analysed the review findings. All authors read the drafts, provided comments and agreed on the final version of the manuscript.

Funding: This study was supported by the Economic and Social Research Council (ESRC) as part of a Fuse funded pump prime small project grant (Research Centre Grant, UKCRC, Res 590-25-0004). Fuse is a UK Clinical Research Collaboration (UKCRC) Public Health Research Centre of Excellence. Funding for Fuse from the British Heart Foundation, Cancer Research UK, National Institute of Health Research, Economic and Social Research Council, Medical Research Council, Health and Social Care Research and Development Office, Northern Ireland, National Institute for Social Care and Health Research (Welsh Assembly Government) and the Wellcome Trust, under the auspices of the UKCRC, is gratefully acknowledged. The views expressed in this paper do not necessarily represent those of the funders or UKCRC. The funders had no role in study design, data collection and analysis, decision to publish, or preparation of the manuscript.

Acknowledgments: The authors wish to thank Fiona Beyer for technical assistance in setting up the systematic review. We would also like to thank the Joanna Briggs Institute (Australia) for allowing us to use JBI SUMARI as well as associated data extraction and quality appraisal tools.

Conflicts of Interest: The authors declare no conflict of interest.

References

1. World Health Organisation. *Global Status Report on Alcohol and Health*; WHO: Geneva, Switzerland, 2014.
2. World Health Organisation. *Global Health Risks. Mortality and Burden of Disease Attributable to Selected Major Risks*; WHO: Geneva, Switzerland, 2009.
3. Gore, F.M.; Bloem, P.J.N.; Patton, G.C.; Ferguson, J.; Joseph, V.; Coffey, C.; Sawyer, S.M.; Mathers, C.D. Global burden of disease in young people aged 10–24 years: A systematic analysis. *Lancet* **2011**, *377*, 2093–2102. [CrossRef]
4. Ng, M.; Fleming, T.; Robinson, M.; Thomson, B.; Graetz, N.; Margono, C.; Mullany, E.C.; Biryukov, S. Global, regional, and national prevalence of overweight and obesity in children and adults during 1980–2013: A systematic analysis for the global burden of disease study 2013. *Lancet* **2014**, *384*, 766–781. [CrossRef]
5. Hunger, J.M.; Major, B.; Blodorn, A.; Miller, C.T. Weighed down by stigma: How weight-based social identity threat contributes to weight gain and poor health. *Soc. Personal. Psychol. Compass* **2015**, *9*, 255–268. [CrossRef]
6. Donoghue, K.; Rose, H.; Boniface, S.; Deluca, P.; Coulton, S.; Alam, M.F.; Gilvarry, E.; Kaner, E.; Lynch, E.; Maconochie, I.; et al. Alcohol consumption, early-onset drinking, and health-related consequences in adolescents presenting at emergency departments in england. *J. Adolesc. Health* **2017**, *60*, 438–446. [CrossRef]
7. Healey, C.; Rahman, A.; Faizal, M.; Kinderman, P. Underage drinking in the UK: Changing trends, impact and interventions. A rapid evidence synthesis. *Int. J. Drug Policy* **2014**, *25*, 124–132. [CrossRef]
8. Norström, T.; Rossow, I.; Pape, H. Social inequality in youth violence: The role of heavy episodic drinking. *Drug Alcohol Rev.* **2018**, *37*, 162–169. [CrossRef]

9. Jackson-Roe, K.; Murray, C.; Brown, G. Understanding young offenders' experiences of drinking alcohol: An interpretative phenomenological analysis. *Drugs Educ. Prev. Policy* **2015**, *22*, 77–85. [CrossRef]
10. Beccaria, F.; Rolando, S.; Ascani, P. Alcohol consumption and quality of life among young adults: A comparison among three European countries. *Subst. Use Misuse* **2012**, *47*, 1214–1223. [CrossRef]
11. Tsiros, M.D.; Olds, T.; Buckley, J.D.; Grimshaw, P.; Brennan, L.; Walkley, J.; Hills, A.P.; Howe, P.; Coates, A.M. Health-related quality of life in obese children and adolescents. *Int. J. Obes.* **2009**, *33*, 387. [CrossRef]
12. Griffiths, L.J.; Parsons, T.J.; Hill, A.J. Self-esteem and quality of life in obese children and adolescents: A systematic review. *Int. J. Pediatr. Obes.* **2010**, *5*, 282–304. [CrossRef]
13. Reece, L.J.; Bissell, P.; Copeland, R.J. 'I just don't want to get bullied anymore, then I can lead a normal life'; insights into life as an obese adolescent and their views on obesity treatment. *Health Expect.* **2016**, *19*, 897–907. [CrossRef]
14. Puhl, R.M.; Wall, M.M.; Chen, C.; Bryn Austin, S.; Eisenberg, M.E.; Neumark-Sztainer, D. Experiences of weight teasing in adolescence and weight-related outcomes in adulthood: A 15-year longitudinal study. *Prev. Med.* **2017**, *100*, 173–179. [CrossRef]
15. Hart, C.L.; Morrison, D.S.; Batty, G.D.; Mitchell, R.J.; Davey Smith, G. Effect of body mass index and alcohol consumption on liver disease: Analysis of data from two prospective cohort studies. *BMJ* **2010**, *340*, c1240. [CrossRef]
16. Pinto Pereira, S.M.; van Veldhoven, K.; Li, L.; Power, C. Combined early and adult life risk factor associations for mid-life obesity in a prospective birth cohort: Assessing potential public health impact. *BMJ Open* **2016**, *6*, e011044. [CrossRef]
17. Kipping, R.R.; Smith, M.; Heron, J.; Hickman, M.; Campbell, R. Multiple risk behaviour in adolescence and socio-economic status: Findings from a UK birth cohort. *Eur. J. Public Health* **2014**, *25*, 44–49. [CrossRef]
18. Rossow, I.; Kuntsche, E. Early onset of drinking and risk of heavy drinking in young adulthood. A 13-year prospective study. *Alcohol Clin. Exp. Res.* **2013**, *37* (Suppl. 1), 304. [CrossRef]
19. Degenhardt, L.; O'Loughlin, C.; Swift, W.; Romaniuk, H.; Carlin, J.; Coffey, C.; Hall, W.; Patton, G. The persistence of adolescent binge drinking into adulthood: Findings from a 15-year prospective cohort study. *BMJ Open* **2013**, *3*, e003015. [CrossRef]
20. Craigie, A.M.; Lake, A.A.; Kelly, S.A.; Adamson, A.J.; Mathers, J.C. Tracking of obesity-related behaviours from childhood to adulthood: A systematic review. *Maturitas* **2011**, *70*, 266–284. [CrossRef]
21. Wymond, B.; Dickinson, K.; Riley, M. Alcoholic beverage intake throughout the week and contribution to dietary energy intake in Australian adults. *Public Health Nutr.* **2016**, *19*, 2592–2602. [CrossRef]
22. White, G.E.; Richardson, G.A.; Mair, C.; Courcoulas, A.P.; King, W.C. Do associations between alcohol use and alcohol use disorder vary by weight status? Results from the national epidemiological survey on alcohol and related conditions-III. *Alcohol Clin. Exp. Res.* **2019**, *43*, 1498–1509.
23. Yeomans, M.R. Short term effects of alcohol on appetite in humans. Effects of context and restrained eating. *Appetite* **2010**, *55*, 565–573. [CrossRef] [PubMed]
24. Public Health England. *National Diet and Nutrition Survey Years 1 to 9 of the Rolling Programme (2008/2009–2016/2017): Time Trend and Income Analyses*; Public Health England: London, UK, 2019.
25. Public Health England. *National diet and Nutrition Survey Results from Years 7 and 8 (Combined) of the Rolling Programme (2014/2015 to 2015/2016)*; Public Health England: London, UK, 2018.
26. Kwok, A.; Dordevic, A.L.; Paton, G.; Page, M.J.; Truby, H. Effect of alcohol consumption on food energy intake: A systematic review and meta-analysis. *Br. J. Nutr.* **2019**, *121*, 481–495. [CrossRef] [PubMed]
27. Albani, V.; Bradley, J.; Wrieden, W.L.; Scott, S.; Muir, C.; Power, C.; Fitzgerald, N.; Stead, M.; Kaner, E.; Adamson, A.J. Examining associations between body mass index in 18–25 year-olds and energy intake from alcohol: Findings from the health survey for England and the Scottish health survey. *Nutrients* **2018**, *10*, 1477. [CrossRef] [PubMed]
28. Giles, E.L.; Brennan, M. Trading between healthy food, alcohol and physical activity behaviours. *BMC Public Health* **2014**, *14*, 1231. [CrossRef] [PubMed]
29. Thompson, C.; Cummins, S.; Brown, T.; Kyle, R. Contrasting approaches to 'doing' family meals: A qualitative study of how parents frame children's food preferences. *Crit. Public Health* **2016**, *26*, 322–332. [CrossRef] [PubMed]

30. MacArthur, G.; Jacob, N.; Pound, P.; Hickman, M.; Campbell, R. Among friends: A qualitative exploration of the role of peers in young people's alcohol use using bourdieu's concepts of habitus, field and capital. *Sociol. Health Illn.* **2016**, *39*, 30–46. [CrossRef] [PubMed]
31. Jones, S.C.; Andrews, K.; Berry, N. Lost in translation: A focus group study of parents' and adolescents' interpretations of underage drinking and parental supply. *BMC Public Health* **2016**, *16*, 1–10. [CrossRef]
32. Wills, W.J.; Lawton, J. Attitudes to weight and weight management in the early teenage years: A qualitative study of parental perceptions and views. *Health Expect.* **2014**, *18*, 775–783. [CrossRef]
33. Fielding-Singh, P.; Wang, J. Table talk: How mothers and adolescents across socioeconomic status discuss food. *Soc. Sci. Med.* **2017**, *187*, 49–57. [CrossRef]
34. Clare, P.; Julie, M.P.; Miranda, C.; Lyndsey, W.; Gia, D.A.; Gayle, L.; Carole, S.; Andrew, W.; Richard, A. Engaging homeless individuals in discussion about their food experiences to optimise wellbeing: A pilot study. *Health Educ. J.* **2017**, *76*, 557–568.
35. Østergaard, J.; Andrade, S.B. Who pre-drinks before a night out and why? Socioeconomic status and motives behind young people's pre-drinking in the United Kingdom. *J. Subst. Use* **2014**, *19*, 229–238. [CrossRef]
36. Scott, S.; Muirhead, C.; Shuckhsmith, J.; Tyrrell, R.; Kaner, E. Does industry-driven alcohol marketing influence adolescent drinking behaviour? A systematic review. *Alcohol Alcohol.* **2017**, *52*, 84–94. [CrossRef] [PubMed]
37. McCreanor, T.; Barnes, H.; Kaiwai, H.; Borell, S.; Gregory, A. Creating intoxigenic environments: Marketing alcohol to young people in Aotearoa New Zealand. *Soc. Sci. Med.* **2008**, *67*, 938–946. [CrossRef] [PubMed]
38. Watson, P.; Wiers, R.W.; Hommel, B.; Ridderinkhof, K.R.; de Wit, S. An associative account of how the obesogenic environment biases adolescents' food choices. *Appetite* **2016**, *96*, 560–571. [CrossRef] [PubMed]
39. Tyrrell, R.L.; Greenhalgh, F.; Hodgson, S.; Wills, W.J.; Mathers, J.C.; Adamson, A.J.; Lake, A.A. Food environments of young people: Linking individual behaviour to environmental context. *J. Public Health* **2016**, *39*, 95–104. [CrossRef] [PubMed]
40. Stead, M.; McDermott, L.; MacKintosh, A.M.; Adamson, A. Why healthy eating is bad for young people's health: Identity, belonging and food. *Soc. Sci. Med.* **2011**, *72*, 1131–1139. [CrossRef]
41. Wills, W.J.; Backett-Milburn, K.; Gregory, S.; Lawton, J. 'If the food looks dodgy I dinnae eat it': Teenagers' accounts of food and eating practices in socio-economically disadvantaged families. *Sociol. Res. Online* **2008**, *13*, 15. [CrossRef]
42. Fry, M. Seeking the pleasure zone: Understanding young adult's intoxication culture. *Australas. Mark. J.* **2011**, *19*, 65–70. [CrossRef]
43. Ander, B.; Abrahamsson, A.; Bergnehr, D. 'It is ok to be drunk, but not too drunk': Party socialising, drinking ideals, and learning trajectories in Swedish adolescent discourse on alcohol use. *J. Youth Stud.* **2017**, *20*, 1–14. [CrossRef]
44. Sweeting, H.; Smith, E.; Neary, J.; Wright, C. 'Now I care': A qualitative study of how overweight adolescents managed their weight in the transition to adulthood. *BMJ Open* **2016**, *6*, e010774. [CrossRef]
45. Savell, E.; Fooks, G.; Gilmore, A.B. How does the alcohol industry attempt to influence marketing regulations? A systematic review. *Addiction* **2016**, *111*, 18–32. [CrossRef] [PubMed]
46. Munt, A.E.; Partridge, S.R.; Allman-Farinelli, M. The barriers and enablers of healthy eating among young adults: A missing piece of the obesity puzzle: A scoping review. *Obes. Rev.* **2016**, *18*, 1–17. [CrossRef] [PubMed]
47. Scott, S.; Reilly, J.; Giles, E.L.; Hillier-Brown, F.; Ells, L.; Kaner, E.; Adamson, A. Socio-ecological influences on adolescent (aged 10–17) alcohol use and linked unhealthy eating behaviours: Protocol for a systematic review and synthesis of qualitative studies. *Syst. Rev.* **2017**, *6*, 180. [CrossRef] [PubMed]
48. Moher, D.; Liberati, A.; Tetzlaff, J.; Altman, D.G. Preferred reporting items for systematic reviews and meta-analyses: The prisma statement. *PLoS Med.* **2009**, *6*, e1000097. [CrossRef] [PubMed]
49. Cooke, A.; Smith, D.; Booth, A. Beyond pico: The spider tool for qualitative evidence synthesis. *Qual. Health Res.* **2012**, *22*, 1435–1443. [CrossRef] [PubMed]
50. Thomas, J.; Harden, A. Methods for the thematic synthesis of qualitative research in systematic reviews. *BMC Med. Res. Methodol.* **2008**, *8*, 45. [CrossRef] [PubMed]
51. Lee, R.P.; Hart, R.I.; Watson, R.M.; Rapley, T. Qualitative synthesis in practice: Some pragmatics of meta-ethnography. *Qual. Res.* **2015**, *15*, 334–350. [CrossRef]

52. Campbell, R.; Pound, P.; Pope, C.; Britten, N.; Pill, R.; Morgan, M.; Donovan, J. Evaluating meta-ethnography: A synthesis of qualitative research on lay experiences of diabetes and diabetes care. *Soc. Sci. Med.* **2003**, *56*, 671–684. [CrossRef]
53. Fraga, S.; Sousa, S.; Ramos, E.; Dias, S.; Barros, H. Alcohol use among 13-year-old adolescents: Associated factors and perceptions. *Public Health* **2011**, *125*, 448–456. [CrossRef]
54. Petrilli, E.; Beccaria, F.; Prina, F.; Rolando, S. Images of alcohol among Italian adolescents. Understanding their point of view. *Drugs Educ. Prev. Policy* **2014**, *21*, 211–220. [CrossRef]
55. Samardzik, S.; Bujsic, G.; Kozul, K.; Tadijan, D. Drinking in adolescents—Qualitative analysis. *Coll. Antropol.* **2011**, *35*, 123–126.
56. Katainen, A.; Lehto, A.-S.; Maunu, A. Adolescents' sense-making of alcohol-related risks: The role of drinking situations and social settings. *Health* **2015**, *19*, 542–558. [CrossRef] [PubMed]
57. Jonsson, L.; Larsson, C.; Berg, C.; Korp, P.; Lindgren, E.-C. What undermines healthy habits with regard to physical activity and food? Voices of adolescents in a disadvantaged community. *Int. J. Qual. Stud. Health Well-Being* **2017**, *12*, 1333901. [CrossRef] [PubMed]
58. Watts, A.W.; Lovato, C.Y.; Barr, S.I.; Hanning, R.M.; Mâsse, L.C. Experiences of overweight/obese adolescents in navigating their home food environment. *Public Health Nutr.* **2015**, *18*, 3278–3286. [CrossRef] [PubMed]
59. Harrison, M.; Jackson, L.A. Meanings that youth associate with healthy and unhealthy food. *Can. J. Diet. Pract. Res.* **2009**, *70*, 6–12. [CrossRef]
60. Taylor, N.L. Negotiating popular obesity discourses in adolescence. *Food Cult. Soc.* **2011**, *14*, 587–606. [CrossRef]
61. Harvey, S.A.; McKay, M.T. Perspectives on adolescent alcohol use and consideration of future consequences: Results from a qualitative study. *Child Care Pract.* **2017**, *23*, 104–120. [CrossRef]
62. Katainen, A.; Rolando, S. Adolescents' understandings of binge drinking in southern and northern European contexts—Cultural variations of 'controlled loss of control'. *J. Youth Stud.* **2015**, *18*, 151–166. [CrossRef]
63. Scott, S.; Shucksmith, J.; Baker, R.; Kaner, E. 'Hidden habitus': A qualitative study of socio-ecological influences on drinking practices and social identity in mid-adolescence. *Int. J. Environ. Res. Public Health* **2017**, *14*, 611. [CrossRef]
64. Ander, B.; Abrahamsson, A.; Gerdner, A. Changing arenas of underage adolescent binge drinking in Swedish small towns. *Nord. Stud. Alcohol Drugs* **2015**, *32*, 427–442. [CrossRef]
65. Dodson, J.L.; Hsiao, Y.-C.; Kasat-Shors, M.; Murray, L.; Nguyen, N.K.; Richards, A.K.; Gittelsohn, J. Formative research for a healthy diet intervention among inner-city adolescents: The importance of family, school and neighborhood environment. *Ecol. Food Nutr.* **2009**, *48*, 39–58. [CrossRef] [PubMed]
66. Yoon, S.; Lam, W.W.T.; Sham, J.T.L.; Lam, T.-H. Learning to drink: How Chinese adolescents make decisions about the consumption (or not) of alcohol. *Int. J. Drug Policy* **2015**, *26*, 1231–1237. [CrossRef] [PubMed]
67. Acier, D.; Kindelberger, C.; Chevalier, C.; Guibert, E. "I always stop before I get sick": A qualitative study on French adolescents alcohol use. *J. Subst. Use* **2015**, *20*, 262–267. [CrossRef]
68. Van Exel, J.; Koolman, X.; de Graaf, G.; Brouwer, W. *Overweight and Obesity in Dutch Adolescents: Associations with Health Lifestyle, Personality, Social Context and Future Consequences: Methods and Tables.* Report 06.82; Institute for Medical Technology Assessment: Rotterdam, The Netherlands, 2006.
69. Bech-Larsen, T.; Boutrup Jensen, B.; Pedersen, S. An exploration of adolescent snacking conventions and dilemmas. *Young Consum.* **2010**, *11*, 253–263. [CrossRef]
70. Chan, K.; Tse, T.; Tam, D.; Huang, A. Perception of healthy and unhealthy food among Chinese adolescents. *Young Consum.* **2016**, *17*, 32–45. [CrossRef]
71. Ensaff, H.; Coan, S.; Sahota, P.; Braybrook, D.; Akter, H.; McLeod, H. Adolescents' food choice and the place of plant-based foods. *Nutrients* **2015**, *7*, 4619–4637. [CrossRef]
72. Gavaravarapu, S.M.; Rao, K.M.; Nagalla, B.; Avula, L. Assessing differences in risk perceptions about obesity among "normal-weight" and "overweight" adolescents—A qualitative study. *J. Nutr. Educ. Behav.* **2015**, *47*, 488–497. [CrossRef] [PubMed]
73. He, C.; Breiting, S.; Perez-Cueto, F.J.A. Effect of organic school meals to promote healthy diet in 11–13 year old children. A mixed methods study in four Danish public schools. *Appetite* **2012**, *59*, 866–876. [CrossRef]
74. Hunsberger, M.; McGinnis, P.; Smith, J.; Beamer, B.A.; O'Malley, J. Calorie labeling in a rural middle school influences food selection: Findings from community-based participatory research. *J. Obes.* **2015**, *2015*, 7. [CrossRef]

75. Protudjer, J.L.P.; Marchessault, G.; Kozyrskyj, A.L.; Becker, A.B. Children's perceptions of healthful eating and physical activity. *Can. J. Diet. Pract. Res.* **2010**, *71*, 19–23. [CrossRef]
76. Rakhshanderou, S.; Ramezankhani, A.; Mehrabi, Y.; Ghaffari, M. Determinants of fruit and vegetable consumption among tehranian adolescents: A qualitative research. *J. Res. Med. Sci.* **2014**, *19*, 482–489. [PubMed]
77. Ridder, M.A.; Heuvelmans, M.A.; Visscher, T.L.; Seidell, J.C.; Renders, C.M. We are healthy so we can behave unhealthily: A qualitative study of the health behaviour of Dutch lower vocational students. *Health Educ.* **2010**, *110*, 30–42. [CrossRef]
78. Silva, D.C.D.A.; Frazão, I.D.S.; Osório, M.M.; Vasconcelos, M.G.L.D. Perception of adolescents on healthy eating. *Ciencia Saude Coletiva* **2015**, *20*, 3299–3308. [CrossRef] [PubMed]
79. Stevenson, C.; Doherty, G.; Barnett, J.; Muldoon, O.T.; Trew, K. Adoelscents' views of food and eating: Identifying barriers to healthy eating. *J. Adolesc.* **2007**, *30*, 417–434. [CrossRef] [PubMed]
80. Stephens, L.D.; McNaughton, S.A.; Crawford, D.; Ball, K. Nutrition promotion approaches preferred by Australian adolescents attending schools in disadvantaged neighbourhoods: A qualitative study. *BMC Pediatr.* **2015**, *15*, 61. [CrossRef] [PubMed]
81. Bakken, S.A.; Sandøy, T.A.; Sandberg, S. Social identity and alcohol in young adolescence: The perceived difference between youthful and adult drinking. *J. Youth Stud.* **2017**, *20*, 1380–1395. [CrossRef]
82. Johnson, P. 'You just get blocked'. Teenage drinkers: Reckless rebellion or responsible reproduction? *Child. Soc.* **2011**, *25*, 394–405. [CrossRef]
83. Davies, E.L.; Martin, J.; Foxcroft, D.R. Young people talking about alcohol: Focus groups exploring constructs in the prototype willingness model. *Drugs Educ. Prev. Policy* **2013**, *20*, 269–277. [CrossRef]
84. Romo-Avilés, N.; Marcos-Marcos, J.; Tarragona-Camacho, A.; Gil-García, E.; Marquina-Márquez, A. "I like to be different from how I normally am": Heavy alcohol consumption among female Spanish adolescents and the unsettling of traditional gender norms. *Drugs Educ. Prev. Policy* **2018**, *25*, 262–272. [CrossRef]
85. Parder, M.-L. What about just saying "no"? Situational abstinence from alcohol at parties among 13–15 year olds. *Drugs Educ. Prev. Policy* **2018**, *25*, 189–197. [CrossRef]
86. Lunnay, B.; Ward, P.; Borlagdan, J. The practise and practice of bourdieu: The application of social theory to youth alcohol research. *Int. J. Drug Policy* **2011**, *22*, 428–436. [CrossRef] [PubMed]
87. Ioannou, S. 'Eating beans . . . that is a "no-no" for our times': Young Cypriots' consumer meanings of 'healthy' and 'fast' food. *Health Educ. J.* **2009**, *68*, 186–195. [CrossRef]
88. Ronto, R.; Ball, L.; Pendergast, D.; Harris, N. Adolescents' perspectives on food literacy and its impact on their dietary behaviours. *Appetite* **2016**, *107*, 549–557. [CrossRef] [PubMed]
89. Ashcraft, P.F. Explanatory models of obesity of inner-city African-American adolescent males. *J. Pediatric Nurs.* **2013**, *28*, 430–438. [CrossRef] [PubMed]
90. Witmer, L.; Bocarro, J.N.; Henderson, K. Adolescent girls' perception of health within a leisure context. *J. Leis. Res.* **2011**, *43*, 334–354. [CrossRef]
91. Sandberg, S.; Skjælaaen, Ø. "Shoes on your hands": Perceptions of alcohol among young adolescents in Norway. *Drugs Educ. Prev. Policy* **2018**, *25*, 449–456. [CrossRef]
92. Knox, K.; Schmidtke, D.J.; Dietrich, T.; Rundle-Thiele, S. "Everyone was wasted"! Insights from adolescents' alcohol experience narratives. *Young Consum.* **2016**, *17*, 321–336. [CrossRef]
93. Jørgensen, M.H.; Curtis, T.; Christensen, P.H.; Grønbæk, M. Harm minimization among teenage drinkers: Findings from an ethnographic study on teenage alcohol use in a rural Danish community. *Addiction* **2007**, *102*, 554–559. [CrossRef]
94. Frederiksen, N.J.S.; Bakke, S.L.; Dalum, P. "No alcohol, no party": An explorative study of young Danish moderate drinkers. *Scand. J. Public Health* **2012**, *40*, 585–590. [CrossRef]
95. Johnson, P. 'You think you're a rebel on a big bottle': Teenage drinking, peers and performance authenticity. *J. Youth Stud.* **2013**, *16*, 747–758. [CrossRef]
96. Trujillo, E.M.; Suárez, D.E.; Lema, M.; Londoño, A. How adolescents learn about risk perception and behavior in regards to alcohol use in light of social learning theory: A qualitative study in Bogota, Colombia. *Int. J. Adolesc. Med. Health* **2015**, *27*, 3–9. [CrossRef] [PubMed]
97. Järvinen, M.; Østergaard, J. Governing adolescent drinking. *Youth Soc.* **2009**, *40*, 377–402. [CrossRef]
98. Hjelkrem, K.; Lien, N.; Wandel, M. Perceptions of slimming and healthiness among Norwegian adolescent girls. *J. Nutr. Educ. Behav.* **2013**, *45*, 196–203. [CrossRef] [PubMed]

99. Szmigin, I.; Griffin, C.; Mistral, W.; Bengry-Howell, A.; Weale, L.; Hackley, C. Re-framing 'binge drinking' as calculated hedonism: Empirical evidence from the UK. *Int. J. Drug Policy* **2008**, *19*, 359–366. [CrossRef] [PubMed]
100. Gunnell, D.; Kidger, J.; Elvidge, H. Adolescent mental health in crisis. *BMJ* **2018**, *361*, K2608. [CrossRef] [PubMed]
101. Hager, A.D.; Leadbeater, B.J. The longitudinal effects of peer victimization on physical health from adolescence to young adulthood. *J. Adolesc. Health* **2016**, *58*, 330–336. [CrossRef] [PubMed]
102. Richards, D.; Caldwell, P.H.; Go, H. Impact of social media on the health of children and young people. *J. Paediatr. Child Health* **2015**, *51*, 1152–1157. [CrossRef] [PubMed]
103. Bugge, A.B. Food advertising towards children and young people in Norway. *Appetite* **2016**, *98*, 12–18. [CrossRef] [PubMed]
104. Freeman, B.; Kelly, B.; Vandevijvere, S.; Baur, L. Young adults: Beloved by food and drink marketers and forgotten by public health? *Health Promot. Int.* **2015**, *31*, 954–961. [CrossRef]
105. Scott, S.; Baker, R.; Shucksmith, J.; Kaner, E. Autonomy, special offers and routines: A Q methodological study of industry-driven marketing influences on young people's drinking behaviour. *Addiction* **2014**, *109*, 1833–1844. [CrossRef]
106. Visram, S.; Crossley, S.J.; Cheetham, M.; Lake, A. Children and young people's perceptions of energy drinks: A qualitative study. *PLoS ONE* **2017**, *12*, e0188668. [CrossRef] [PubMed]
107. Visram, S.; Cheetham, M.; Riby, D.M.; Crossley, S.J.; Lake, A.A. Consumption of energy drinks by children and young people: A rapid review examining evidence of physical effects and consumer attitudes. *BMJ Open* **2016**, *6*, e010380. [CrossRef] [PubMed]
108. Pitt, H.; Thomas, S.L.; Bestman, A. Initiation, influence, and impact: Adolescents and parents discuss the marketing of gambling products during Australian sporting matches. *BMC Public Health* **2016**, *16*, 967. [CrossRef] [PubMed]
109. Laghi, F.; Liga, F.; Baumgartner, E.; Baiocco, R. Time perspective and psychosocial positive functioning among Italian adolescents who binge eat and drink. *J. Adolesc.* **2012**, *35*, 1277–1284. [CrossRef] [PubMed]
110. Macdonald, L.; Olsen, J.R.; Shortt, N.K.; Ellaway, A. Do 'environmental bads' such as alcohol, fast food, tobacco, and gambling outlets cluster and co-locate in more deprived areas in Glasgow city, Scotland? *Health Place* **2018**, *51*, 224–231. [CrossRef] [PubMed]
111. Katikireddi, S.V.; Whitley, E.; Lewsey, J.; Gray, L.; Leyland, A.H. Socioeconomic status as an effect modifier of alcohol consumption and harm: Analysis of linked cohort data. *Lancet Public Health* **2017**, *2*, e267–e276. [CrossRef]

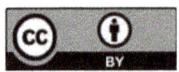

© 2019 by the authors. Licensee MDPI, Basel, Switzerland. This article is an open access article distributed under the terms and conditions of the Creative Commons Attribution (CC BY) license (http://creativecommons.org/licenses/by/4.0/).

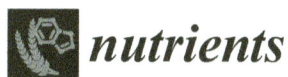

Article

The 'Voice' of Key Stakeholders in a School Food and Drink Intervention in Two Secondary Schools in NE England: Findings from a Feasibility Study

Lorraine McSweeney [1], Jen Bradley [1], Ashley J. Adamson [1,2] and Suzanne Spence [1,2,*]

1. Human Nutrition Research Centre, Population Health Sciences Institute, Faculty of Medical Sciences, Newcastle University, Framlington Place, Newcastle upon Tyne NE2 4HH, UK; lorraine.mcsweeney@newcastle.ac.uk (L.M.); jen.bradley@newcastle.ac.uk (J.B.); ashley.adamson@newcastle.ac.uk (A.J.A.)
2. Fuse, UKCRC Centre for Translational Research in Public Health, UK
* Correspondence: suzanne.spence@newcastle.ac.uk; Tel.: +44-(0)-191-2087739

Received: 9 October 2019; Accepted: 7 November 2019; Published: 12 November 2019

Abstract: Background: Overweight/obesity affects one-third of UK 11–15-year olds. Individually focussed interventions alone have limited effectiveness. Food choice architecture approaches increase the visibility and convenience of foods to facilitate the choice of 'healthier' foods and reduce 'unhealthy' foods. This qualitative component of a School Food Architecture (SFA) study aimed to determine the perceptions of pupils and staff in relation to school food provision and their perceptions of the intervention. **Methods**: Pupil focus groups and staff one-to-one interviews. Topic guides were developed from literature and in consultation with a Young Person's Advisory Group. Thematic analysis was applied. Results: Focus group ($n = 4$) themes included: dining hall practices, determinants of choice, and aspects of health. Interview themes ($n = 8$) included: catering practices, health awareness, education, and knowledge of intervention. Pupils liked to purchase hand-held, quick to purchase foods potentially limiting the access to fruits and vegetables. Pupils were aware of 'healthier' food choices but would choose other options if available. **Conclusions**: Schools provide a daily school meal for large numbers of pupils, with time and dining environment constraints. Pupils consume 35–40% of their daily energy intake at school, therefore interventions enabling healthier eating in school are essential, including making healthier choices readily available and accessible.

Keywords: school food; pupils; food choice

---

1. Introduction

One-third of the 11–15-year olds in the UK are overweight or obese [1]. This has consequences for their emotional, behavioural and physical health and may result in morbidity and premature mortality in adulthood [2–4]. The UK government aims to halve childhood obesity rates by 2030 [5]. Chapter two of the Childhood Obesity plan sets out strategies to address this goal; including a commitment 'to support all children with high quality nutrition' [5]. Given the proportion of food that children eat at school [6], focusing on schools as an environment for promoting healthier food choices [5] has the potential to influence a substantial proportion of food intake across all social groups and offers the potential to form new food habits [7]. However, the reduction of overweight/obesity is a complex challenge. Major areas of concern are high intakes of energy, fat and sugar-sweetened beverages and low intake of fibre, fruit and vegetables [7]. The UK National Diet and Nutrition survey [8] reports that free sugars make up 14.1% of the 11–18-year olds daily calorie intake and sugar sweetened beverages amount for 22% of their diet. Fruit and vegetable consumption averages at 2.7 portions per day.

Encouraging healthy eating in children and young people is multifaceted and influenced by a myriad of external factors. Food-related decision-making processes are thought to be governed by a two-way system: the reflective system is driven by values and intentions; it requires thought [9]. The second, an automatic system requires little or no thought and is motivated by feelings and our environment [9].

The World Health Organisation (WHO) advocate population-based strategies which seek to change the social norm by encouraging a change in behaviour to improve health, however, behaviour change has proved challenging [10]. Current evidence suggests that changing the number of available food options or altering the positioning of foods could contribute to positive changes in behaviour. To enable more certain and generalisable conclusions about these potentially important effects, further research is warranted in real-world settings [11]. One approach to facilitate behaviour change is food choice architecture; that is increasing the visibility and convenience of foods to encourage the purchase and uptake of 'healthier' foods and reduce 'unhealthy' foods [12], and may reduce inequalities [13]. Reducing the cognitive demands of healthy food choice at the point of purchase has the potential to affect health behaviours [14].

This study aims to explore the perceptions of pupils, teaching and catering staff to school food provision, and the perceived impact of an intervention which repositioned drinks, cookies and fruit in the school dining hall.

2. Materials and Methods

2.1. Study Design and Setting

Two secondary schools in North East England participated. The intervention focused on the placement of fruit, cakes/cookies and drinks. Fruit was placed in front of cakes/cookies and drinks were positioned according to sugar content, with water now positioned at eye level. Pupils participated in age-appropriate focus groups and school staff (teaching and catering) in one-to-one semi-structured interviews. Pupil focus-groups and staff interviews were conducted during the school day on school premises. Focus groups were facilitated by L.M. and S.S. and lasted approximately 1 h. Staff interviews were approximately 30 min and facilitated by L.M.

2.2. Participants, Recruitment and Consent

Named contacts for the school were contacted by lead researcher (S.S.) by email or telephone to request help in organising the recruitment of pupils. A purposive sample [15] of pupils aged 11–16 years were provided with a study information sheet and invited to take part in one of the two focus groups (per school): ages 11–13 years and 14–16 years. Parent and pupil written consent was required prior to participating.

A sample of teaching and catering staff were invited by email or telephone to take part in the one-to-one interview. Written consent was obtained before participation.

2.3. Materials

The focus group and interview topic guides were developed from the literature and in consultation with the Young Person's Advisory Group-North East (YPAG). The topic guides can be found in Appendices A and B. Participants were asked to discuss topics related to day-to-day practices of school food provision, satisfaction of school foods, perceptions of school regulations relating to school food provision, perceptions of health, and awareness, if any, of the intervention.

2.4. Data Management and Statistical Analysis

Interviews and focus groups were digitally recorded with the participant's consent and transcribed verbatim. Data was analysed using thematic analysis. NVivo software was used to aid indexing and charting [16]. Guided by the principles of grounded theory [17], the data was repeatedly read and coded independently by L.M. within a framework of a priori issues identified from the topic guide and by participants or which emerged from the data. Regular discussion and review of the analysis by L.M. and S.S. acted as a quality control measure.

3. Results

3.1. Focus Groups

Eight pupils from each of the two schools (four in each age category; total $n = 16$) took part in an age separated focus group discussion. Three themes and 15 sub-themes were identified (Table 1).

Table 1. Themes and sub-themes from pupil focus groups.

Theme	Sub-Themes
Dining hall day-to-day practices	■ Perceptions of dining hall rules ■ Dining hall atmosphere ■ Having to wait in long queues ■ Knowing the daily menu and offers ■ Use of meal deals ■ Pre-ordering of food items ■ Pupils can buy snack foods ■ Some food items sell out quickly ■ Monitoring of pupil eating
Aspects of 'healthy' eating	■ Consumption of fruit, vegetables and salad ■ Strategies that would inspire pupils to eat healthier ■ Consumption, restriction and selling of 'unhealthy' food options ■ Drink consumption ■ Pupil perception of healthier eating
School food architecture intervention implementation	■ Pupils' perception of dining room changes

3.2. Dining Hall Day-to-Day Practices

Overall pupils were accepting of dining hall practices though there was some frustration over the length of queues and time they had to wait to be served. The necessity of having to queue often impacted on pupil's knowledge of daily menus. Although many items such as sandwiches, pasta pots and pizza were available daily, pupils found it difficult to know what the hot meals/special offers would be:

'You can have a look. When you go in, there's a big one (menu) on the side but sometimes it's hard to track what day it is. When you actually get there (hot food counter), there is a piece of paper and it says what's on today's meal deals (FG4)'.

Although the hot meal deals appeared to be popular among the pupils, as they represented good value, some pupils reported buying the items such as pizza or pasta pots daily for a speedy decision and purchase. Despite the popularity of the meal deals, some felt the choice was limited; every day the deal included a small drink and a cookie but an alternate type of dessert or fruit was classed as extra which not all pupils had the budget for:

'I think we should be allowed to get fruit and a drink because otherwise you're only allowed to get your meal and fruit. I don't think that's right because I think people could be dying of thirst but they want to be really healthy and they don't want to get a cookie. That means if you've got a drink, you would have to pay extra for it'. (FG4)

Many pupils purchased food at the morning break, some would keep the item to eat at lunch-time thus removing the pressure to join the lunch-time queue. Items for sale at mid-morning included bacon rolls, sausage sandwiches and paninis. Pupils who ate a hot snack at break said that this often influenced what they might want to purchase at lunch-time:

'I just like taking a cookie and then a drink. Sometimes you don't want a big meal. You just want something little to snack on'. (FG2)

In one school the purchase of sweet items, such as the cookies, was limited to one a day, the other school did not appear to impose such limits. Staff reported they were not always able to monitor the pupil's purchases because of the multiple till points in the dining hall and separate hall where sandwiches were sold.

3.3. Aspects of 'Healthy' Eating

Pupils of all ages were aware of the importance of eating fruit for health, however, the availability, price and quality of the provided fruit was not always an incentive:

'I'm only allowed to spend £ 2.00 a day and like if I want a meal and some fruit I've got to pay extra'. (FG1)

Whilst some of the younger pupils said they did not worry about their diet for health ...

'Like with me being a younger kid I know what's healthy and what's not and I'll admit I do eat unhealthy food, but yes, you can say, "Oh eat this instead of this," but I'll be honest, we won't listen because we just think, "Oh we're young, we can do whatever we want"'. (FG1)

Pupils were aware of the disconnect between what they were being told and taught and what happened in reality:

'I think they have unhealthy foods on display. It's like you're telling us to be healthy but you're showing us unhealthy food, of course we're going to choose the unhealthy one instead of the healthy choice which you're trying to make us choose. It's pointless telling us to choose healthy stuff when you're putting out unhealthy stuff for us to buy I think'. (FG2)

One school regularly took part in charity fund-raising initiatives whereby staff and pupils were selling sweets and cakes:

'Yes, they sell anything that they can make money out of. So at the minute my form has just been selling ice pops because it's been really hot. But some are selling donuts, cookies, chocolate, pick 'n' mix'. (FG3)

Pupils were generally open for the school implementing strategies to encourage healthier choices and had some ideas:

'Lower the unhealthy stuff I think. Like, maybe not make it not every day. Instead of cookies one day have the fruit pots instead and then one day have the cookies have fruit pots so you're like, "I might as well have something healthy since that's all there is"'. (FG4)

However, when asked if further restrictions should be made such as the blanket banning of certain foods there was strong opposition, especially in one school where 'unhealthier' items were not already restricted. Pupils said they would just go to the local shops or bring in items from home. Although pupils understood that fizzy drinks were considered unhealthy, the consumption of 'juice' (diluting juice) was thought to be an everyday necessity:

'I think you drink juice anyway in your normal day ... I think it's unfair if they went no juice because you're drinking juice anyway so that's not really going to make a difference. I think it's more the food that you're taking in'. (FG4)

The pupils appeared satisfied with the choice of the current school drink provision and would not make any changes. Less acceptable was the current provision of free water. Although pupils in both schools reported the availability of water fountains there was reluctance to use them:

'It's (water fountain) not like one of those ones where you put your cup underneath and press it, which I think would be such a good idea. There are other ones and it's like a tiny little bowl about that big with a tap coming out of it and you press the button and it just trickles out of the top. But people put their mouth around it, so I've never got a drink out of there'. (FG3)

3.4. School Food Architecture Intervention Implementation

The pupils were asked if they had noticed any changes to the dining hall in recent weeks. Pupils spoke of tables being moved around, walls being decorated and different cheese on the pasta. It was only with prompting that the pupils spoke about the introduction of the fruit pots:

'The fruit used to be put on a plate whereas now they make some effort with presentation, like all cut up and . . . they do little fruit pots as well'. (FG1)

No other observations were made.

3.5. Staff Interviews

One member of the teaching staff and three catering staff members were interviewed from each school (total $n = 8$). Eight themes and 25 sub-themes were identified (Table 2).

Table 2. Themes and sub-themes from school staff interviews.

Theme	Sub-Themes
School food provision is important	■ Pupils have the opportunity of a daily hot meal ■ Pupils have access to healthy food ■ School food influences pupil's eating behaviour
School catering practices	■ Development of menus ■ Complying with school food regulations ■ Responding to pupil requests and demands
Types of foods pupils buy	■ Snack foods ■ Fruit, vegetables and salads ■ Things that influence pupil choice
Day-to-day serving practices and issues	■ Food pricing and information ■ Serving food methods ■ Dining hall atmosphere ■ Queuing and time limits ■ School rules
Drinks and foods considered to be less healthy	■ Drink availability ■ The consumption of less healthy foods ■ The school has rules restricting 'junk' foods
Nutrition, health awareness and education	■ Pupil's nutritional needs ■ Educating pupils about nutrition
Perceptions and knowledge of the school foods intervention	■ Staff understanding of the intervention ■ Views of the intervention ■ Impact of the intervention ■ Negative effects of the intervention
How school food provision could be improved or enhanced	■ School plans to improve school food provision ■ School foods improvement 'wish-list'

3.6. School Food Provision Is Important

There was an overwhelming consensus that providing pupils with 'good' food was vital. It was acknowledged that for certain pupils, a school meal may be the only hot meal they received that day:

'The school cares about the food here, they're always trying to improve and do better—give better stuff and that—everything is fresh'. (ST03)

Showing pupils a different side to food and diet was considered an important aspect:

'There is a different world of taste and nourishment and healthy eating, and we need to be showing them—you know, for some children who've never sat in a restaurant and eaten good quality restaurant food, that if we can be that representation in school as much as we can be, with different flavours, different cultural foods'. (ST01)

3.7. School Catering Practices

Interviewees spoke of the need to comply with the local council school food regulations. Menus were developed through development chefs. The importance of knowing what the pupils liked and would eat was stressed:

'I think you've got to know your kids and your kitchen and know what's going to sell that day'. (ST02)

Staff recognised that despite restrictions being put in place, for example, the amount of sugar that cakes, cookies and drinks were allowed to contain, it was not practical to enforce:

'However, where it falls down, is that, for example, you might see a homemade muffin, which has been made directly to the (regulated) recipe, but then a student can buy three of them. So there is no restriction on quantity. A student can buy, what a student wants'. (ST05)

3.8. Types of Foods Pupils Buy

It was acknowledged that many pupils made use of the opportunity to buy hot snack items and sandwiches at break-time, this often impacted on their lunch-time choices:

'You have to be careful, because they might have had a bacon sandwich at break and then they want a biscuit at lunch. There's still that bit about, "I can have three slabs of cake". So I think there needs to be a bit more work done on volume and quantity of what they're actually buying and do you introduce a healthier way of choices'. (ST05)

The staff too were aware that many pupils would choose 'easy' options for speed and familiarity.

3.9. Day-to-Day Serving Practices and Issues

The complexity of dealing with the sheer volume of pupils at one lunch sitting was an everyday challenge:

'Yes, we've got a pasta area which is separate. We've got a hot service area, which is your main food, a chicken area, and a pizza area. It does take the pressure off the main hatch, but there is still a massive queue at the main hatch'. (ST03)

'It's pretty busy, because we haven't got a massive dining hall. Obviously, we're getting more and more kids. We only have one sitting at the moment. I think they're getting rushed with their food. I think it's like trying to get them in, fed, and out ready for more people coming in'. (ST04)

The number of pupils being catered for made it impossible to monitor individual purchases, the school with purchasing restrictions in place suggested they found this difficult to enforce:

'I think it might just be in the school, you know, and that's them saying no, one item, breakfast one item, one drink. And I have seen the children say, "I want two". "No, you can't, you're only allowed one". Send their friend back up or the other one, you know. Like sometimes you watch them and think, "You've just got that cookie for him", but you can't sort of stand there and argue and say, "No, that's not for him"'. (ST02)

3.10. Drinks and Food Considered to Be Less Healthy

One school which had 'junk food' restrictions tried to adhere to their policy:

'Yes, so we've obviously got food policy in place. We, on a general- around the corridors, at break and lunch, will take pop and anything like big packs of biscuits, big bags of sweets. We will go into assembly ... just to remind- they're non-negotiable, they'll be taken off you or parents can come and collect them ... we monitor it that way'. (ST01)

Nonetheless, catering staff found the restrictions conflicting:

'That's it, there is nothing stopping them going into the quad (separate school food purchasing area) and getting a cake and a cookie, and then coming back into the dining hall and saying, "I'll have another cake, I'll have a cookie and a flapjack"'. (ST03)

3.11. Nutrition, Health Awareness and Education

The attitudes and pupil's knowledge of diet were highlighted as being key:

'I think we are aware that being in a deprived area, there might be a number of students who haven't eaten anything in the morning. There are also a lot of students, even if they could eat anything in the morning, they don't and they don't think that's a problem. There is still the issue where they might think a packet of crisps is fine for breakfast'. (ST05)

Providing dietary education to pupils of all ages was considered important:

'I think it would be better, almost if it was a curriculum requirement within PHSE (personal, social, health and economic: a school curriculum subject), in every year group, until they leave school'. (ST05)

3.12. Perception and Knowledge of the School Foods Intervention

The catering staff were able to describe the changes that had been requested of them during the intervention and reported being happy to comply. There was some surprise expressed by the staff as the intervention had made them more aware of the drinks being sold and the high level of sugar contained in some:

'No, I think everything that they did was great because it opened my eyes, because of the sugar content, which I was so surprised at'. (ST02)

The subtlety of the intervention was praised:

'I think the fact that it was subtly done, I think the children weren't really- it was obviously subconscious decisions they were making, which I think is about product placement, isn't it? And preparation for selling that type of thing'. (ST05)

The introduction of the fruit pots sparked interest and extra consumption:

'The kids were asking, "Why are you getting all these pots?" Many of the kids did ask, "Oh, are you starting to do fruit up here. We never used to take fruit up to any other point, bar the main hatch. I think they noticed, "Oh, I'll have fruit." When it's there, they were taking it'. (ST03)

The increase in fruit purchases was thought to be due to the novelty factor:

'Sort of ... Yes. Because it was amazing because they said, "How is it?" And I went, "Absolutely great." They did 40 pots, you know, to start off with. Keep on the 40 pots, and then all of a sudden it was like 20 pots, and I'm saying, "Well, what's happening? They're not taking it, they're (catering staff) just bringing it back"'. (ST02)

There was some concern that the fruit pots would take longer to prepare, however, it was conceded that once in a routine the preparation was not onerous.

There were fewer comments regarding the changes in the drink positioning although one school felt the quantities of water being sold had changed:

'I thought there was more water, because I'll tell you why. I was doing the orders and I would get, say, six cases of water. I upped it to eight'. (ST02)

3.13. How School Food Provision Could Be Improved or Enhanced

At the end of the interview staff were asked to describe their ideas or future plans to improve school food provision.

'I'd suggested recently with student council that we give a reward system (for choosing healthier options) if we see good practice in place ... ... like through a prize at the end of term or something like that could be put into place for that'. (ST01)

4. Discussion

Several barriers to pupils making healthier choices were identified. In both schools, pupils and staff spoke of the long queues and lack of time to sit and enjoy what was purchased; these issues have been reported in previous studies and negatively influence the eating experience [7]. There appeared to be an active intent by schools to provide more convenience hand-held type foods in several locations that would be quick to access and encourage pupils to leave the dining area quicker. Both schools sold hot sandwich type items at morning break which appeared to be popular. Some pupils stated that they would eat/keep these items as a lunch replacement and then purchase an additional snack/biscuit/drink at lunchtime. This practice potentially limits the pupil's access to fruit, vegetables and salads. Also highlighted was the occurrence of individual pupils purchasing the same types of foods on daily basis such as pizza slices, paninis and pasta, again limiting the consumption of fruit and vegetables. Reasons for these habitual purchases were lack of awareness of the daily menu, speed of purchase and familiarity with prices. Regardless of the schools complying with the local council guidelines with regards to sugar content in recipes, the pupils' capacity to purchase more than one 'regulated' item means they could exceed the daily recommendations.

Pupils were aware of the health reasons behind the restrictions though and stated that if unhealthier items were available to buy then they would do so. It has been reported that children may be less able than adults to resist temptations in choosing unhealthier options if available [7]. It has been suggested that even adult study participants would be more likely to buy food items that are directly available to them as opposed to pictures or description of items [18]. Furthermore, it is established that having knowledge of 'healthier/unhealthier' foods alone is unlikely to influence pupil food choice [19]. Both staff and pupils felt there was too much availability of cookies/sweet items. Previous work with much younger pupils (kindergarten to 10 years) [20] suggests that the involvement of pupils in the design and promotion of healthy eating promotion materials may help to establish group norms about attitudes and preferences towards healthy food consumption.

Despite pupils' awareness of healthy eating guidelines there was opposition of an all-out ban of certain foods and drinks; especially for juice (diluting juice); juice was considered to be an essential component of the daily diet. Mâsse et al. (2014) [21] suggested that having access to sugar sweetened beverages (SSB) at school may disproportionately affect pupils from a less healthy home environment, as they are likely to consume SSB both at home and school. There were suggestions that if certain food items were removed, such as pizzas, pupils would just bring in packed-lunches or buy items from out-with school. There were examples of conflicting practices; one school regularly hosted charity fund-raising schemes by selling confectionery, cakes, etc. to pupils at discounted prices (cheaper than items sold in the dining room). This conflict did not go unnoticed with pupils commenting on the disconnect of healthy eating messages being promoted by the school and the availability of such foods. In older pupils, such as those in this study, perceived eating norms may act as a form of normative social influence whereby they may copy the behaviour of others when they are concerned with feeling socially accepted or establishing a relationship with the source of the influence [22].

With respect to the intervention, implementation did not seem to cause many difficulties for the staff. Some staff expressed surprise in the amount of sugar some of the drinks offered to pupils contained. The increased sale of the fruit pots was seen as a positive development by staff, despite a decline after two weeks. Pupils were not aware of the changes being made to the positioning of drinks and cookies, although with some prompting, they reported being aware of the introduction of the fruit pots.

5. Limitations

The data collected in this study were from two schools in the North East of England; the pupils who consented were selected purposively from the school council, therefore, opinions may not be representative of the general 'school' population or generalisable to other areas.

6. Conclusions

Secondary schools face many barriers and challenges in providing a school food service. As highlighted in the childhood obesity plan [5], the healthiest choice should be the easiest choice. However, as demonstrated in this study, the everyday practicalities of implementing this in a school setting is challenging. Pupils are receiving mixed messages in terms of education and the types and number of 'unhealthy' items they are able to buy, not just at lunch-time, but throughout the school day. Moreover, reducing unhealthier options but also giving pupils choice does not guarantee they will choose the healthier options [19]. As suggested by the pupils themselves, reducing the availability of 'unhealthier' options, by not selling cakes/cookies/pizza every day but limiting to once or twice a week, may be a more pragmatic approach.

Author Contributions: Conceptualization S.S. and L.M.; methodology S.S. and L.M.; validation, S.S., L.M., and J.B.; formal analysis, L.M.; writing—original draft preparation, L.M., S.S., J.B.; writing—review and editing, L.M., S.S., J.B. and A.J.A.; supervision, A.J.A.; project administration, S.S.; funding acquisition, S.S.

Funding: This study was funded by The Academy of Medical Sciences Springboard Health of the Public 2040 award.

Acknowledgments: AJA is funded by the National Institute of Health Research as a senior investigator. The authors would like to thank Wendy Wrieden, Population Health Sciences Institute, Newcastle University, and Christine Crowe, Judith MacMorran, David Stobbs and Roz Rigby, Public Health Newcastle City Council, for their contribution to this study. Thanks are also given to the schools, staff and pupils who consented to participate and share their views.

Conflicts of Interest: The authors declare no conflict of interest.

Appendix A Focus Group Topic Guide

1. *Experience of taking school lunches*

    - Can you tell me about your experience of having a school lunch?
        - Timing
        - Atmosphere
        - Organisation
        - Payment method/system
    - What sort of food and drink do you normally select for your school lunch?
    - What influences your decision on what food and drink to choose?
        - Dining hall layout
        - Food availability
        - Card Vs cash
        - Other lunchtime commitments?
        - Any 'unspoken rules'?

2. *Satisfaction of available foods*

    - What do you think about the food and drink choices available in your school?
    - Are there other types of foods/drinks/snacks you would like to be available?
        - Meal deals?
    - Are there any changes you would like to be made to the available food and drinks?
        - Why?
        - What?
        - Availability of water?
        - Cost of drinks?

3. *Knowledge and views of food and health*

    - (Can you tell me what you know about healthy eating?) Younger group only
        - What do you think are healthy food and drinks in school?
    - Do you think young people want to make healthier food and drink choices?
        - Why?

- How do you think pupils can be helped to make healthier food and drink choices when buying food and drinks at school?

4. *Views of school food regulations*

    - Do you know of any rules in your school about the food and drinks on offer?
        - Any 'unspoken rules'?
    - How would you feel if certain foods and drinks were banned in school?
        - What do you think about schools being able to restrict the types of foods available for you to buy?
    - Can you tell me about any changes you might have noticed in your school canteen recently?
        - Relating to how certain foods and drinks were promoted

    Relating to how certain food and drinks were positioned

Appendix B Staff Interview Topic Guide

1. Importance of school food

    - Can you tell me your views of school food provision?
        - In relation to other school activities/priorities
        - In relation to pupil's health
            - Whose role is it to promote health to pupils?
        - In relation to pupil's behaviour
    - What do you feel about the restriction of certain types of foods and drinks in schools?
        - Is it feasible/acceptable to do so?

2. School practices

    - Can you describe how your school food provision operates?
        - Policies
        - Menus
            - Sugar awareness
            - Compliant drinks—what does this mean?
        - Food purchasing
        - Pupil payment system
        - Day-to-day practice
        - Kitchen/dining facilities
        - Pupil use/uptake
            - Pupil involvement in decision-making?
        - Pupil adherence to 'rules'/practices
            - How is it organised/applied?
            - Who is responsible?
        - Monitoring of practices/processes

- ○ Staff involvement/practice in the dining room
3. School food intervention

    - Can you describe the food/drink intervention that recently took place in your school?
        - ○ What changes were made?
        - ○ Who was responsible for making the changes?
        - ○ Were the changes noticed by anyone?
            - ■ Who? Comments?
        - ○ Were the changes practical/feasible?
            - ■ Describe any difficulties/issues
            - ■ Can you describe any unexpected findings?
    - Positive and negative?
        - ○ How could the intervention have been done differently?
        - ○ If you were able to make *any* changes you wanted to school food provision what would they be and why?

References

1. Public Health England. *Patterns and Trends in Child Obesity*; Gov. uk: London, UK, 2018.
2. Public Health England. Childhood Obesity: Applying All Our Health. Available online: https://www.gov.uk/government/publications/childhood-obesity-applying-all-our-health (accessed on 9 October 2019).
3. Wien, M.; Biro, F.M. Childhood obesity and adult morbidities. *AJCN* **2010**, *91*, 1499S–1505S. [CrossRef]
4. Reilly, J.J.; Kelly, J. Long-term impact of overweight and obesity in childhood and adolescence on morbidity and premature mortality in adulthood: Systematic review. *Int. J. Obes.* **2010**, *35*, 891. [CrossRef] [PubMed]
5. Department of Health and Social Care. Global Public Health Directorate: Obesity Food and Nutrition/10800. In *Childhood Obesity: A Plan for Action, Chapter 2*; Gov. uk: London, UK, 2018.
6. Neumark-Sztainer, D.; French, S.A.; Hannan, P.J.; Story, M.; Fulkerson, J.A. School lunch and snacking patterns among high school students: Associations with school food environment and policies. *Int. J. Behav. Nutr. Phys. Act.* **2005**, *2*, 14. [CrossRef] [PubMed]
7. Oostindjer, M.; Aschemann-Witzel, J.; Wang, Q.; Skuland, S.E.; Egelandsdal, B.; Amdam, G.V.; Schjøll, A.; Pachucki, M.C.; Rozin, P.; Stein, J.; et al. Are school meals a viable and sustainable tool to improve the healthiness and sustainability of children's diet and food consumption? A cross-national comparative perspective. *Crit. Rev. Food Sci. Nutr.* **2017**, *57*, 3942–3958. [CrossRef] [PubMed]
8. Public Health England. *National Diet and Nutrition Survey Results from Years 7 and 8 (Combined) of the Rolling Programme (2014/2015 to 2015/2016)*; Gov. uk: London, UK, 2018.
9. Marteau, T.M.; Ogilvie, D.; Roland, M.; Suhrcke, M.; Kelly, M.P. Judging nudging: Can nudging improve population health? *BMJ* **2011**, *342*, d228. [CrossRef] [PubMed]
10. World Health Organisation. *Global Health Risks: Mortality and Burden of Disease Attributable to Selected Major Risks*; WHO Library Cataloguing-in-Publication Data: Geneva, Switzerland, 2009.
11. Hollands, G.J.; Carter, P.; Anwer, S.; King, S.E.; Jebb, S.A.; Ogilvie, D.; Shemilt, I.; Higgins, J.P.T.; Marteau, T.M. Altering the availability or proximity of food, alcohol, and tobacco products to change their selection and consumption. *Cochrane Database Syst. Rev.* **2019**, *9*. [CrossRef]
12. Ensaff, H.; Homer, M.; Sahota, P.; Braybrook, D.; Coan, S.; McLeod, H. Food Choice Architecture: An Intervention in a Secondary School and its Impact on Students' Plant-based Food Choices. *Nutrients* **2015**, *7*, 4426–4437. [CrossRef] [PubMed]
13. Marteau, T.; Hollands, G.; Fletcher, P. Changing human behaviour to prevent disease: The importance of targeting automatic processes. *Science* **2012**, *337*, 1492–1495. [CrossRef] [PubMed]
14. Allan, J.L.; Johnston, M.; Campbell, N. Snack purchasing is healthier when the cognitive demands of choice are reduced: A randomised controlled trial. *Health Psychol.* **2015**, *34*, 750–755. [CrossRef] [PubMed]

15. Tongco, D. Purposive Sampling as a Tool for Informant Selection. *Ethnobot. J.* **2007**, *5*, 147–158. [CrossRef]
16. NVIVO 12 Pro. 2011. Available online: https://www.qsrinternational.com/nvivo/nvivo-products/nvivo-12-pro (accessed on 9 October 2019).
17. Corbin, J.; Strauss, A. Grounded Theory Research: Procedures, Canons, and Evaluative Criteria. *Qual. Sociol.* **1990**, *13*, 3–21. [CrossRef]
18. Bushong, B.; King, L.M.; Camerer, C.F.; Rangel, A. Pavlovian Processes in Consumer Choice: The Physical Presence of a Good Increases Willingness-to-Pay. *Am. Econ. Rev.* **2010**, *100*, 1556–1571. [CrossRef]
19. Waddingham, S.; Shaw, K.; Van Dam, P.; Bettiol, S. What motivates their food choice? Children are key informants. *Appetite* **2018**, *120*, 514–522. [CrossRef] [PubMed]
20. Gustafson, C.R.; Abbey, B.M.; Heelan, K.A. Impact of schoolchildren's involvement in the design process on the effectiveness of healthy food promotion materials. *Prev. Med. Rep.* **2017**, *6*, 246–250. [CrossRef] [PubMed]
21. Mâsse, L.C.; de Niet-Fitzgerald, J.E.; Watts, A.W.; Naylor, P.J.; Saewyc, E.M. Associations between the school food environment, student consumption and body mass index of Canadian adolescents. *IJBNPA* **2014**, *11*, 29. [CrossRef] [PubMed]
22. Sharps, M.; Robinson, E. Perceived eating norms and children's eating behaviour: An informational social influence account. *Appetite* **2017**, *113*, 41–50. [CrossRef] [PubMed]

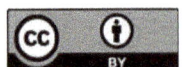

© 2019 by the authors. Licensee MDPI, Basel, Switzerland. This article is an open access article distributed under the terms and conditions of the Creative Commons Attribution (CC BY) license (http://creativecommons.org/licenses/by/4.0/).

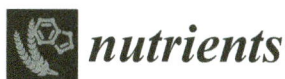

Article

Factors Influencing British Adolescents' Intake of Whole Grains: A Pilot Feasibility Study Using SenseCam Assisted Interviews

Maya Kamar [1], Charlotte Evans [1,*] and Siobhan Hugh-Jones [2]

[1] Nutritional Epidemiology Group (NEG), School of Food Science and Nutrition, University of Leeds, Leeds LS2 9JT, UK; mayakamar@gmail.com
[2] School of Psychology, Faculty of Medicine and Health, University of Leeds, Leeds LS2 9JT, UK; s.hugh-jones@leeds.ac.uk
* Correspondence: c.e.l.evans@leeds.ac.uk; Tel.: +44-(0)113-343-3956

Received: 22 July 2019; Accepted: 17 October 2019; Published: 1 November 2019

Abstract: High whole grain intake is beneficial for health. However, adolescents consume low levels of whole grain and the understanding of the underpinning reasons for this is poor. Using a visual, participatory method, we carried out a pilot feasibility study to elicit in-depth accounts of young people's whole grain consumption that were sensitive to their dietary, familial and social context. Furthermore, we explored barriers and suggested facilitators to whole grain intake and assessed the feasibility of using SenseCam to engage adolescents in research. Eight British adolescents (aged 11 to 16 years) wore a SenseCam device which auto-captured images every twenty seconds for three consecutive days. Participants then completed traditional 24-hour dietary recalls followed by in-depth interviews based on day three SenseCam images. Interview data were subjected to thematic analysis. Findings revealed that low adolescent whole grain intake was often due to difficulty in identifying whole grain products and their health benefits; and because of poor availability in and outside of the home. The images also captured the influence of parents and online media on adolescent daily life and choices. Low motivation to consume whole grains, a common explanation for poor diet quality, was rarely mentioned. Participants proposed that adolescent whole grain consumption could be increased by raising awareness through online media, improved sensory appeal, increased availability and variety, and tailoring of products for young people. SenseCam was effective in engaging young people in dietary research and capturing data relevant to dietary choices, which is useful for future research.

Keywords: whole grain; fibre; adolescents; SenseCam; interviews

1. Introduction

Whole grains are a source of dietary fibre and are rich in protein, vitamins, minerals, and phyto-chemicals [1–3]. Systematic reviews indicate that high whole grain consumption may lead to improved insulin sensitivity and reductions in blood pressure, total and low density lipoprotein (LDL) cholesterol, colorectal cancer, breast cancer, cardiovascular disease (CVD) risk [4–11], although the evidence on improved weight status and reduced waist circumference is less consistent [12]. It has been suggested that a daily intake of around one to three 30 g servings of whole grain foods substantially reduces the risk of disease outcomes [3,13,14]. Although the U.S. Department of Agriculture (USDA) recommends three or more ounce-equivalents/day of whole grain for adults and 1.5 to 4 ounce-equivalents/day for children/adolescents [15], national data show that the mean intake among American adults and children/adolescents is much lower, at around 0.82 and 0.57 ounce-equivalents/day, respectively [16]. Similarly low levels of intake are reported in the United Kingdom (UK). The UK's

National Dietary Survey of British Adults (NDNS) (2008–2011) reported that 18% of adults and 15% of children/adolescents do not consume any whole grain foods, with the median intake for adults and children/adolescents being around 20 g/day and 13 g/day, respectively [17,18]. In the UK, adolescents and individuals from lower socio-economic groups appear to have the lowest levels of intake [17–19].

Most studies exploring whole grain intake correlates have been conducted on other age groups or on non-UK adolescents [20,21]. Previous research has reported the following as possible barriers to whole grain intake: lack of awareness and misconceptions about whole grain food products; inability to identify them; lack of awareness of the health benefits; perceived or experienced negative sensory properties; high price; low availability and accessibility; and lack of knowledge of preparation techniques [22]. National studies clearly reveal the need to target UK adolescents to improve their whole grain intake. Doing so could have significant benefits to health in the short- and long-term and potentially the health of their own families in the future [23–25].

There are challenges when researching factors influencing adolescent eating habits. Focus groups with adolescents have revealed a strong effect of peer influence but may have led to a restricted expression of views based on the group as a whole rather than views of individuals. In addition, the difficulties associated with whole grain identification has prompted a need for in-depth exploration of the topic [22]. Furthermore, traditional methods of surveys or interviews have been critiqued as inadequate for capturing the complexity of factors influencing dietary behaviour [26]. Adolescents' dietary behaviour is shaped by everyday contexts, such as family and school. We need to develop methods to engage young people in dietary research and to capture the key contextual influences on their dietary behaviour to better understand barriers to consumption and potential opportunities for intervention. Visual methods of data collection and analysis are gaining popularity in health research [27], and are advocated by The Lancet Commission on adolescent health to increase engagement and participant-led research and the potential for new insights. This study aimed to explore the feasibility of young people using a camera called SenseCam (developed by Microsoft®Research, Cambridge, UK; see Figure 1) to enhance the exploratory interviews. SenseCam is a wearable camera which hangs from the neck and auto-captures approximately 3600 first-person point-of-view digital images per day.

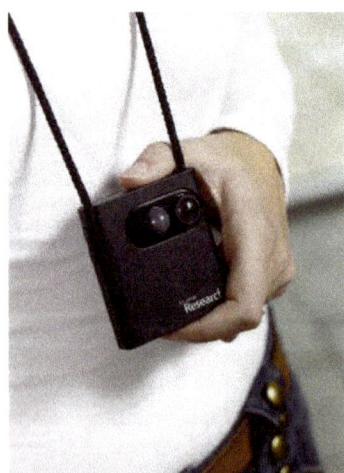

Figure 1. The Microsoft® SenseCam digital camera and how it is worn by participants.

This technology was initially used in research with memory-impaired patients to capture and aid in recalling details of daily life [28]. SenseCam has since been used in a variety of health research projects, including physical activity and nutrition mainly with adults [29–32]. A few SenseCam studies have involved adolescents, some of which included documenting and measuring active and sedentary behavior [33], as well as measuring built environmental features that impact physical activity [34]. These studies offered quantitative analysis of the SenseCam images and feasibility testing of the technology. One recent study used focus groups to understand adolescents' experiences of using SenseCam, in a study measuring daily exposure to food marketing across media to explore determinants of health [35]. However, to date, no studies have explored the potential of SenseCam to help us understand influences on adolescent whole grain intake. SenseCam images can be used to scaffold interviews, helping people to remember dietary choices, and to provide and explain context. This could generate novel insights into the real-world dietary behaviour of adolescents. Our pilot feasibility study aimed to generate new insights into whole grain intake in ways that are sensitive to lived experience and context, explore barriers and suggested facilitators to whole grain intake and assess the feasibility of using SenseCam to engage and work with adolescents.

2. Methods

2.1. Ethics and Participant Recruitment

The University of Leeds MEEC Faculty Research Ethics Committee approved the study protocol (MEEC 13-015, date of approval 9 April 2014). This study adhered to the guidelines laid down in the Declaration of Helsinki. Head teachers and all adolescent participants provided written informed consent, along with parental/carer assent. Guidelines and recommendations on ethical use of SenseCam were utilised from previous studies [36].

Participants were recruited via school contacts and word of mouth. Participants interested in taking part were given an overview of the study and information sheets, and were invited to email or telephone the researcher if they were interested in participating. The maximum number for recruitment was ten adolescents due to the availability of one SenseCam device. Moreover, saturation would be expected to be reached by this number based on similar research in other areas [28–30,32–35]. Therefore, recruitment was stopped after ten participants expressed interest in the project.

2.2. Using SenseCam

The study was single-blinded, in that participants were told that the researcher was interested in adolescent lifestyle and the factors that influence this. Interest in dietary intake and the focus on whole grain was not revealed to the participants in order to limit bias and the possibility of altered behaviour.

The device used in this study was the Microsoft® SenseCam, which auto-captured images every 20–30 s. One device was available throughout the study, and participants used it in turn. After signing the consent forms at the first meeting with the researcher, the participants were briefed on the study and SenseCam. They used the SenseCam for three days, followed by an interview on day four. Participants were advised that they could use the pause button on the SenseCam device, which freezes image auto-capture for five minutes. They were allowed to remove it in situations of discomfort or locations where objection or unwanted attention would occur, such as in private gatherings or places of worship. Participants were requested to ask permission to use SenseCam at school and were encouraged to explain the purpose of the camera if asked. They were provided with a script with details of the research and data confidentiality to use in these situations.

2.3. In-Depth Interviews

At interview start, traditional 24-hour dietary recalls of day three were conducted, with the aid of the Food Standard Agency's (FSA) Photographic Atlas of Food Portion Sizes [37,38]. Results of the 24-hour recalls are not reported here. Following the 24-hour recalls, the SenseCam images were uploaded to a secure, password-protected study file. In line with our ethical protocol, participants were given time to privately check and remove any of the uploaded SenseCam images before proceeding to the interview.

Interviews were semi-structured (see Supplementary Materials (Table S1) for the interview schedule), and directly assisted by the participant approved SenseCam images from day three. Day three was chosen as participants' memory of the day was likely to be more reliable and participant behavior more natural as they adjusted to SenseCam wear over the three days. Approximately 1900 day three images were available per participant for use in the interview. The interview began by focusing on broad questions about adolescent lifestyle. Early in the interview, the true focus of the research was revealed and the interview focused in on dietary choice. SenseCam images were displayed on a computer screen and participants scrolled through images and either chose to stop at a particular image or were asked to stop at one by the researcher (often related to meals or discussed topics). The interviewer encouraged participants to express their opinions freely and used open, non-leading questions and interviews oscillated between researcher-led and participant-led questions and comments. At a later point in the interview, and in order to encourage participants to express opinions on how to increase whole grain intake, information on the definition and health benefits of whole grains was provided. Upon completion of the interviews, participants were provided with vouchers and a certificate to thank them for their contribution to the research project. Interviews were audio-recorded and lasted approximately 75 min each.

2.4. Data Analysis

The interview recordings were transcribed by the first author, with all identifying information removed. Data were analysed using inductive thematic analysis as described by Braun and Clarke [39]. NVivo software was used to aid in management of data analysis (NVivo qualitative data analysis Software, 2012). First, transcripts were read carefully line by line and assigned descriptive labels. Second, units of text containing common labels were assigned provisional codes. Interviews and coding continued until no new codes were generated (data saturation). This was reached after eight interviews. At this point, codes (linked to the original text) were screened and those relevant to the research question were grouped into common themes. Emergent themes were discussed with the second and third authors and credibility checks were conducted (i.e., that the interpretation of the data were credible for their assignment to a theme and that there was sufficient evidence to support a theme). The third and final stage of analysis involved a review and refinement of the themes for ease of data presentation.

3. Results

Ten participants were recruited. Two participants dropped out due to family concern over SenseCam use with regards to privacy issues and the possibility of negative attention. The final sample of eight participants were aged 11 to 16 years old (median age: 13.5 years; see Table 1). Participants were British adolescents with a mixture of ethnic backgrounds, and there were equal numbers of males and females. Only three out of eight participants were given permission to use SenseCam at school, and the remaining participants used it outside school hours and during the weekend.

Table 1. Descriptive details of participants using pseudonyms ($n = 8$).

Participant	Gender	Age	Ethnicity
Participant 1—Nathan	Male	13	British Asian—Indian
Participant 2—Dylan	Male	11	British White
Participant 3—Hannah	Female	15	British Black/African
Participant 4—Olivia	Female	14	British White
Participant 5—Peter	Male	13	British Asian—Chinese
Participant 6—Sasha	Female	12	British White
Participant 7—Liam	Male	16	British Mixed White background
Participant 8—Emma	Female	14	British White

3.1. Factors Influencing Whole Grain Consumption

This sample of young people appeared relatively interested in health. Five out of eight participants spontaneously reported that they tried to eat healthily although they felt this was hard to do in practice. Their motivation to eat well was driven by looking and feeling good, weight management and longer-term health. Factors influencing whole grain consumption have been categorised under five themes: confusion and uncertainty, taste, home availability and influence, availability and accessibility beyond home, peer and social norms.

3.1.1. Confusion and Uncertainty

When asked about whole grain foods, most participants (by "most" we mean six or seven participants out of eight) perceived them as a *"healthier version of something [they] already ate"* (Sasha, F., 12 years). However, most participants were unsure about how to identify a whole grain product, and were confused about what made it a whole grain food and why it had health benefits. Two images of participants choosing food revealed this confusion. First, in reference to Figure 2a, the participant described seeded white bread as wholemeal toast, and second, in reference to Figure 2b, the participant thought her rice cake (and all rice cakes) were whole grain by default.

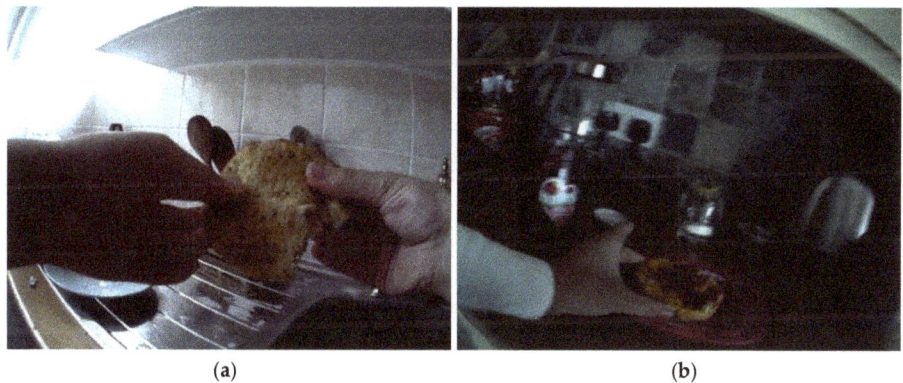

Figure 2. SenseCam images highlighting confusion in whole grain identification (Sasha and Emma) including seeded white bread (**a**) and rice cakes (**b**).

Five participants thought that colour was the main identification marker of whole grain products, and seven thought of wholemeal bread as the most obvious form of whole grain food.

"I try to go for the brown-looking varieties, as I've heard that brown bread is healthier, but that's it. I don't know why it is healthier and what's healthy about it" (Liam, M., 16 years).

There was an assumption that whole grain was bread with added seeds or made with organic wheat which increased its fibre content. Another participant thought that whole grain products must contain less sugar, which was why it was healthier and recommended for people with diabetes, unlike "white bread". Another participant mentioned that his father ate *"those healthy breads with fibre which filled you up right away"* (Peter, M, 13 years). Participants who mentioned fibre (five out of eight) stated it was better for digestion and *"helped food travel in the intestines"*, but were generally unsure of this. Only one participant said they might examine the product ingredient label to assess its whole grain status (without knowing the research was on whole grains): *"here I was reading the labels. It would usually say whole grain somewhere on the front. Because if it was whole grain then the company is like (sic) proud and literally wants everyone to know"* (Peter, M., 13 years).

Overall, participants were confused about what constituted a whole grain product, why it was healthy and how to identify whole grain foods. At this point in the interview, all participants were taught by the interviewee how to identify a whole grain product.

3.1.2. Taste

Although participants expressed various opinions about whole grain foods, they all stated that the texture was dry—mainly as they had wholemeal bread in mind. Negative perceptions of texture were often combined with negative taste perceptions, and participants felt that these would need to be overcome to improve consumption: *"I would only think of eating whole grain one day in the future if I wanted to be healthy. But I don't see myself liking it any time soon"* (Nathan, M., 13 years). One participant said that mixed varieties, such as 50-50 breads, were more acceptable in terms of taste and texture. Three participants expressed a preference for wholemeal vs. white bread for toasting, a preference stemming from habit through home availability (see Theme 3): It was a *"habit that became personal preference really"* (Olivia, F., 14 years). Some participants cited their preference for wholemeal bread as it was tastier, more "special", filling, and healthier as white bread could *"make [her] fat"* (Hannah, F., 15 years). Following clarification of other whole grain foods, participants expressed favourable attitudes towards products such as wholemeal rolls, wraps, chapattis and rotis, and whole grain breakfast cereals. Most participants were pleasantly surprised to learn that other products such as bulgur wheat, brown rice, brown pasta, quinoa and popcorn were whole grain foods and expressed positive attitudes towards these based on taste and health benefits: *"Oh I love bulgur wheat, it's so good! It has a really nice consistency because it's slightly chewy but crunchy and nutty. It's nice!"* (Olivia, F., 14 years); *"Ummm I've actually had some of it (whole grain pasta). I really like it because now I know it's healthy and it still tastes nice at the same time!"* (Peter, M., 13 years). Thus, negative perceptions of whole grains were driven largely by the taste and texture of wholemeal bread, but more positive attitudes emerged when a broader range of foods were considered.

3.1.3. Home Availability and Influence

SenseCam images indicated that home was still the main source of food for these young people, including food to be taken to school. The high number of SenseCam images capturing family meals led to discussions about the influence of the home environment and availability of whole grains on young people's consumption. Reported home availability of whole grains ranged from a constant supply to little availability. One participant said, *"There is always a brown loaf in the house. There's more often brown bread than white bread"* (Olivia, F., 14 years). An image of her mother cutting wholemeal bread, prompted the participant to explain how increased availability made her more likely to consume this type of whole grain food. Good availability of whole grain was also linked to parents of participants being described as health-conscious and who regularly provided whole grain foods at mealtimes. However, in the case of a few participants (by "few" we mean one or two participants), one or both parents preferred lower fibre varieties and this was cited as the reason for low availability in the home. Additionally, parental concern about food waste was perceived as a further factor that reduced whole grain purchases and availability.

Cultural factors also influenced whole grain consumption as ethnic whole grain options were accepted and enjoyed by some participants (by "some" we mean three to five participants). Examples included rotis and chapattis, consumed by participants having South Asian origins, bulgur wheat by those having Turkish origins, and teff by those having African origins. Cultural varieties were described as fundamental to many family meals and were often the sole source of whole grain. While viewing the image of a homemade bulgar-based omelette (Figure 3), the interviewer asked the participant to explain the food shown in the image. This led to the discussion that he enjoyed this type of food, and that he had not been aware it was whole grain.

"I'd have a chapatti or a roti with my dinner—I like those. But I wouldn't go for the whole grain option otherwise like, say, in a sandwich or to school. I prefer white bread" (Nathan, M., 13 years).

The home environment was influential not just through availability but also, for some, through parental modelling and expectations. Although two participants were sceptical of parental "advice", e.g., *"my mum would tell me something because theoretically it is the "right" thing to do or heard it from culture."* (Hannah, F., 15 years), most participants rated their family as their number one trusted source of health and dietary advice. The behaviour and beliefs of parents appeared influential to the dietary intake of the young participants. For example, in relation to consumption of fruit and vegetables, one participant stated: *"I guess it all eventually sinks in and becomes your own priority too."* (Olivia, F., 14 years).

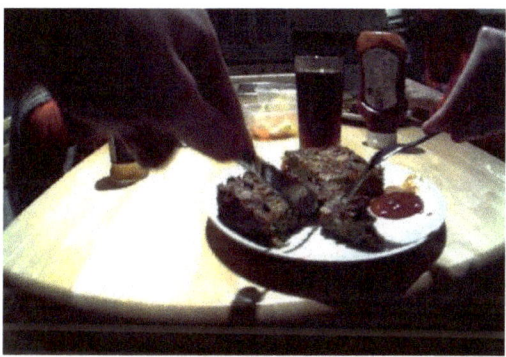

Figure 3. An example of cultural whole grain varieties consumed by participants at home: a bulgur-based omelette.

3.1.4. Availability and Accessibility beyond Home

SenseCam images capturing food shopping prompted discussion of the availability and accessibility of whole grain foods in public spaces. Five participants reported that it was *"cheaper and easier to get white bread"* (Dylan, M., 11 years) than whole grain varieties and that this was a key factor limiting the participants' ability to consume the recommended three portions per day. However, they felt that, compared to refined products, whole grain products were not as visible or *"out there"*, and that *"whole grain [varieties] would be somewhere at the top of the shelf or something, where you don't notice them as much"* (Liam, M., 16 years). An image of supermarket shelves showing a dominance of white products lead the participants to reflect on this: *"If you go to the big supermarkets, you won't see anything of that sort of stuff. You'd see the small stuff that are cultural, like a few pittas, maybe some roti. The bread section is just like being one whole shelf of white bread and then maybe, less visible, a few loaves of brown bread"* (Dylan, M., 11 years).

Most participants stated that it was difficult to access whole grain products in public. *"When you're eating out I don't think it's available enough at all! Because when you see things like fast food or just general restaurants, if they do any kind of bread it's always white bread."* (Emma, F., 14 years). Another participant explained that, when eating out, *"You have to ask them to bring whole grain bread. And only a few places might have it"* (Hannah, F., 15 years). Accessing whole grain snacks in public spaces was seen as very difficult, as most vending machines in schools, hospitals, and public places *"never have whole grain cereal bars or the like"* (Nathan, M., 13 years). When asked about the availability of whole grain varieties in school, all participants stated that it was very hard or impossible to find them: *"school food is always pre-packed stuff, then they're just ovened or microwaved. You would find croissants and, say, toast with butter. So it's not usually proper food or even freshly cooked."* (Peter, M., 13 years). Whole grain snack options (including cereal bars) were perceived to be limited in number and overpriced.

Discussions on the cost of food, and its influence on choice, was mixed. Most participants perceived white bread as cheaper, based on high demand and market competition, and whole grain foods as more expensive, but were unsure what processing methods were increasing the cost. For a few participants, item price was the dominant determinant of food choice outside the home, followed (according to one of the participant) by brand, sugar content and additives: *"people want the tastiest and the cheapest"* (Hannah, F., 15 years).

3.1.5. Peer and Social Norms

Although the participants claimed that peers rarely directly influenced their food choice, some influence was reported following probing. According to one of the participants, in the back of one's mind, there might be a fear of behaving outside of norms: *"They might start asking what is this stuff you're eating there? And just the fact that you might be questioned or the slightest possibility of teased or mocked, especially by the boys, makes you think twice before doing anything that is remotely different than others"* (Olivia, F., 14 years). This also included consumption of more ethnic food types, as two of the participants pointed out. A participant stopped at the image of a takeaway outlet where he was buying a meal with his friends: *"You need to be the same as everyone else. Everything and anything that is different might be mocked"* (Nathan, M., 13 years). Participants reported that pressure to conform to norms dissipated somewhat during later adolescence. One participant explained changes during the last two years of secondary education: *"You start embracing the things you were taught and your own beliefs and hang around people who think similarly"* (Liam, M., 16 years). This participant reported his friends' support (manifesting as lack of jeering) when ordering a salad or asking for the whole grain option.

SenseCam images of social media (e.g., Instagram photos) as well as clothes shopping prompted discussions about social norms for body shape (Figure 4). Carbohydrates were talked about in a negative way by participants of both genders, and participants felt that whole grains were carbohydrates they are meant to avoid. One young participant had engaged in carbohydrate-free dieting before deciding to manage her weight in a healthy way with an emphasis on whole grain: *"I eat whole grain when I am in diet-mode. It keeps me full and helps me lose weight. I read it online."* (Sasha, F., 12 years). Several participants spoke of similar "days of feeling healthy", where whole grains featured more predominantly, but it was nonetheless perceived as optional.

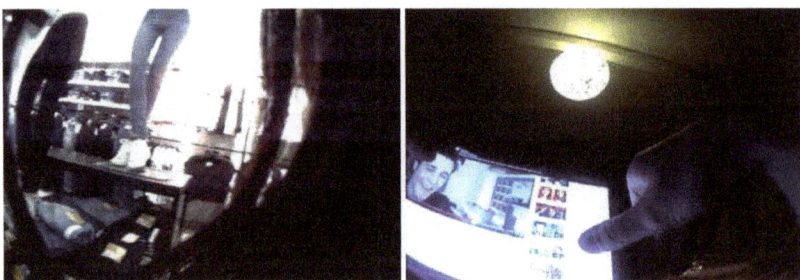

Figure 4. Clothes shopping and social media images prompted discussions around body image and the negative perceptions of carbohydrates.

3.2. Improving Adolescent Whole Grain Consumption

Towards the final part of the interview, participants were asked to imagine that they were whole grain teenage ambassadors with the power and budget to intervene at any level to promote whole grain consumption among adolescents. Their suggestions spanned three themes.

3.2.1. Promote Knowledge and Awareness

Participants believed that young people would consume more whole grain foods if they were more knowledgeable of their health benefits and were more aware of their nature: *"So that they actually know that whole grain is much better for you even though it may be more expensive or less 'out there'... I don't think most of them know about HOW much healthier it may be. And I think that would make them try to eat more whole grain"* (Peter, M., 13 years). They felt there should be more awareness of other whole grain products other than wholemeal bread, such as brown rice, brown pasta, wholemeal wraps, bulgur wheat and quinoa. Participants recommended persuasive media (spanning radio, TV, and online) to promote knowledge, including celebrity endorsement (although the credibility of this might be questioned by some): *"You have to do something really catchy to get people to see it or care. It has to be catchy enough or funny to be talked about or shared with friends so people would remember it."* (Nathan, M., 13 years). Others suggested paying famous YouTubers with high numbers of young followers to promote whole grains as part of their healthy food blogging. According to the participants, this would spark interest and discussion: *"I watch a lot of YouTubers. they're all eating more healthily and it's like—quinoa! Wait, what is quinoa? Is that actually a healthy thing? Then I go ask my mum and look it up online and find out all about it."* (Olivia, F., 14 years). One participant suggested that whole grain companies should sponsor sports events: *"If McDonald's [is doing] it, then Kellogg's certainly can!"* (Liam, M., 16 years).

Targeted campaigns to promote knowledge and awareness were advocated for some settings, for example, using public spaces where people were *"in the mood for being healthy"*, such as gyms and hospitals. However, prompting intake via school-based activities presented mixed views. Simply trying to promote whole grain intake in the form of posters or leaflets was perceived as ineffective, as students will *"look at it and just scoff or make fun of it"* (Hannah, F., 15 years). However, educating young people about whole grains was seen to be more promising, although experiences to date were poor. Most participants reported that they had, at some point, probably heard that *"Brown bread was better than any other bread—that's what they said in school"* (Sasha, F., 12 years) but felt that there was inadequate coverage and discussion of how to identify whole grain products and understand their health benefits. Participants also complained that such sessions were too general, lecture-like, repetitive, and did not involve enough activities to provoke their interest or make the content memorable. However, school-based education which debunked myths about carbohydrates (and the dangers of cutting them) was reported as necessary and likely to be effective. *"Some teenagers think that healthier means almost no food, or no carbohydrates. Tell them to eat the right carbohydrates, not to eliminate them!"* (Hannah, F., 15 years). This was suggested as part of more engaging and informative education: *"I think a whole session in class should tackle this whole grain issue. It makes more sense in every single way: less processing, healthier, more environmentally friendly. It is convincing in every way, and it would lead to lots of discussions on how industry makes something less healthy the norm and people just follow through. These things don't get discussed in class and I feel they should. I hadn't even heard half the things I learnt about fibre today in school!"* (Sasha, F., 12 years).

3.2.2. Changing Norms

Although increased knowledge and awareness was felt to be important, five out of eight participants stressed that the current perception of whole grains as *"special foods for extra health-conscious individuals"* (Liam, M., 16 years) limited consumption by young people. Participants emphasised the importance of shifting norms instead: *"Make it seem like a normal thing, rather than a special thing like only for healthy people... Make it dominate the market. Create varieties too... Get parents to give it to children when they're little. Like white bread should get the special 'white bread' label and not whole grain, because whole grain is the norm of bread. Just like that"* (Olivia, F., 14 years). Improving availability was described as an important way to change norms, particularly in terms of removing less healthy choices. One participant argued that this is more important than knowledge in improving consumer choice: *"I think if I had that kind of budget and that kind of power I'd sort of force shops to reduce stocks of white bread, increase stock of brown bread and make that more often on the shelf and more obvious than white bread. I want white bread to be a lot rarer in shops. I don't care if people don't know what brown bread is and the benefits of it, I just want it to be available. It sort of makes it the norm."* (Dylan, M., 11 years). Changing what is provided in schools was also recommended: *"I think the easiest way would be to get them to change the restaurant venues around the school which students flood out for lunch for to have brown bread. Oh and change the canteen!"* (Emma, F., 14 years). Shaping norms through changed availability could also be managed through cost. Participants suggested that white bread should be made more expensive than whole grain, and the money that is made through sales of white bread would offset the extra cost of increased whole grain production.

3.2.3. Improving Appeal

Making whole grain products more appealing in their packaging was suggested as a key mechanism to promote the chances of young people choosing it. Currently, whole grain products are perceived as serious and boring, for people with special interests or who are fussy eaters, and are associated with "free-from" products. Whole grain products, they suggested, needed re-branding as normal and appealing for the average consumer: *"We want flashy colours, big fonts, and loads of colour. Why does the whole grain cereal look so much more dull and serious than a chocolate cereal?"* (Liam, M., 16 years). Packaging should also be improved in terms of clear labelling: *"Why should it be such a riddle to figure it out? There should be a large clear stamp, like a government-regulated thing, that says whole grain."* (Nathan, M., 13 years). Improved appeal was also suggested in the form of integrating whole grains in products that adolescents already enjoyed: *"Maybe they should make a pizza with whole grain dough, whole grain ice cream cone, or oatmeal chocolate wafers. More whole grain choco-puffs and tea biscuits too—and don't make them the more expensive ones. They should think of more subtle and exciting ways to fit it in our everyday life!"* (Hannah, F., 15 years).

3.3. The SenseCam Experience

Apart from initial parental concern in the case of some participants, all participants approached were keen to take part in the research, expressing interest in SenseCam. They described it as "original", "exciting", and "cool" to be the first to try something new. When asked during the interviews about using SenseCam, they expressed favourable attitudes and felt this is the type of research that adolescents would engage in. They were also pleased at the notion that research was "using their language", as a large portion of their daily life revolved around communicating with and around photos of their day: *"For us it's all about [communicating with] pictures and uploading loads of them every day. And we just do it for fun, so it's great to see that science is also catching up!"* (Sasha, F., 12 years). These positive appraisals were supported by observations during the interview, as the adolescents' engagement with the picture-viewing and commenting on contextual settings was high. Participants reported they did not mind wearing the SenseCam for three days and were not concerned about privacy or unwanted attention (which few of them reported) as reporting on everyday life in photos was a norm in this age group due to the popularity of social media. These findings confirmed that SenseCam is feasible and acceptable to use in this age group to explore dietary behaviour.

4. Discussion

This pilot feasibility study aimed to increase understanding of young people's whole grain consumption by using a visual, participatory method to elicit novel data and determine the feasibility and acceptability of using SenseCam technology. Findings highlighted the complex interplay of factors shaping the adolescents' consumption, from education to family behaviour to sensory appeal. Images captured the impact of parents and online media on participants' daily life and choices. While many poor dietary practices are explained by low motivation, this study showed that low adolescent whole grain intake may be due to the difficulty of identifying whole grain products and their health benefits as well as poor availability in and outside of the home. The participants offered creative ideas on raising awareness through online media, improved sensory appeal, increased availability and variety, and tailoring of products for young people. The findings also suggest that SenseCam was a feasible method of researching diet in young people and effective in engaging them in research; in order to capture routine but important dietary practices in everyday life, and in scaffolding a participant-led interview.

4.1. Adolescents, Health and Whole Grains

The adolescents were generally aware of whole grain foods, and despite a few misconceptions and issues in identification, they knew that whole grain was healthier than refined grain but were unsure why. During the interview, learning about the different varieties of whole grain and their health benefits was of significant interest to participants; learning that a certain desirable food type was in fact whole grain seemed to motivate them to try it more often in the future. Learning about different varieties of whole grain foods (other than wholemeal bread) may improve the appeal of whole grain foods and increase consumption. This is particularly important, given the centrality of taste and sensory appeal to this age group [20,21]. Although sensory appeal was ranked highly by adolescents, an appreciation of the healthiness of food did emerge [40], especially among the older participants. Their views on healthy foods were largely based on processed vs. less processed/fresh food, being preservative- and artificial colouring-free. This may be attributed to the trends being promoted online and in schools regarding preservatives and processing of foods. These findings seem to be in line with those from focus groups with adolescents [22]. It may be useful to promote whole grain to this age group by focusing on it being less processed than its refined counterpart.

4.2. Family as Highly Influential

When it came to food habits and nutritional information, most participants were influenced by their family members who were reported as encouraging them to improve the quality of their diet, albeit only minimally or occasionally in some cases. Pro-active or absent parental influence appeared to impact home availability of whole grain foods, knowledge, attitudes, and habitual consumption although this needs confirmation through a larger study. Participants also cited accompanying their parents to food shopping, evident in most participants' SenseCam photos. Therefore, with the right incentives for both parents and adolescents, an active participation in shaping family (and personal) meals could be developed and directed towards an increased whole grain food availability and consumption. The conclusions drawn from these data are in line with those of existing studies on whole grain with adolescents, where habitual consumption, home availability of whole grain foods and family meal frequency were positively associated with whole grain food intake [20,21].

The participants' statements, along with the observed patterns with whole grain consumption in different households, may contradict the common belief that peers were the most influential group for adolescents—at least when it comes to health and nutritional information [23]. Accessibility of whole grain foods at home was better than outside the home, including school. Reduced availability of whole grain and healthier food choices outside the home and at school was reported in the literature [23,40]. Participants reported a difference in whole grain consumption between weekends and weekdays, and home versus eating out. They were more likely to eat healthy at home than at school, and certainly more than eating out. This points to the need to provide a wider range of choices of whole grain foods for adolescents to purchase in school and in venues around schools.

4.3. School as a Starting Point for Whole Grain Promotion

In addition to increasing whole grain product availability in school canteens, schools would be a perfect setting to encourage whole grain awareness discussions and as an example to lead discussions on food processing, product normalising and low carbohydrate diets. Participants criticised the school system for lack of focus on useful well-being knowledge, a problem noted in other studies [41].

4.4. Teenage Culture and Importance of Social Media

Our findings suggest that peers are influential although not as much as parents; a point also highlighted in a systematic review on adolescent healthy eating interventions [23]. In our study, it was unclear why peers were not considered a major source for dietary influence, but a greater level of peer pressure was reported by younger adolescents, where desire to adhere to social norms appeared strongest. Older adolescence was marked by emergence of "interest" groups, which allowed for less pressure to conform and an increased level of autonomy and friendships based on shared values and lifestyles, including food choices [42]. These trends or differences between adolescence age-stages should be accounted for in interventions targeting younger compared with older adolescents.

Social media creates trends and priorities through celebrities sharing live images of their daily life and giving advice on YouTube and Instagram. There is a substantial focus on exercising, healthy eating, and fitness on these channels, sometimes to extremes. As teenagers are receptive to and trust their social media celebrities it would be helpful to make use of their credibility to pass a healthier whole grain message that could counteract some of the extreme diet tips and fads being promoted. Normalising or integrating whole grain promotion in an appealing way for this age group should include it being a food that would help empower their efforts in healthy weight maintenance or physical activity/sports programmes—an intervention element suggested in a systematic review on adolescents and healthy eating [23]. Moreover, efforts to promote whole grain foods based on general healthiness may be hindered by misconceptions or rumours surrounding the avoidance of all "carbohydrates" in the media, as mentioned by the participants. Acknowledging the body-image challenges facing this age group as well as the abundance of low-carbohydrate dietary advice in the media is important, and efforts to increase whole grain intake in this age group needs to address these issues.

4.5. SenseCam as a Valuable Tool to be Used with Adolescents

Perhaps one of the interesting findings from the use of SenseCam images during the interviews was the challenge of whole grain identification for the participants. There were instances where participants reported consuming whole grain foods, but the images would reveal otherwise. These difficulties are mainly attributed to wider challenges in the various definitions of wholegrain across the globe and reinforcing official recommendations [6,43,44]. An official definition and recommended intakes for whole grains in the UK have not yet been established nor promoted, thus such misconceptions and difficulties are to be expected [3,14]. The current study, with its use of SenseCam images, highlights the potential for this tool to explain and further understand the magnitude and complexities related to whole grain identification, as well as in the case of other food categories.

The SenseCam interviews began with participants declaring autonomy in food choice, a view which was prominent in focus groups with adolescents on whole grain intake [22]. However, the SenseCam images revealed details of daily life that shifted the conversations towards acknowledging the substantial family and home influence on food choices. They helped remind participants of instances where they had unknowingly consumed whole grains and revealed their liking of it. The images also helped remind them of details of the day, such as time spent on social media or instances of label reading, starting new interesting discussions on lifestyle and behavioural influences that may have been unlikely otherwise. SenseCam-assisted interviews therefore have the potential to overcome some of the limitations associated with traditional research methods in this age group and provide a more complete picture of barriers and enhancers. The feedback on SenseCam-assisted interviews was very positive in this age group, specifically in relation to it being a novel technology that included use of images. They also recommended using innovative technology for purposes of scientific research, to encourage adolescents to engage in research. This preference among young people to trying new technologies had been cited in previous studies [35,45], and the integration of technology in research with adolescents may allow for higher enjoyment and participation in an age group often seen as reluctant to engage in research.

4.6. Study Limitations

The main limitations of this study were related to the small sample of participants. Although the study is qualitative and does not claim to be representative of UK adolescents, the type of adolescent taking part in this research may not be representative of all adolescents. Furthermore, adolescents from low SES backgrounds were underrepresented. There are also limitations to the use of SenseCam.

The process of obtaining ethical approval for under 18 year olds was particularly challenging, due to the multitude of privacy, confidentiality and participant inconvenience concerns [36]. There were concerns over privacy raised by some participants' schools and family members, which had to be dealt with. This led to only three out of eight participants being able to wear the SenseCam to school and resulted in loss of information and data at school. From a practical perspective, participants also complained about the short battery life of the SenseCam which seemed to be shorter than previously reported [46] and the length of the strap which was probably designed for adults rather than children. At times this meant the camera was not at the ideal height. For this reason and also due to obstructions such as items of clothing or hair blocking the lens it is recommended that the design of SenseCam is refined for use in younger participants and clear instructions are provided to reduce the risk of poor quality images.

5. Conclusions

This innovative pilot study provided insight into adolescent daily life and contexts surrounding dietary choices, with particular emphasis on whole grain awareness, attitudes and consumption. Adolescents in this study were pro-active, interested and receptive to health messages and expressed the need to be targeted in ways which are relevant to their world. This could include factors related to branding, taste and texture. Participants trusted their family and their social media celebrities, and availability of whole grain foods at home was a key to increased consumption. This study established the feasibility of using SenseCam technology with young people to research their dietary practices. Young people explained their reason for participating was the chance to use an interesting visual based approach that reflected the realities of their lives. The study also shows that a one-size-fits-all approach is unlikely to be effective with adolescents, and tailored approaches for different age groups are recommended. A lack of motivation should not be assumed in this age group but an understanding of the microelements of their daily lives are necessary in order to design successful programmes to improve dietary behavior.

Supplementary Materials: The following are available online at http://www.mdpi.com/2072-6643/11/11/2620/s1, Table S1. Framework of concepts used as guidance and prompts during the interviews. Concepts/ideas inspired from literature on whole grain, adolescent diet, and adolescent lifestyle [21,47–55].

Author Contributions: M.K., C.E. and S.H.-J. planned the study. M.K. undertook the study and analysis. C.E. and S.H.-J. reviewed and refined the work. M.K. wrote the first draft of the paper. All authors were involved in subsequent and final drafts.

Funding: This research has no source of external funding.

Acknowledgments: We wish to thank the schools and young people for participating in this study. We thank Microsoft Research and the SenseCam steering committee for the loan of the camera to support this research.

Conflicts of Interest: This research has no source of external funding and therefore no conflict of interest.

References

1. Slavin, J.; Jacobs, D.; Marquart, L.; Weimer, K. The role of whole grains in disease prevention. *J. Am. Diet. Assoc.* **2001**, *101*, 780–786. [CrossRef]
2. Slavin, J. Why whole grains are protective: Biological mechanisms. *Proc. Nutr. Soc.* **2003**, *62*, 129–134. [CrossRef] [PubMed]
3. Seal, C.J.; Nugent, A.P.; Tee, E.-S.; Thielecke, F. Whole-grain dietary recommendations: The need for a unified global approach. *Br. J. Nutr.* **2016**, *115*, 2031–2038. [CrossRef] [PubMed]
4. Chanson-Rolle, A.; Meynier, A.; Aubin, F.; Lappi, J.; Poutanen, K.; Vinoy, S.; Braesco, V. Systematic review and meta-analysis of human studies to support a quantitative recommendation for whole grain intake in relation to type 2 diabetes. *PLoS ONE* **2015**, *10*, e0131377. [CrossRef] [PubMed]

5. Aune, D.; Keum, N.; Giovannucci, E.; Fadnes, L.T.; Boffetta, P.; Greenwood, D.C.; Tonstad, S.; Vatten, L.J.; Riboli, E.; Norat, T. Whole grain consumption and risk of cardiovascular disease, cancer, and all cause and cause specific mortality: Systematic review and dose-response meta-analysis of prospective studies. *BMJ* **2016**, *353*, i2716. [CrossRef] [PubMed]
6. Ferruzzi, M.G.; Jonnalagadda, S.S.; Liu, S.; Marquart, L.; McKeown, N.; Reicks, M.; Riccardi, G.; Seal, C.; Slavin, J.; Thielecke, F. Developing a standard definition of whole-grain foods for dietary recommendations: Summary report of a multidisciplinary expert roundtable discussion. *Adv. Nutr. Int. Rev. J.* **2014**, *5*, 164–176. [CrossRef]
7. Ye, E.Q.; Chacko, S.A.; Chou, E.L.; Kugizaki, M.; Liu, S. Greater whole-grain intake is associated with lower risk of type 2 diabetes, cardiovascular disease, and weight gain. *J. Nutr.* **2012**, *142*, 1304–1313. [CrossRef]
8. Aune, D.; Chan, D.S.; Lau, R.; Vieira, R.; Greenwood, D.C.; Kampman, E.; Norat, T. Dietary fibre, whole grains, and risk of colorectal cancer: Systematic review and dose-response meta-analysis of prospective studies. *BMJ* **2011**, *343*, d6617. [CrossRef]
9. Lei, Q.; Zheng, H.; Bi, J.; Wang, X.; Jiang, T.; Gao, X.; Tian, F.; Xu, M.; Wu, C.; Zhang, L. Whole grain intake reduces pancreatic cancer risk: A meta-analysis of observational studies. *Medicine* **2016**, *95*, e2747. [CrossRef]
10. Mourouti, N.; Kontogianni, M.D.; Papavagelis, C.; Psaltopoulou, T.; Kapetanstrataki, M.G.; Plytzanopoulou, P.; Vassilakou, T.; Malamos, N.; Linos, A.; Panagiotakos, D.B. Whole grain consumption and breast cancer: A case-control study in women. *J. Am. Coll. Nutr.* **2016**, *35*, 143–149. [CrossRef]
11. Jacobs, D.R.; Marquart, L.; Slavin, J.; Kushi, L.H. Whole-grain intake and cancer: An expanded review and meta-analysis. *Nutr. Cancer* **1998**, *30*, 85–96. [CrossRef] [PubMed]
12. Sadeghi, O.; Sadeghian, M.; Rahmani, S.; Maleki, V.; Larijani, B.; Esmaillzadeh, A. Whole-grain consumption does not affect obesity measures: An updated systematic review and meta-analysis of randomized clinical trials. *Adv. Nutr.* **2019**. [CrossRef]
13. Bjorck, I.; Ostman, E.; Kristensen, M.; Anson, N.M.; Price, R.K.; Haenen, G.R.M.M.; Havenaar, R.; Knudsen, K.E.B.; Frid, A.; Mykkanen, H.; et al. Cereal grains for nutrition and health benefits: Overview of results from in vitro, animal and human studies in the healthgrain project. *Trends Food Sci. Technol.* **2012**, *25*, 87–100. [CrossRef]
14. Seal, C.J.; Brownlee, I.A. Whole-grain foods and chronic disease: Evidence from epidemiological and intervention studies. *Proc. Nutr. Soc.* **2015**, *74*, 313–319. [CrossRef]
15. U.S. Department of Health and Human Services; U.S. Department of Agriculture. 2015–2020 Dietary Guidelines for Americans. Available online: http://health.gov/dietaryguidelines/2015/guidelines/ (accessed on 20 October 2019).
16. Reicks, M.; Jonnalagadda, S.; Albertson, A.M.; Joshi, N. Total dietary fiber intakes in the us population are related to whole grain consumption: Results from the national health and nutrition examination survey 2009 to 2010. *Nutr. Res.* **2014**, *34*, 226–234. [CrossRef]
17. Mann, K.; Pearce, M.; McKevith, B.; Thielecke, F.; Seal, C. Whole grain intake in the uk remains low: Results from the national diet and nutrition survey rolling programme years 1, 2 and 3. *Proc. Nutr. Soc.* **2015**, *74*, E60. [CrossRef]
18. Mann, K.D.; Pearce, M.S.; McKevith, B.; Thielecke, F.; Seal, C.J. Low whole grain intake in the uk: Results from the national diet and nutrition survey rolling programme 2008–11. *Br. J. Nutr.* **2015**, *113*, 1643–1651. [CrossRef]
19. Nelson, M.; Erens, B.; Bates, B.; Church, S.; Boshier, T. *Low Income Diet and Nutrition Survey: Summary of Key Findings*; The Stationery Office: London, UK, 2007.
20. Pohjanheimo, T.; Luomala, H.; Tahvonen, R. Finnish adolescents' attitudes towards wholegrain bread and healthiness. *J. Sci. Food Agric.* **2010**, *90*, 1538–1544. [CrossRef]
21. Larson, N.I.; Neumark-Sztainer, D.; Story, M.; Burgess-Champoux, T. Whole-grain intake correlates among adolescents and young adults: Findings from project eat. *J. Am. Diet. Assoc.* **2010**, *110*, 230–237. [CrossRef]
22. Kamar, M.; Evans, C.; Hugh-Jones, S. Factors influencing adolescent whole grain intake: A theory-based qualitative study. *Appetite* **2016**, *101*, 125–133. [CrossRef]
23. Shepherd, J.; Harden, A.; Rees, R.; Brunton, G.; Garcia, J.; Oliver, S.; Oakley, A. Young people and healthy eating: A systematic review of research on barriers and facilitators. *Health Educ. Res.* **2006**, *21*, 239–257. [CrossRef] [PubMed]

24. Croll, J.K.; Neumark-Sztainer, D.; Story, M. Healthy eating: What does it mean to adolescents? *J. Nutr. Educ.* **2001**, *33*, 193–198. [CrossRef]
25. Story, M.; Neumark-Sztainer, D.; French, S. Individual and environmental influences on adolescent eating behaviors. *J. Am. Diet. Assoc.* **2002**, *102*, S40–S51. [CrossRef]
26. Pain, H. A literature review to evaluate the choice and use of visual methods. *Int. J. Qual. Methods* **2012**, *11*, 303–319. [CrossRef]
27. Glegg, S.M. Facilitating interviews in qualitative research with visual tools: A typology. *Qual. Health Res.* **2019**, *29*, 301–310. [CrossRef] [PubMed]
28. Berry, E.; Kapur, N.; Williams, L.; Hodges, S.; Watson, P.; Smyth, G.; Srinivasan, J.; Smith, R.; Wilson, B.; Wood, K. The use of a wearable camera, sensecam, as a pictorial diary to improve autobiographical memory in a patient with limbic encephalitis: A preliminary report. *Neuropsychol. Rehab.* **2007**, *17*, 582–601. [CrossRef] [PubMed]
29. Gemming, L.; Doherty, A.; Kelly, P.; Utter, J.; Mhurchu, C.N. Feasibility of a sensecam-assisted 24-h recall to reduce under-reporting of energy intake. *Eur. J. Clin. Nutr.* **2013**, *67*, 1095–1099. [CrossRef]
30. Chen, J.; Marshall, S.J.; Wang, L.; Godbole, S.; Legge, A.; Doherty, A.; Kelly, P.; Oliver, M.; Patterson, R.; Foster, C. Using the Sensecam as an Objective Tool for Evaluating Eating Patterns. In Proceedings of the 4th International SenseCam & Pervasive Imaging Conference, San Diego, CA, USA, 18–19 November 2013; ACM: New York, NY, USA, 2013; pp. 34–41. [CrossRef]
31. Kelly, P.; Doherty, A.; Berry, E.; Hodges, S.; Batterham, A.M.; Foster, C. Can we use digital life-log images to investigate active and sedentary travel behaviour? Results from a pilot study. *Int. J. Behav. Nutr. Phys. Act.* **2011**, *8*, 44. [CrossRef]
32. Gemming, L.; Rush, E.; Maddison, R.; Doherty, A.; Gant, N.; Utter, J.; Mhurchu, C.N. Wearable cameras can reduce dietary under-reporting: Doubly labelled water validation of a camera-assisted 24 h recall. *Br. J. Nutr.* **2015**, *113*, 284–291. [CrossRef]
33. Kelly, P.; Doherty, A.R.; Hamilton, A.; Matthews, A.; Batterham, A.M.; Nelson, M.; Foster, C.; Cowburn, G. Evaluating the feasibility of measuring travel to school using a wearable camera. *Am. J. Prev. Med.* **2012**, *43*, 546–550. [CrossRef]
34. Sheats, J.L.; Winter, S.J.; Padilla-Romero, P.; Goldman-Rosas, L.; Grieco, L.A.; King, A.C. Comparison of Passive Versus Active Photo Capture of built Environment Features by Technology Naïve Latinos Using the Sensecam and Stanford Healthy Neighborhood Discovery Tool. In Proceedings of the 4th International SenseCam & Pervasive Imaging Conference, San Diego, CA, USA, 18–19 November 2013; ACM: New York, NY, USA; pp. 8–15. [CrossRef]
35. Barr, M.; Signal, L.; Jenkin, G.; Smith, M. Capturing exposures: Using automated cameras to document environmental determinants of obesity. *Health Promot. Int.* **2015**, *30*, 56–63. [CrossRef] [PubMed]
36. Kelly, P.; Marshall, S.J.; Badland, H.; Kerr, J.; Oliver, M.; Doherty, A.R.; Foster, C. An ethical framework for automated, wearable cameras in health behavior research. *Am. J. Prev. Med.* **2013**, *44*, 314–319. [CrossRef] [PubMed]
37. Nelson, M.; Atkinson, M.; Meyer, J.; (on Behalf of the Food Standards Agency). *A Photographic Atlas of Food Portion Sizes*; Food Standards Agency: London, UK, 1997.
38. Nelson, M.; Atkinson, M.; Meyer, J.; (on Behalf of the Food Standards Agency). *Food Portion Sizes: A User's Guide to the Photographic Atlas*; Food Standards Agency: London, UK, 1997.
39. Braun, V.; Clarke, V. Using thematic analysis in psychology. *Qual. Res. Psychol.* **2006**, *3*, 77–101. [CrossRef]
40. O'Neil, C.E.; Nicklas, T.A.; Zanovec, M.; Cho, S.S.; Kleinman, R. Consumption of whole grains is associated with improved diet quality and nutrient intake in children and adolescents: The national health and nutrition examination survey 1999–2004. *Public Health Nutr.* **2011**, *14*, 347–355. [CrossRef]
41. Moon, A.; Mullee, M.; Rogers, L.; Thompson, R.; Speller, V.; Roderick, P. Helping schools to become health-promoting environments—an evaluation of the wessex healthy schools award. *Health Promot. Int.* **1999**, *14*, 111–122. [CrossRef]
42. Contento, I.R.; Williams, S.S.; Michela, J.L.; Franklin, A.B. Understanding the food choice process of adolescents in the context of family and friends. *J. Adolesc. Health* **2006**, *38*, 575–582. [CrossRef]
43. Ross, A.B.; Kristensen, M.; Seal, C.J.; Jacques, P.; McKeown, N.M. Recommendations for reporting whole-grain intake in observational and intervention studies. *Am. J. Clin. Nutr.* **2015**, *101*, 903–907. [CrossRef]

44. Mozaffarian, R.S.; Lee, R.M.; Kennedy, M.A.; Ludwig, D.S.; Mozaffarian, D.; Gortmaker, S.L. Identifying whole grain foods: A comparison of different approaches for selecting more healthful whole grain products. *Public Health Nutr.* **2013**, *16*, 2255–2264. [CrossRef]
45. Boushey, C.J.; Kerr, D.A.; Wright, J.; Lutes, K.D.; Ebert, D.S.; Delp, E.J. Use of technology in children's dietary assessment. *Eur. J. Clin. Nutr.* **2009**, *63*, S50–S57. [CrossRef]
46. Gemming, L.; Utter, J.; Mhurchu, C.N. Image-assisted dietary assessment: A systematic review of the evidence. *J. Acad. Nutr. Dietet.* **2015**, *115*, 64–77. [CrossRef]
47. O'Dea, J.A. Why do kids eat healthful food? Perceived benefits of and barriers to healthful eating and physical activity among children and adolescents. *J. Am. Diet. Assoc.* **2003**, *103*, 497–501. [CrossRef] [PubMed]
48. Bissonnette, M.M.; Contento, I.R. Adolescents' perspectives and food choice behaviors in terms of the environmental impacts of food production practices: Application of a psychosocial model. *J. Nutr. Educ.* **2001**, *33*, 72–82. [CrossRef]
49. Dennison, C.M.; Shepherd, R. Adolescent food choice: An application of the theory of planned behaviour. *J. Hum. Nutr. Diet.* **1995**, *8*, 9–23. [CrossRef]
50. Krolner, R.; Rasmussen, M.; Brug, J.; Klepp, K.-I.; Wind, M.; Due, P. Determinants of fruit and vegetable consumption among children and adolescents: A review of the literature. Part ii: Qualitative studies. *Int. J. Behav. Nutr. Phys. Activ.* **2011**, *8*, 112. [CrossRef] [PubMed]
51. Zeinstra, G.G.; Koelen, M.A.; Kok, F.J.; De Graaf, C. Cognitive development and children's perceptions of fruit and vegetables; a qualitative study. *Int. J. Behav. Nutr. Phys. Activ.* **2007**, *4*, 30. [CrossRef] [PubMed]
52. Kubik, M.Y.; Lytle, L.; Fulkerson, J.A. Fruits, vegetables, and football: Findings from focus groups with alternative high school students regarding eating and physical activity. *J. Adolesc. Health* **2005**, *36*, 494–500. [CrossRef]
53. McMackin, E.; Dean, M.; Woodside, J.V.; McKinley, M.C. Whole grains and health: Attitudes to whole grains against a prevailing background of increased marketing and promotion. *Public Health Nutr.* **2012**, *1*, 1–9. [CrossRef]
54. McKinley, M.; Lowis, C.; Robson, P.; Wallace, J.; Morrissey, M.; Moran, A.; Livingstone, M. It's good to talk: Children's views on food and nutrition. *Eur. J. Clin. Nutr.* **2005**, *59*, 542–551. [CrossRef]
55. Wind, M.; Bobelijn, K.; de Bourdeaudhuij, I.; Klepp, K.-I.; Brug, J. A qualitative exploration of determinants of fruit and vegetable intake among 10-and 11-year-old schoolchildren in the low countries. *Ann. Nutr. Metab.* **2005**, *49*, 228–235. [CrossRef]

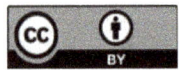

© 2019 by the authors. Licensee MDPI, Basel, Switzerland. This article is an open access article distributed under the terms and conditions of the Creative Commons Attribution (CC BY) license (http://creativecommons.org/licenses/by/4.0/).

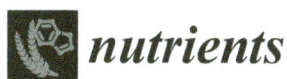

Article

Food Consumption in Adolescents and Young Adults: Age-Specific Socio-Economic and Cultural Disparities (Belgian Food Consumption Survey 2014)

Lucille Desbouys [1,*], Karin De Ridder [2], Manon Rouche [1] and Katia Castetbon [1]

1. Research Center in "Epidemiology, Biostatistics and Clinical Trials", School of Public Health, Université libre de Bruxelles (ULB), 1070 Brussels, Belgium
2. Sciensano, Department of Epidemiology and Public Health and Surveillance, Unit "Lifestyle and chronic diseases", 1050 Brussels, Belgium
* Correspondence: lucille.desbouys@ulb.ac.be

Received: 7 June 2019; Accepted: 3 July 2019; Published: 4 July 2019

Abstract: A key issue in nutritional public health policies is to take into account social disparities behind health inequalities. The transition from adolescence toward adulthood is a critical period regarding changes in health behaviors. This study aimed to determine how consumption of four emblematic food groups (two to favor and two to limit) differed according to socio-economic and cultural characteristics of adolescents and young adults living in Belgium. Two non-consecutive 24-h dietary recalls were carried out in a nationally representative sample of 10–39 year old subjects ($n = 1505$) included in the Belgian food consumption survey 2014. Weighted daily mean consumption of "fruits and vegetables", "whole grain bread and cereals", "refined starchy food", and "sugary sweetened beverages" (SSB) was calculated and explored in multivariable linear regressions stratified into four age groups. After adjustment, 10–13 year old adolescents living in less educated households daily consumed lower amounts of "fruits and vegetables" (adjusted mean: 165.6 g/day (95% CI: 125.3–206.0)) and "whole grain bread and cereals" (40.4 g/day (22.9–58.0)), and higher amounts of SSB (309.7 g/day (131.3–488.1)) than adolescents of same ages living in more educated households (220.2 g/day (179.8–260.7); 59.0 g/day (40.3–77.8); and 157.8 g/day (1.7–314.0), respectively). The same trends were observed in older groups, along with strong consumption disparities according to region of residency, country of birth, and occupation, with specificities according to age. Our findings suggest the need to better explore such disparities by stage of transition to adulthood, and to adapt nutritional health programs.

Keywords: diet; food; nutrition survey; socio-economic factors; adolescent; young adult

1. Introduction

Nutrition may play an important role in the increasing burden of cancer, obesity, diabetes, and cardiovascular diseases. In addition to physical activity, a diet rich in vegetables, fruits, and fibers is recommended, along with limited consumption of processed foods high in fat, refined starches and sugars, red and processed meat, sugary sweetened beverages (SSB), and alcohol [1,2]. In Belgium, recent analyses identified the group of 14–17 year old adolescents as having the worst dietary habits when considering adhesion to dietary guidelines [3]. In the 18–39 year old group, conclusions were mitigated: consistent with adolescents, these adults had the highest consumption of nutrient-poor foods (comprising SSB, alcoholic drinks, biscuits and pastries, confectionary and chocolates, salty and fried snacks, etc.) than the youngest and oldest groups, while they also increased consumption of vegetables, fruits, and whole grain bread in comparison to youngest.

Dietary habits are acquired at adolescence and during the transition toward adulthood. Over the past few decades, this key period has increasingly occupied a greater portion of the life course: biological factors related to earlier puberty precede a longer and later appropriation of the adult social role, going beyond the current limit of 19 years [4]. Moreover, the health-related behavior of future adults may be influenced by socio-economic living conditions, family, the school and work environment, and development of a social network [4–8]. To better understand the different factors involved in acquisition of dietary habits, a comparison of adolescent and young adult behavioral determinants is therefore of interest.

In high-income countries, dietary disparities in food group consumption have been widely pointed out in the general population. For instance, whole grains, fresh fruits and vegetables, lean meats, and low-fat dairy products are more likely to be consumed by adults of higher socio-economic status (SES) [9]. As recent literature reviews concluded, food group consumption disparities also involve adolescents. Fruit, vegetable, and dairy intake is higher when parental SES is more favorable [10–15], while consumption of SSB and salty or sugary energy-dense products is higher when socio-economic living conditions are lower [10,12,13]. Other disparities according to birthplace, length of time living in a country [16], migration generation [17], and urban/rural place of living [10] have been observed in different countries. However, available information from quality studies on food group consumption disparities in adolescents is scattered, and the variety of studied determinants is limited. Literature focusing on diet disparities in young adults is extremely scarce.

The aim of the present research is to determine how consumption of food groups to favor (fruits and vegetables, whole grain bread, and cereals) and to limit (SSB, refined starchy food) differed according to socio-economic and cultural characteristics of adolescents (according to the common definition, i.e., 10–13 and 14–17 years), young adults (end of adolescence, i.e., 18–25 years), and adults (26–39 years).

2. Materials and Methods

2.1. Sampling

We analyzed 10–39 year old subject data from the 2014 Belgian food consumption survey (BFCS), a nationally representative cross-sectional survey conducted in the general population living in Belgium. The BFCS (methods described in detail elsewhere [18]) is part of the "European union (EU) Menu" project coordinated by the European food safety authority (EFSA). To summarize, persons aged 3–64 years were randomly selected from the Belgian national population register, following a multistage stratified sampling procedure. Geographic stratification according to the 11 provinces was used. The number of interviews to be carried out in each province was proportional to the size of each province, and divided into 50 to define the number of municipalities to be selected. Then, within each sampled municipality, individuals were selected by stratifying into 10 age-gender strata following the EFSA age group cut-off recommendations [19]. Data collection was divided equally over the four seasons and seven days of the week so as to integrate seasonal and day-to-day variations in food intake.

2.2. Dietary Assessment

A country-specific version of GloboDiet, a computerized 24-h dietary recall (24h-R) program developed and maintained by the international agency for research on cancer, was used [19,20]. Each 24h-R interview was conducted by a trained dietician. The multipass 24h-R method was used with a rapid and consecutive list of consumed foods and recipes at each eating occasion; a description and quantification of such foods and recipes, a summary of the 24h-R, and a description and quantification of dietary supplements. Each recipe was broken down into a list of foods.

All foods were classified according to the FoodEx2 food classification system developed by EFSA [19,21]. For the present analysis, some adaptations were made: for example, the "starchy food" group was divided into "whole grain bread and cereal" and "refined starchy food", the latter including potatoes and tubers. An SSB group was formed and included all non-alcoholic beverages containing intrinsic sugar, added sugar, flavored milks, and sugary milk substitutes. Mean daily consumption of "fruits and vegetables", "whole grain bread and cereals", "refined starchy food", and SSB was calculated by subject.

Food consumption was linked to the Belgian food composition data (Nubel) and to the Dutch food composition data (NEVO) to estimate total energy intake. The Black method and Goldberg cut-off [22] were used to identify 18–39 year old under-reporters: the mean energy intake of each subject was compared to the basal metabolic rate (BMR), estimated by the Schofield equation [23]. A mean physical activity level of 1.55 was used. Energy intake day-to-day variations, a between-subject BMR variation of 8.5%, and a between-subject physical activity level variation of 15% were considered. Among 10–17 year olds, since the Black method does not take into account energy needs related to growth, under-reporters were those declaring mean energy intake below two standard deviations of the mean energy intake of the sample.

2.3. Socio-Economic Status and Cultural Characteristics

Variables related to household type and education level were adapted to adolescents and young adults. Whatever the age, if the subject was still in school during the survey, the number of children in the household included the subject, while the highest education level of the household was the parental education level. If the subject was 18 years old or older and not schooled, the highest education level in the household was defined according to the education level of the subject and his/her partner if applicable. Occupation (of the mother and the 26–39 year old adult subject) was divided into 5 categories, with "inactive" status including students, retired persons, the unemployed, those on sick leave, and the disabled. Working status was grouped into "student", "active", and "inactive" categories, as to be adapted to the 18–25 year old group. In addition, household type, country of birth, and main language spoken at home were considered.

2.4. Statistical Analyses

Pregnant and breastfeeding women were excluded from analyses; energy under-reporters were included. A weighting factor calculated according to age, gender, day of first dietary recall (weekday or weekend), season, and province of residency, along with sample design, were taken into account in statistical analyses (using the "svyset" function, Stata®). All analyses were stratified into four age groups: 10–13 years, 14–17 years, 18–25 years, and 26–39 years. For each food group, mean consumption of the two observation days was calculated. Univariate linear regressions of daily mean consumptions, with SES variables, gender, and region, were systematically adjusted for total energy intake (Table S1). Those variables with a significance level under 0.20 were included in initial multivariable models. After a manual backward stepwise process, final multivariate linear regressions included variables significantly associated with daily mean consumption (p-value <0.05), along with confounding variables (i.e., that is, variables whose removal increased or decreased consumed amounts by more than 10% for other variables included in the model). In addition, once an explanatory variable was retained for an age group, even though it was not significantly associated with the outcome or was not a confounder, this variable (or the one(s) concerning the same topic in other age groups) was also kept for all age groups. Adjusted mean daily consumption was post-estimated using predictive margins, with co-variates being treated as non-fixed [24]. The absence of co-linearity between variables included in multivariate models, normal distribution, homoscedasticity, and linearity of residuals, along with the absence of influence of potential outliers, were graphically verified in unweighted models. All analyses were performed using Stata® version 14 (StataCorp, College Station, TX, USA).

3. Results

The total sample under study was composed of 1505 subjects having completed two non-consecutive 24h-R, stratified into 447 10–13, 470 14–17, 233 18–25, and 355 26–39 year olds

(Table S2). One (0.2%) under-reporter was identified among the 10–13 year olds, 3 (0.6%) among the 14–17 year olds, 47 (20.2%) among the 18–25 year olds, and 68 (19.2%) among the 26–39 year olds. Mean total energy intake during the two days of study was 1,783.2 kcal/day (SEM: 28.3), 1979.9 kcal/day (35.7), 2056.2 kcal/day (70.1), and 2033.9 kcal/day (42.4), respectively.

Nearly all adolescents and young adults consumed "fruits and vegetables" and "refined starchy food" at least once during the two days of recall (Table 1). The mean daily consumption of "fruits and vegetables" was statistically higher among 18–25 and 26–39 year olds than among 10–13 year olds. The consumption of "whole grain bread and cereals" and contribution to total starchy food intake were statistically higher among 26–39 year olds than among 10–13 year olds. "Refined starchy food" and SSB consumptions were the highest among 14–17 year olds. "Refined starchy food" contribution to total starchy food intake and SSB contribution to total beverage intake were significantly lower among 26–39 year olds than among 10–13 year olds.

Table 1. Consumption, at least once during the two days of recall, mean daily consumption, and contribution to total intake of four food groups according to age group. Belgian food consumption survey 2014.

Food Groups	Age Category				p [a]
	10–13 years $n = 447$	14–17 years $n = 470$	18–25 years $n = 233$	26–39 years $n = 355$	
Fruits and vegetables					
Consumption at least once during the 2 days (%)	97.8	98.1	98.5	99.5	
Mean daily consumption (g/day (SEM))	190.2 (6.8) *	196.7 (7.6)	221.1 (12.1)	**269.6 (11.5)**	<0.001
Whole grain bread and cereals					
Consumption at least once during the 2 days (%)	51.6	52.0	55.9	62.5	
Mean daily consumption (g/day (SEM))	37.3 (3.2) *	42.0 (3.3)	43.1 (4.9)	**63.5 (4.9)**	<0.001
Mean contribution to total starchy food intake (% (SEM))	16.6 (1.2) *	15.5 (1.1)	16.9 (1.8)	**24.0 (1.6)**	<0.001
Refined starchy food					
Consumption at least once during the 2 days (%)	99.4	100.0	99.8	99.2	
Mean daily consumption (g/day (SEM))	188.4 (4.9) *	**226.6 (6.0)**	220.7 (10.9)	203.4 (7.4)	<0.001
Mean contribution to total starchy food intake (% (SEM))	83.4 (1.2) *	84.5 (1.1)	83.1 (1.8)	**76.0 (1.6)**	<0.001
Sugary sweetened beverages					
Consumption at least once during the 2 days (%)	71.9	74.4	74.1	60.3	
Mean daily consumption (g/day (SEM))	258.7 (17.4) *	**327.8 (17.5)**	322.4 (33.3)	240.3 (21.1)	<0.01
Mean contribution to total beverage intake (% (SEM))	24.3 (21.4) *	26.9 (1.3)	20.2 (1.9)	**14.1 (1.1)**	<0.001

[a] Test of difference in means compared with the reference group; * Reference group; bold: category for which consumption statistically significantly differed from the reference category ($p < 0.05$).

3.1. Fruits and Vegetables

Among 10–13 and 14–17 year olds, and after adjustment, "fruit and vegetable" consumption was lower in households with a secondary or lower education level than households with postgraduate education (Table 2). Regional disparities were observed to the detriment of Wallonia (in 10–13 year olds) and the Brussels-Capital region (in 14–17 year olds) inhabitants, which consumed lower amounts of "fruits and vegetables" than the Flemish. In the 14–17 year old group only, boys, adolescents whose mothers were manual workers and those born in Belgium consumed significantly fewer "fruits and vegetables" daily than girls, subjects whose mothers had a managerial or academic occupation and those born in EU and outside the EU, respectively. Finally, among 26–39 year olds, subjects living in a single-parent family and those born in Belgium had lower "fruit and vegetable" consumption than those couples without children and born outside the EU, respectively.

Table 2. Adjusted [a] mean consumption (g/day) of fruits and vegetables according to socio-economic, cultural characteristics, and age group. Belgian food consumption survey 2014.

Characteristics	10–13 years, n = 435 Mean (95%CI) [b]	p	14–17 years, n = 460 Mean (95%CI) [c]	p	18–25 years, n = 229 Mean (95%CI) [d]	p	26–39 years, n = 352 Mean (95%CI) [e]	p
Gender		0.80		<0.01		0.34		0.39
Male	183.7 (145.3–222.0)		187.8 (137.5–238.2)		211.6 (179.9–243.4)		244.5 (205.2–283.8)	
Female	187.0 (149.3–224.7) *		234.1 (184.0–284.1) *		234.6 (198.9–270.4) *		266.6 (238.3–294.9) *	
Household type		0.93		0.41				<0.01
Two-parent family	185.1 (146.4–223.8) *		213.9 (164.9–262.9) *		-		-	
Single–parent family	186.4 (154.0–218.8)		201.4 (153.3–249.6)		-		-	
Single					184.2 (91.6–276.8)	0.37	195.7 (140.1–251.2)	
Single–parent family					185.4 (130.9–239.9)		196.8 (142.5–251.2) *	
Couple without children					265.4 (190.6–340.2)		281.9 (219.6–344.1) *	
Two-parent family	-		-		227.5 (189.5–265.5) *		263.0 (235.8–290.1)	
Other					202.9 (135.9–270.0)		329.6 (230.7–428.5)	
Highest education level in the household		<0.01		0.02		0.07		
2dary education or lower	165.6 (125.3–206.0)		184.6 (135.8–233.4)		182.9 (141.7–224.2)			
Bachelor's degree or equivalent	169.2 (128.1–210.3)		223.8 (172.0–275.6)		231.8 (189.8–273.8)			
Postgraduate education	220.2 (179.8–260.7) *		224.9 (172.1–277.7) *		256.9 (207.9–305.9) *			
Education level of the responder								0.27
2dary education or lower	-		-		-		236.4 (199.3–273.5)	
Bachelor's degree or equivalent							259.8 (221.8–297.9)	
Postgraduate education							283.0 (241.4–324.7) *	
Maternal occupation		0.54		<0.01				
Inactive	182.1 (151.6–212.6)		185.4 (159.7–211.2)					
Manual worker	178.4 (137.0–219.8)		136.7 (107.2–166.2)					
Self-employed	193.6 (156.7–230.4)		205.4 (164.9–245.8)					
Employee or intermediate	209.1 (188.7–229.4)		204.4 (184.4–224.4)		-		-	
Managerial or academic	198.7 (149.2–248.2) *		243.6 (146.2–341.0) *					
No mother declared	182.5 (139.6–225.4)		214.8 (157.6–272.1)					
Working status						0.68		
Student	-		-		216.7 (184.6–248.8)		-	
Inactive					202.9 (133.9–272.0)			
Active					234.3 (195.8–272.9) *			

Table 2. Cont.

Characteristics	10–13 years, n = 435		14–17 years, n = 460		18–25 years, n = 229		26–39 years, n = 352	
	Mean (95%CI) [b]	p	Mean (95%CI) [c]	p	Mean (95%CI) [d]	p	Mean (95%CI) [e]	p
Occupation								0.24
Inactive							228.1 (180.2–276.0)	
Manual worker							228.9 (177.5–280.3)	
Self-employed	-		-		-		271.0 (211.2–330.8)	
Employee or intermediate							286.8 (252.3–321.3)	
Managerial or academic							260.6 (195.8–325.4) *	
Country of birth		0.28		<0.001		0.69		**0.02**
Belgium	184.6 (148.6–220.6) *		203.3 (155.7–250.9) *		222.9 (197.4–248.4) *		246.6 (220.6–272.7) *	
EU	174.5 (121.7–227.3)		255.5 (190.0–320.9)		200.6 (145.5–255.8)		281.7 (197.4–366.0)	
Outside the EU	215.4 (159.4–271.4)		350.6 (257.0–444.2)		257.0 (127.3–386.8)		**389.7 (293.8–485.6)**	
Language spoken at home		0.97		0.32		0.18		0.21
French and/or Dutch	185.8 (149.7–221.9) *		207.5 (160.1–255.0) *		217.9 (193.2–242.5) *		261.8 (236.8–286.9) *	
Mixed incl. French or Dutch	182.3 (136.2–228.4)		238.1 (169.9–306.3)		297.1 (217.3–377.0)		198.0 (94.7–301.2)	
Language other than French or Dutch	180.2 (90.5–270.0)		260.0 (158.7–361.3)		238.5 (84.3–392.8)		166.3 (60.5–272.1)	
Region of residency		**<0.001**		**0.04**		0.14		0.09
Flanders	202.6 (164.3–240.9) *		220.1 (170.2–270.1) *		235.6 (204.9–266.4) *		270.5 (242.1–298.8) *	
Brussels	191.9 (136.8–247.0)		170.1 (114.1–226.0)		237.4 (129.2–345.6)		245.2 (122.6–367.8)	
Wallonia	**148.1 (110.5–185.6)**		205.2 (156.2–254.2)		193.1 (155.7–230.4)		227.5 (197.4–257.6)	

[a] Adjusted for total energy intake and other variables included in the model; [b] $R^2 = 13.6\%$; [c] $R^2 = 17.3\%$; [d] $R^2 = 12.1\%$; [e] $R^2 = 11.9\%$; * reference category; bold: category for which consumption statistically significantly differed from reference category ($p < 0.05$); -: variable not concerning the age group.

3.2. Whole Grain Bread and Cereals

After adjustment, the region of residency was associated with daily mean consumption of "whole grain bread and cereals", with Wallonia (in all age groups) and Brussels-Capital region (in 10–13 and 14–17 year old groups) residents consuming smaller amounts than the Flemish (Table 3). Among 10–13 and 14–17 year olds, "whole grain bread and cereal" consumption was lower in households with secondary or lower education levels than households with postgraduate education. Among 14–17 and 18–25 year olds, subjects born in Belgium ate significantly fewer "whole grain bread and cereals" than those born elsewhere in the EU. In the 14–17 year old group only, adolescents whose mothers had a managerial or academic occupation consumed significantly fewer "whole grain bread and cereals" daily than subjects whose mothers were manual workers, employees, or with an intermediate occupation.

3.3. Refined Starchy Food

After adjustment, in all age groups, except in the 18–25 year old group, subjects living in Wallonia consumed higher amounts of "refined starchy food" than the Flemish (Table 4). Males consumed generally higher amounts of "refined starchy food" than females, significantly only among 14–17 and 26–39 year olds. In the 18–25 year old group, subjects speaking mixed languages, including French or Dutch, consumed higher amounts of "refined starchy food" than those speaking exclusively French and/or Dutch.

3.4. Sugary Sweetened Beverages

In all age groups and after adjustment, households or responders with a secondary education level or less consumed higher amounts of SSB daily than those with a postgraduate education, or a bachelor's degree depending on the age group (Table 5). Indeed, education level gradients were observed in the 10–13 and 14–17 year old groups. Among 14–17 and 18–25 year olds, subjects born in Belgium significantly consumed higher amounts of SSB than those born outside the EU. Among 18–25 year olds, subjects living in Flanders significantly consumed higher amounts of SSB than those living in the Brussels-Capital region. Among 26–39 year olds, inactive and manual workers showed higher consumption of SSB than employees or those with an intermediate occupation.

Table 3. Adjusted [a] mean consumption (g/day) of whole grain bread and cereals according to socio-economic and cultural characteristics, and age group. Belgian food consumption survey 2014.

Characteristics	10–13 years, n = 435		14–17 years, n = 463		18–25 years, n = 229		26–39 years, n = 352	
	Mean (95%CI) [b]	p	Mean (95%CI) [c]	p	Mean (95%CI) [d]	p	Mean (95%CI) [e]	p
Highest education level in the household		0.02		0.03		0.16		0.77
2dary education or lower	40.4 (22.9–58.0)		46.6 (25.7–67.5)		32.5 (21.4–43.6)		53.5 (35.0–72.1)	
Bachelor's degree or equivalent	49.2 (32.0–66.4)		57.1 (35.6–78.5)		42.1 (27.8–56.5)		61.0 (45.1–76.8)	
Postgraduate education	59.0 (40.3–77.8) *		64.8 (43.7–85.9) *		53.3 (32.9–73.6) *		65.2 (45.2–85.2) *	
Education level of the responder								
2dary education or lower	-		-		-		-	
Bachelor's degree or equivalent	-		-		-		-	
Postgraduate education	-		-		-		-	
Maternal occupation		0.12		0.02				
Inactive	39.6 (25.7–53.6)		35.9 (24.2–47.5)					
Manual worker	28.8 (19.3–38.3)		39.6 (27.2–52.0)					
Self-employed	54.3 (28.4–80.1)		31.7 (16.3–47.2)					
Employee or intermediate	38.4 (31.4–45.4)		44.7 (36.2–53.2)					
Managerial or academic	25.4 (7.4–43.5) *		17.7 (2.0–33.5) *					
No mother declared	50.9 (32.5–69.4)		58.2 (36.1–80.3)					
Working status						0.65		
Student					38.6 (28.9–48.4)			
Inactive					35.7 (10.4–61.1)			
Active					47.2 (29.6–64.7) *			
Occupation								0.25
Inactive							48.2 (29.9–66.5)	
Manual worker							65.1 (35.2–95.0)	
Self-employed							38.8 (9.4–68.1)	
Employee or interm.							68.3 (53.0–83.6) *	
Managerial or academic							61.2 (34.9–87.6)	
Country of birth		0.30		0.02		0.02		0.86
Belgium	47.5 (31.5–63.5) *		52.2 (33.4–71.1) *		39.3 (28.6–50.1) *		59.8 (50.4–69.2) *	
EU	69.4 (26.1–112.8)		94.1 (56.2–131.9)		104.1 (60.0–148.2)		52.8 (17.5–88.2)	
Outside the EU	62.3 (31.2–93.4)		84.7 (33.1–136.3)		31.6 (11.6–51.7)		50.6 (10.7–90.5)	
Region of residency		<0.001		<0.001		<0.001		<0.001
Flanders	60.1 (42.9–77.4) *		66.0 (45.8–86.3) *		55.3 (43.5–67.0) *		72.0 (59.2–84.7) *	
Brussels	39.8 (20.5–59.2)		40.9 (17.3–64.6)		35.2 (11.2–59.2)		50.6 (18.5–82.6)	
Wallonia	30.7 (13.2–48.2)		40.6 (19.2–61.9)		18.6 (3.0–34.2)		33.6 (20.9–46.3)	

[a] Adjusted for total energy intake and other variables included in the model; [b] two influent outliers excluded, $R^2 = 18.1\%$; [c] $R^2 = 16.3\%$; [d] $R^2 = 22.8\%$; [e] $R^2 = 12.0\%$, * reference category; bold: category for which consumption statistically significantly differed from reference category ($p < 0.05$); -: variable not concerning the age group.

Table 4. Adjusted [a] mean consumption (g/day) of refined starchy food according to socio-economic and cultural characteristics, and age group. Belgian food consumption survey 2014.

Characteristics	10–13 years, n = 447 Mean (95%CI) [b]	p	14–17 years, n = 470 Mean (95%CI) [c]	p	18–25 years, n = 233 Mean (95%CI) [d]	p	26–39 years, n = 355 Mean (95%CI) [e]	p
Gender		0.77		<0.001		0.08		0.04
Male	198.1 (185.2–211.0)		**239.0 (223.9–254.1)**		225.2 (195.5–254.8)		**208.6 (186.9–230.2)**	
Female	195.6 (182.7–208.5) *		198.7 (185.5–211.8) *		193.0 (176.4–209.7) *		180.1 (165.2–194.9) *	
Language spoken at home		0.13		0.09		0.02		0.45
French and/or Dutch	194.0 (183.9–204.1) *		219.3 (208.5–230.2) *		205.3 (189.0–221.5) *		196.8 (183.2–210.3) *	
Mixed incl. French or Dutch	209.1 (182.1–236.1)		234.0 (201.5–266.4)		**271.1 (225.8–316.4)**		188.6 (142.5–234.7)	
Language other than French or Dutch	248.3 (192.1–304.6)		175.8 (133.9–217.8)		195.5 (106.6–284.4)		138.8 (51.4–226.1)	
Region of residency		<0.001		<0.01		0.80		0.04
Flanders	183.5 (171.5–195.5) *		204.3 (192.1–216.4) *		205.2 (180.8–229.6) *		182.8 (168.0–197.6) *	
Brussels	212.8 (183.3–242.2)		243.0 (201.0–284.9)		209.7 (173.4–246.0)		189.6 (134.8–244.4)	
Wallonia	**218.4 (204.1–233.8)**		**239.5 (221.8–257.2)**		216.4 (196.4–236.5)		**219.0 (194.4–243.4)**	

[a] Adjusted for total energy intake and other variables included in the model; [b] $R^2 = 23.1\%$; [c] $R^2 = 29.9\%$; [d] $R^2 = 40.1\%$; [e] $R^2 = 20.9\%$; * reference category; bold: category for which consumption statistically significantly differed from reference category ($p < 0.05$); -: variable not concerning the age group.

Table 5. Adjusted [a] mean consumption (g/day) of sugary sweetened beverages according to socio-economic and cultural characteristics, and age group. Belgian food consumption survey 2014.

Characteristics	10–13 years, n = 435 Mean (95%CI) [b]	p	14–17 years, n = 460 Mean (95%CI) [c]	p	18–25 years, n = 229 Mean (95%CI) [d]	p	26–39 years, n = 352 Mean (95%CI) [e]	p
Household type		0.33		0.92		0.26		0.35
Two–parent family	234.5 (72.0–396.9) *		360.9 (252.4–469.4) *		-		-	
Single–parent family	270.3 (109.0–431.5)		356.3 (263.6–448.9)					
Single					585.6 (194.1–977.1)		288.9 (196.6–381.2)	
Single–parent family					382.6 (220.0–545.1)		162.8 (53.2–272.5) *	
Couple without children	-		-		267.0 (58.0–476.1)		307.6 (223.1–392.1)	
Two–parent family					250.9 (178.2–323.6) *		260.2 (186.5–334.0)	
Other					417.5 (201.2–633.7)		286.8 (140.8–432.8)	
Highest education level in the household		<0.001		<0.01		0.02		
2dary education or lower	309.7 (131.3–488.1)		403.9 (283.7–524.2)		398.1 (291.9–504.2)		-	
Bachelor's degree or equivalent	260.6 (101.3–420.0)		402.8 (292.2–513.4)		225.8 (141.3–310.3) *		-	
Postgraduate education	157.8 (1.7–314.0) *		275.5 (167.5–383.4) *		300.5 (181.6–419.5)			

Table 5. Cont.

Characteristics	10–13 years, n = 435		14–17 years, n = 460		18–25 years, n = 229		26–39 years, n = 352	
	Mean (95%CI) [b]	p	Mean (95%CI) [c]	p	Mean (95%CI) [d]	p	Mean (95%CI) [e]	p
Education level of the responder		0.33		0.46				0.03
2dary education or lower	-		-		-		336.6 (241.2–432.0)	
Bachelor's degree or equivalent	-		-		-		221.7 (167.8–275.7)	
Postgraduate education	-		-		-		195.6 (139.2–251.9) *	
Maternal occupation								
Inactive	263.1 (206.9–319.3)		356.9 (282.9–431.0)					
Manual worker	338.0 (245.7–430.3)		405.8 (255.4–556.2)					
Self-employed	205.6 (121.3–290.0)		320.3 (213.8–426.7)					
Employee or intermediate	289.2 (242.7–335.6)		291.4 (245.5–337.3)					
Managerial or academic	242.5 (133.6–351.3) *		251.9 (117.8–386.1) *				-	
No mother declared	233.5 (40.2–426.7)		369.2 (248.8–489.7)					
Working status						0.76		
Student					287.6 (200.5–374.8)			
Inactive					391.0 (134.0–647.9)		-	
Active					295.1 (200.8–389.4) *			
Occupation								0.01
Inactive							345.5 (209.0–481.9)	
Manual worker							311.6 (200.3–422.9)	
Self-employed							289.5 (167.0–412.0)	
Employee or intermediate							181.8 (139.8–223.7) *	
Managerial or academic							215.3 (119.3–311.2)	
Country of birth		0.27		0.02		<0.01		0.62
Belgium	242.2 (83.1–401.3) *		369.7 (270.0–469.5) *		318.5 (245.7–391.3) *		257.2 (201.2–313.2) *	
EU	187.6 (−1.8–377.0)		267.2 (121.6–412.8)		327.2 (38.4–616.0)		314.6 (179.6–449.6)	
Outside the EU	292.9 (97.2–488.5)		237.0 (98.8–375.1)		85.0 (−73.6–243.5)		334.2 (114.7–553.6)	
Region of residency		0.08		0.23		<0.01		0.05
Flanders	248.9 (91.4–406.5) *		381.7 (279.9–483.5) *		346.1 (256.3–435.9) *		265.7 (216.2–315.2)	
Brussels	167.5 (11.1–324.0)		332.5 (203.4–461.5)		111.0 (−13.8–235.8)		175.0 (81.0–269.1)	
Wallonia	247.9 (71.9–424.0)		323.0 (210.8–435.3)		297.5 (197.2–397.8)		291.6 (199.6–383.7) *	

[a] Adjusted for total energy intake and other variables included in the model; [b] $R^2 = 21.7\%$; [c] $R^2 = 14.6\%$; [d] $R^2 = 24.7\%$; [e] $R^2 = 26.2\%$; * reference category; bold: category for which consumption statistically significantly differed from reference category ($p < 0.05$); -: variable not concerning the age group.

4. Discussion

Our aim was to determine differences in consumption of four food groups according to socio-economic and cultural characteristics of adolescents and young adults living in Belgium. In a representative sample in which diet was measured with two non-consecutive 24h-R, consumption of food groups to favor (fruits and vegetables, whole-grain products) increased with age. Moreover, consumption of food groups to limit (refined starchy food and SSB) was the highest among older adolescents (14–17 years), then decreased with adult age. As in other high-income countries, diet disparities in fruit, vegetable, and SSB consumption were observed, to the detriment of less well-educated subjects. In addition, our study provides new findings on whole grain product consumption disparities in all age groups. Strong regional disparities were found, independently of SES and for all food groups. Furthermore, our results indicate that oldest adolescents and young adults who were born in Belgium had less favorable consumption than those born abroad, either within or outside of the EU. Overall, the socio-economic and cultural influences upon food group consumption differ according to age group.

Overall, findings related to education and occupation are consistent with disparities observed in other high-income countries [10–13,15]. Education is considered to reflect health and nutrition literacy, i.e., the ability to appropriate nutritional information and to implement behavior accordingly [6]. Occupation is associated with the potential influence upon dietary behavior of the work environment, conditions, and the social network, along with social standing [25]. In addition, education is a determinant of occupation (and income, unavailable in our study); thus, all these indicators are interrelated, but are independently involved in dietary disparities [9,26,27]. In all age groups, and particularly among adolescents in the studied sample, less-well-educated households and subjects ate smaller amounts of healthy products and higher amounts of unhealthy products than the more educated. These results are consistent with recent studies among adolescents [10–13] and young adults [28]. However, disparities in whole grain product consumption had rarely been studied previously: one German study reported no significant association with parental education [29]. In line with previous studies [9,11,12,26], occupation was involved in certain dietary disparities, but not in all age or food groups. Manual workers and inactive subjects, and older adolescents with such parents, were more likely to have an unhealthy diet (higher amounts of SSB and smaller amounts of fruits and vegetables, respectively) than other occupational and active categories. However, older adolescents whose mothers had the highest occupational status were those least consuming whole grain products, which would require further investigations in order to be explained.

Other new insights have emerged from our findings. Wide dietary disparities were encountered according to the region of residency in all age groups and independently of socio-economic conditions. Flanders is socio-economically more advantaged in comparison to Wallonia and the Brussels-Capital region in terms, for instance, of unemployment rate, poverty, and social exclusion [30]. Walloon inhabitants (mainly French-speaking) generally had a less healthy diet than the Flemish (mainly Dutch speakers), which had been previously shown [31]. In multilingual, multiregional Switzerland, substantial differences in diet were found according to linguistic region: indeed, in the 18–75 year old population, weighted daily mean intake of vegetables was significantly higher in German and French regions than in the Italian region, but the daily mean intake of "soft drinks" was higher in the German region than in the French and Italian regions [32]. Authors pointed out the influence of dietary habits from bordering countries: the diet observed in each Swiss region was comparable to that in the neighboring country. Indeed, a parallel could be made between the German community in Switzerland and the Belgian Flanders community, since they consumed higher amounts of vegetables and SSB daily than their French-speaking counterparts. In another study on the diversity of dietary patterns in European countries, the French population consumed fewer soft drinks than other Europeans; in the Netherlands, juice and soft drink consumption was higher than the European mean [20]. Nevertheless, in the Netherlands, vegetable and fruit consumption was lower than in other European countries [33], contradicting the hypothesis of cultural influence from bordering countries on Belgian dietary habits.

Regional dietary specificities in Belgium may therefore be only partly explained by neighboring influences, possibly combined with various changes in regional public health policies.

Furthermore, being born in Belgium, as opposed to the EU or outside the EU (depending on the food group), was globally associated with a less healthy diet (lower amounts of fruits, vegetables, and whole grain products, and higher amounts of SSB), mainly among 14–17 and 18–25 year olds. Previous studies on migration disparities in diet showed that migrants—and especially recent migrants [16]—had higher dietary quality scores [34], healthier patterns [35], and consumed more vegetables than natives or less recent migrants [16]. In one study, foreign-born subjects also ate more SSB than natives [16], while this was not the case in the present study. Here, we only made a distinction between migrants from EU and outside the EU, but more detailed information on country of birth and age at arrival in the host country should also be investigated, so as to better explore potential acculturation phenomena [36–38] in a multicultural country such as Belgium.

We also sought to determine whether dietary disparities were life-stage-specific. We observed that consumption of four emblematic food groups improved with age, being the less favorable among 14–17 year olds. Moreover, in such group of older adolescents, the socio-economic and cultural characteristics of diet disparities were the most diverse. However, complex interpretation of findings in 18–25 year olds and limited sample size made it difficult to identify age specificities. It would be useful to study more in-depth factors involved in dietary behavior during this rather lengthy stage of "semi-dependency" in young adults, i.e., the influence of family transmission, school, or work environment, and individual health and well-being. In addition, changes in diet occurring when the subject becomes responsible for others (partner, children) would be of interest.

For a relevant interpretation of our findings, some limitations should be noted. By definition, collected SES variables differed according to age group, with certain variables specific to life stage. For example, parental occupation was collected in 10–13 and 14–17 year old groups, while that of the subject themselves was collected in adult groups. In the 18–25 year old group, occupational categories such as managerial or academic were not plausible, so the working status was therefore coded into "student", "inactive", and "active". The interpretation of occupational disparities between age groups was therefore limited even if some common trends were observed in the hierarchy of status. In addition, the 18–25 year old group was composed of two-thirds of students living with their parents or dependent on their family (median age = 20.3 years), and one-third of non-students living independently (median age = 23.3 years). This heterogeneity also limited interpretation of potential disparities between food consumption and household type in this age group. Additional stratified analyses according to student status would have been useful, but were not feasible due to the small number of subjects concerned.

Language mainly spoken at home was only associated with refined starchy food consumption in this study. Categorization of this cultural variable aimed to indirectly and partially explore differences in literacy and its potential influence on diet [39]. However, the main language spoken in the household was asked in a semi-open question (Dutch or French option, since they are the two main languages among the three official languages in Belgium according to region of residency vs. another language, with open field to specify). Numerous subjects indicated that they spoke more than one language, without specification of hierarchy; lack of accuracy may therefore be suspected.

Finally, based on two non-consecutive recall days, virtually the entire adolescent and young adult population under study consumed refined starchy food and fruits and vegetables, while up to three-fourths of the sample consumed SSB, and up to two-thirds ate whole grain bread and cereals. In terms of starchy food consumption, the challenge lies in convincing the entire population to more often replace refined product consumption with whole grain products, since overall consumption is low. For fruits, vegetables, and SSB, the wide socio-economic and cultural disparities in all age groups suggest that accessibility [9] and affordability [40] of such products, along with associated perception of availability [41] and benefits to health [42], are factors that must be considered. Less well-educated adolescents and young adults born in Belgium identified as currently consuming fewer fruits, vegetables, and whole grain products, and more SSB, should be specifically targeted.

5. Conclusions

The present study emphasizes socio-economic and cultural disparities in the consumption of four food groups in adolescents and young adults living in Belgium. A healthier diet pattern was observed with age, and our findings suggest that certain disparities may be life-stage-specific. Further analyses addressing other food group consumption (such as for instance meat, fish and eggs, or dairy products) or using a prospective design are needed to better understand changes in dietary behavior occurring between adolescence and young adulthood. Overall, a lower education level, birth in Belgium, and living in Wallonia (excepted for SSB consumption) were independently associated with less healthy dietary habits in all age groups. These characteristics, which had not been previously elucidated, along with regional specificities, should be taken into account in future public nutrition interventions.

Supplementary Materials: The following are available online at http://www.mdpi.com/2072-6643/11/7/1520/s1, Table S1: Adjusted for total energy intake mean consumption (g/day) of four food groups according to socio-economic and cultural characteristics and age group. Belgian food consumption survey 2014, Table S2: Description of the study sample. Adolescents and young adults, Belgian food consumption survey 2014.

Author Contributions: Conceptualization, L.D. and K.C.; methodology, L.D. and K.C.; formal analysis, L.D.; investigation, L.D.; resources, K.D.R.; data curation, K.D.R.; writing—original draft preparation, L.D. and K.C.; writing—review and editing, K.D.R. and M.R.; visualization, L.D.; supervision, K.C.; project administration, K.C.; funding acquisition, L.D. and K.C.

Funding: The Belgian food consumption survey 2014 was the result of a collaboration between the Sciensano (formerly Scientific Institute of Public Health), the Federal Public Service Health, Food Chain Safety and Environment, and the European Food Safety Authority. This research was funded by the French Community of Belgium, as part of the "Actions de Recherche Concertée" funding program. The APC was funded with the support of the University Foundation of Belgium.

Acknowledgments: We thank Jerri Bram for English editing of the manuscript.

Conflicts of Interest: The authors declare no conflict of interest. The funders had no role in the design of the study; in the collection, analyses, or interpretation of data; in the writing of the manuscript, or in the decision to publish the results.

References

1. World Cancer Research Fund; American Institute for Cancer Research. Diet, Nutrition, Physical Activity and Cancer: A Global Perspective: Continuous Update Project Expert Report 2018. Available online: https://www.wcrf.org/dayietandcancer (accessed on 10 December 2018).
2. World Health Organization. Global Status Report on Noncommunicable Diseases 2014. Available online: http://www.who.int/nmh/publications/ncd-status-report-2014/en/ (accessed on 14 January 2018).
3. Bel, S.; De Ridder, K.; Lebacq, T.; Ost, C.; Teppers, E.; Cuypers, K.; Tafforeau, J. Habitual food consumption of the Belgian population in 2014–2015 and adherence to food-based dietary guidelines. *Arch. Public Health* **2019**, *77*, 14. [CrossRef] [PubMed]
4. Sawyer, S.M.; Azzopardi, P.S.; Wickremarathne, D.; Patton, G.C. The age of adolescence. *Lancet Child Adolesc. Health* **2018**, *2*, 223–228. [CrossRef]
5. Sawyer, S.M.; Afifi, R.A.; Bearinger, L.H.; Blakemore, S.-J.; Dick, B.; Ezeh, A.C.; Patton, G.C. Adolescence: A foundation for future health. *Lancet* **2012**, *379*, 1630–1640. [CrossRef]
6. Galobardes, B.; Shaw, M.; Lawlor, D.A.; Lynch, J.W.; Davey Smith, G. Indicators of socioeconomic position (part 1). *J. Epidemiol. Community Health* **2006**, *60*, 7–12. [CrossRef] [PubMed]
7. Galobardes, B.; Shaw, M.; Lawlor, D.A.; Lynch, J.W.; Davey Smith, G. Indicators of socioeconomic position (part 2). *J. Epidemiol. Community Health* **2006**, *60*, 95–101. [CrossRef] [PubMed]
8. Nelson, M.C.; Story, M.; Larson, N.I.; Neumark-Sztainer, D.; Lytle, L.A. Emerging adulthood and college-aged youth: An overlooked age for weight-related behavior change. *Obesity* **2008**, *16*, 2205–2211. [CrossRef] [PubMed]

9. Darmon, N.; Drewnowski, A. Does social class predict diet quality? *Am. J. Clin. Nutr.* **2008**, *87*, 1107–1117. [CrossRef]
10. Grosso, G.; Marventano, S.; Nolfo, F.; Rametta, S.; Bandini, L.; Ferranti, R.; Bonomo, M.C.; Matalone, M.; Galvano, F.; Mistretta, A. Personal eating, lifestyle, and family-related behaviors correlate with fruit and vegetable consumption in adolescents living in sicily, southern Italy. *Int. J. Vitam. Nutr. Res.* **2013**, *83*, 355–366. [CrossRef]
11. Lehto, E.; Ray, C.; Te Velde, S.; Petrova, S.; Duleva, V.; Krawinkel, M.; Behrendt, I.; Papadaki, A.; Kristjansdottir, A.; Thorsdottir, I.; et al. Mediation of parental educational level on fruit and vegetable intake among schoolchildren in ten European countries. *Public Health Nutr. USA* **2015**, *18*, 89–99. [CrossRef]
12. Finger, J.D.; Varnaccia, G.; Tylleskar, T.; Lampert, T.; Mensink, G.B.M. Dietary behaviour and parental socioeconomic position among adolescents: The German Health Interview and Examination Survey for Children and Adolescents 2003–2006 (KiGGS). *BMC Public Health* **2015**, *15*, 498. [CrossRef]
13. Drouillet-Pinard, P.; Dubuisson, C.; Bordes, I.; Margaritis, I.; Lioret, S.; Volatier, J.-L. Socio-economic disparities in the diet of French children and adolescents: A multidimensional issue. *Public Health Nutr.* **2017**, *20*, 870–882. [CrossRef] [PubMed]
14. Drewnowski, A.; Rehm, C.D. Socioeconomic gradient in consumption of whole fruit and 100% fruit juice among US children and adults. *Nutr. J.* **2015**, *14*, 3. [CrossRef] [PubMed]
15. Gopinath, B.; Flood, V.M.; Burlutsky, G.; Louie, J.C.; Baur, L.A.; Mitchell, P. Pattern and predictors of dairy consumption during adolescence. *Asia Pac. J. Clin. Nutr.* **2014**, *23*, 612–618. [PubMed]
16. Llull, R.; Bibiloni, M.; Pons, A.; Tur, J.A. Food consumption patterns of Balearic Islands' adolescents depending on their origin. *J. Immigr. Minor. Health* **2015**, *17*, 358–366. [CrossRef] [PubMed]
17. Rouche, M.; De Clercq, B.; Lebacq, T.; Dierckens, M.; Moreau, N.; Desbouys, L.; Godin, I.; Castetbon, K. Socioeconomic Disparities in Diet Vary According to Migration Status among Adolescents in Belgium. *Nutrients* **2019**, *11*, 812. [CrossRef] [PubMed]
18. Bel, S.; van den Abeele, S.; Lebacq, T.; Ost, C.; Brocatus, L.; Stiévenart, C.; Teppers, E.; Tafforeau, J.; Cuypers, K. Protocol of the Belgian food consumption survey 2014: Objectives, design and methods. *Arch. Public Health* **2016**, *74*, 20. [CrossRef]
19. European Food Safety Authority. Guidance on the EU Menu methodology. *EFSA J.* **2014**, *12*, S58.
20. Slimani, N.; Casagrande, C.; Nicolas, G.; Freisling, H.; Huybrechts, I.; Ocké, M.C.; Niekerk, E.M.; van Rossum, C.; Bellemans, M.; De Maeyer, M.; et al. The standardized computerized 24-h dietary recall method EPIC-Soft adapted for pan-European dietary monitoring. *Eur. J. Clin. Nutr.* **2011**, *65* (Suppl. 1), S5–S15. [CrossRef]
21. European Food Safety Authority. The food classification and description system FoodEx 2 (revision 2). *EFSA Support. Publ.* **2015**, *12*, 84.
22. Black, A.E. Critical evaluation of energy intake using the Goldberg cut-off for energy intake:basal metabolic rate. A practical guide to its calculation, use and limitations. *Int. J. Obes. Relat. Metab. Disord.* **2000**, *24*, 1119–1130. [CrossRef]
23. Schofield, W.N. Predicting basal metabolic rate, new standards and review of previous work. *Hum. Nutr. Clin. Nutr.* **1985**, *39* (Suppl. 1), 5–41. [PubMed]
24. Williams, R. Using the margins command to estimate and interpret adjusted predictions and marginal effects. *Stata J.* **2012**, *12*, 308–331. [CrossRef]
25. Galobardes, B.; Morabia, A.; Bernstein, M.S. Diet and socioeconomic position: Does the use of different indicators matter? *Int. J. Epidemiol.* **2001**, *30*, 334–340. [CrossRef] [PubMed]
26. Méjean, C.; Si Hassen, W.; Lecossais, C.; Allès, B.; Péneau, S.; Hercberg, S.; Castetbon, K. Socio-economic indicators are independently associated with intake of animal foods in French adults. *Public Health Nutr.* **2016**, *19*, 3146–3157. [CrossRef] [PubMed]
27. Si Hassen, W.; Castetbon, K.; Cardon, P.; Enaux, C.; Nicolaou, M.; Lien, N.; Terragni, L.; Holdsworth, M.; Stronks, K.; Hercberg, S.; et al. Socioeconomic Indicators are Independently Associated with Nutrient Intake in French Adults: A DEDIPAC Study. *Nutrients* **2016**, *8*, 158. [CrossRef] [PubMed]
28. Thornton, L.E.; Pearce, J.R.; Ball, K. Sociodemographic factors associated with healthy eating and food security in socio-economically disadvantaged groups in the UK and Victoria, Australia. *Public Health Nutr.* **2014**, *17*, 20–30. [CrossRef] [PubMed]

29. Harris, C.; Flexeder, C.; Thiering, E.; Buyken, A.; Berdel, D.; Koletzko, S.; Bauer, C.-P.; Bruske, I.; Koletzko, B.; Standl, M. Changes in dietary intake during puberty and their determinants: Results from the GINIplus birth cohort study. *BMC Public Health* **2015**, *15*, 841. [CrossRef] [PubMed]
30. Observatoire de la Santé et du Social de Bruxelles-Capitale. Baromètre Social 2018: Rapport Bruxellois sur L'état de la Pauvreté. Available online: http://www.ccc-ggc.brussels/sites/default/files/documents/graphics/rapport-pauvrete/barometre_social_2018.pdf (accessed on 18 April 2019).
31. De Ridder, K.; Bel, S.; Brocatus, L.; Cuypers, K.; Lebacq, T.; Moyersoen, I.; Ost, C.; Teppers, E. Enquête de Consommation Alimentaire 2014–2015. Rapport 4: La Consommation Alimentaire. Available online: https://fcs.wivisp.be/nl/Gedeelde%20%20documenten/FRANS/Rapport%204/Resume_rapport_4_finaal_finaal.pdf (accessed on 5 April 2019).
32. Chatelan, A.; Beer-Borst, S.; Randriamiharisoa, A.; Pasquier, J.; Blanco, J.M.; Siegenthaler, S.; Paccaud, F.; Slimani, N.; Nicolas, G.; Camenzind-Frey, E.; et al. Major Differences in Diet across Three Linguistic Regions of Switzerland: Results from the First National Nutrition Survey menuCH. *Nutrients* **2017**, *9*, 1163. [CrossRef] [PubMed]
33. Slimani, N.; Fahey, M.; Welch, A.A.; Wirfält, E.; Stripp, C.; Bergström, E.; Linseisen, J.; Schulze, M.B.; Bamia, C.; Chloptsios, Y.; et al. Diversity of dietary patterns observed in the European Prospective Investigation into Cancer and Nutrition (EPIC) project. *Public Health Nutr.* **2002**, *5*, 1311–1328. [CrossRef] [PubMed]
34. Martin, M.A.; van Hook, J.L.; Quiros, S. Is socioeconomic incorporation associated with a healthier diet? Dietary patterns among Mexican-origin children in the United States. *Soc. Sci. Med.* **2015**, *147*, 20–29. [CrossRef]
35. Northstone, K.; Smith, A.D.; Cribb, V.L.; Emmett, P.M. Dietary patterns in UK adolescents obtained from a dual-source FFQ and their associations with socio-economic position, nutrient intake and modes of eating. *Public Health Nutr.* **2014**, *17*, 1476–1485. [CrossRef] [PubMed]
36. Pillen, H.; Tsourtos, G.; Coveney, J.; Thodis, A.; Itsiopoulos, C.; Kouris-Blazos, A. Retaining Traditional Dietary Practices among Greek Immigrants to Australia: The Role of Ethnic Identity. *Ecol. Food Nutr.* **2017**, *56*, 312–328. [CrossRef] [PubMed]
37. Osei-Kwasi, H.A.; Powell, K.; Nicolaou, M.; Holdsworth, M. The influence of migration on dietary practices of Ghanaians living in the United Kingdom: A qualitative study. *Ann. Hum. Biol.* **2017**, *44*, 454–463. [CrossRef] [PubMed]
38. Sanou, D.; O'Reilly, E.; Ngnie-Teta, I.; Batal, M.; Mondain, N.; Andrew, C.; Newbold, B.K.; Bourgeault, I.L. Acculturation and nutritional health of immigrants in Canada: A scoping review. *J. Immigr. Minor. Health* **2014**, *16*, 24–34. [CrossRef] [PubMed]
39. Velardo, S. The Nuances of Health Literacy, Nutrition Literacy, and Food Literacy. *J. Nutr. Educ. Behav.* **2015**, *47*, 385–389. [CrossRef] [PubMed]
40. Bihan, H.; Castetbon, K.; Mejean, C.; Peneau, S.; Pelabon, L.; Jellouli, F.; Le Clesiau, H.; Hercberg, S. Sociodemographic factors and attitudes toward food affordability and health are associated with fruit and vegetable consumption in a low-income French population. *J. Nutr.* **2010**, *140*, 823–830. [CrossRef] [PubMed]
41. Williams, L.K.; Thornton, L.; Crawford, D.; Ball, K. Perceived quality and availability of fruit and vegetables are associated with perceptions of fruit and vegetable affordability among socio-economically disadvantaged women. *Public Health Nutr.* **2012**, *15*, 1262–1267. [CrossRef] [PubMed]
42. Pollard, J.; Greenwood, D.; Kirk, S.; Cade, J. Motivations for fruit and vegetable consumption in the UK Women's Cohort Study. *Public Health Nutr.* **2002**, *5*, 146. [CrossRef]

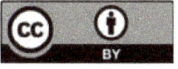

© 2019 by the authors. Licensee MDPI, Basel, Switzerland. This article is an open access article distributed under the terms and conditions of the Creative Commons Attribution (CC BY) license (http://creativecommons.org/licenses/by/4.0/).

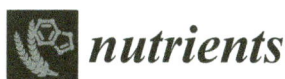

Article

Mapping and Predicting Patterns of Chinese Adolescents' Food Preferences

Shaojing Sun [1], Jinbo He [2,*] and Xitao Fan [2]

[1] School of Journalism, Fudan University, Shanghai 200433, China
[2] School of Humanities and Social Science, the Chinese University of Hong Kong (Shenzhen), Shenzhen 518172, China
* Correspondence: anlfhe@gmail.com or hejinbo@cuhk.edu.cn; Tel.: +86-0755-2351-6572

Received: 25 June 2019; Accepted: 3 September 2019; Published: 6 September 2019

Abstract: This study aimed to examine the patterns of, as well as the predictors for, Chinese adolescents' food preferences. Using the national data of the China Health and Nutrition Survey (CHNS), we analyzed the data of 697 adolescents in the age range of 12 to 17 years. Latent class analysis revealed four types of food preferences: *varied diet* (37.09%, $n = 254$), *avoiding vegetables* (19.69%, $n = 131$), *low appetite* (7.56%, $n = 50$), and *healthy diet* (35.66%, $n = 222$). Major predictors for food preferences included demographic variables (e.g., gender, urban versus rural residence), nutrition knowledge, preference for activities, and social attitudes. Results did not show any significant differences in BMI z-scores among the four latent classes. However, there were significant differences in the number of sleeping hours among the classes.

Keywords: latent class analysis; food preference; Chinese; adolescents

---

1. Introduction

Food preference refers to the degree of liking or disliking food [1]. Ample evidence has indicated that food preference is closely related to a variety of physical health outcomes, such as micronutrient inadequacy [2], obesity [3], cardiovascular disease [4], and cancer [5]. Given the rising rates of obesity and vascular disease [6] and the poor dietary choices in China [7], promoting healthy diet (e.g., fruit and vegetable intake) has become a vital issue for public health [8].

It has been suggested that one important way to improve dietary quality at the population level is to identify behaviors and related characteristics affecting one's adherence to dietary recommendations and guidelines [9]. As such, it would be meaningful to explore potential predictors or risk factors (e.g., food preference) associated with unhealthy dietary patterns. Despite being related to each other, past research has distinguished between dietary patterns and stated preferences for food [10]. The former speaks to one's actual food consumption and dietary history, whereas the latter reflects the underlying attitude and motivation. Our study focused on food preferences, and it differed fundamentally from recent studies on dietary patterns (e.g., Zhen et al. [11]). Specifically, the food preferences were measured with attitude-related questions (e.g., how much do you like fast food?) in our study, while the dietary patterns were measured with questions tapping into children's actual behavior or dietary history (e.g., "whether you had rice, noodles, candy, milk in the past three days") in Zhen et al. [11]. Differentiation of dietary patterns and preferences is particularly important for children and adolescents, as their actual food consumption is often contingent on their parents' decision [12].

Many studies have indicated that food preference is a complex phenomenon, as it is premised on a range of psychological, social, and cultural factors [13,14]. Pearson et al. [13] found that individual habits (e.g., eating while watching TV), social environment (e.g., parental pressure to eat), and physical environment (e.g., availability of fruits and vegetables at home) together influenced young adolescents' preference for consumption of fruits and vegetables. Verstraeten et al. [15], in a sample of 784 school-age

Ecuadorian adolescents, found that both individual factors (e.g., perceived benefits of food) and environmental factors (e.g., school support and parental permissiveness) significantly affected one's eating behaviors (e.g., vegetable intake, unhealthy snacking). Examining the relationship between food consumption and physical activity, Choi and Ainsworth [16] found that active men consumed more grain products, fruits, and vegetables than did the sedentary people. On the other hand, active women tended to consume more legumes and vegetables than did the sedentary ones. Fussner, Luebbe, and Smith [17] showed that disordered eating symptoms were significantly associated with one's sensitivity to social reward and social punishment. More succinctly, de Ridder et al. [18] concluded that individual factors (e.g., intentions, self-regulatory skills) and social/environmental factors (e.g., social norms, availability) are the most important determinants of a healthy diet.

Adolescence, an important transition stage from childhood to adulthood, entails dramatic biological, emotional, and cognitive changes [19]. With these changes, adolescents are particularly susceptible to inadequacies of nutrients [20]. The effects and consequences of dietary patterns during this important transition period have received considerable attention in the research literature. Movassagh et al. [21] identified five types of dietary patterns (i.e., "Vegetarian-style", "Western-like", "High-fat, high-protein", "Mixed" and "Snack") among adolescents. Furthermore, the vegetarian-style dietary pattern during adolescence had a positive long-term impact on one's bone health.

In addition to the dietary issues associated with adolescents, researchers have been paying more attention to the relationships between dietary factors and other related health issues (e.g., body weight, sleep). For the relationship between adolescents' dietary factors and weight change, Laska et al. [22], in a sample of adolescents in Minnesota, found that their diet soda intake was positively related to BMI among females, but not among males. Also, past research supported the linkage between diet and sleep quality, although the mechanism underlying the linkage is not always clear. Peuhkuri, Sihvola, and Korpela [23] summarized past studies and contended that food intake could affect sleep. They pointed out that a balanced and varied diet (e.g., rich in vegetables, fruits, whole grains, low-fat protein) could improve sleep, because such diets might stimulate the synthesis of serotonin and melatonin that were conducive to better sleep. Similarly, St-Onge, Mikic, and Pietrolungo [24] noted that past studies, though mixed and focusing on short-term effects, tended to support the conclusion that some foods (e.g., fish, fruits, vegetables) were sleep-promoting. St-Onge et al. [24], however, called for clinical studies as to exploring the long-term effects of dietary patterns on sleep duration and quality. Notably, recent research has begun to examine the dynamic relationship between diet and sleep duration, as well as the implications for weight-related outcomes, obesity, and other chronic diseases [25].

Given that nutrition intake is a cultural and biological process, rather than a mere physiological and biochemical process [26], prior findings on food consumption in western cultural context might not be readily generalizable to Chinese adolescents. Moreover, to date, little research has been conducted to explore Chinese adolescents' food preferences and the related predictors and health risks thereof [27,28]. For instance, Shi et al. [28] found that more than half of Chinese students reported liking for Western-style fast foods (hamburgers, soft drinks and chocolate). Nonetheless, the studies of Shi et al. [28] and Deng [27] mainly focused on the influences of SES (socioeconomic status) on adolescents' food preferences. As a matter of fact, despite being potentially predictive of Chinese adolescents' food preferences, a broad range of psychological, social, and cultural factors remain understudied.

Overall, past research on adolescents' food preferences mainly focused on the western cultural context. In contrast, food consumption of youngsters is particularly understudied in Asian cultures such as China. In the present study, using a national dataset and the analytic approach of Latent class analysis (LCA) model, we aimed to explore the typology and potential predictors/correlates (e.g., demographics, nutrition knowledge, preference for physical activities, social attitudes, sleep hours) of food preferences.

2. Methods

2.1. Data Description

We used the publicly available data of the "China Health and Nutrition Survey" (CHNS), which was sponsored and designed by the Carolina Population Center at the University of North Carolina at Chapel Hill and the National Institute of Nutrition and Food Safety at the Chinese Center for Disease Control and Prevention. The survey focused on health and nutritional issues of Chinese population. An important goal of the project was to investigate the impact of changes, occurring at community, household, and individual levels, on one's health/nutrition behavior and outcomes.

The first wave of the survey was in 1989, and since then, there have been ten waves of data collection. In this study, we used the most recently released wave of data collected in 2011, covering 289 communities and 5923 families, with 15,725 participants in total. Data for major variables in the present study are available only for those above 12 years old. With this restraint, we identified a total of 697 adolescents between 12 and 17 years old as the sample of this study.

Of the 697 participants, 51.5% were male and 48.5% were female. The average age was 14.25 years old with a standard deviation of 1.65. As for education, 35.6% of the adolescents were elementary school students and 48.8% were middle/high school students. Also, 48.5% of the participants were living in urban regions, whereas 51.5% were living in rural regions at the time of survey. Table 1 presents the descriptive statistics for the total sample.

Table 1. Descriptive statistics for the total sample ($n = 697$).

	Mean ± SD/% (n)	Min-Max	Skewness	Kurtosis
Gender (male = 1)	51.5% (359)	1–2	0.06	−2.01
Education (primary school = 1)	35.6% (248)	1–5	0.64	0.73
Residence (urban = 1)	48.5% (338)	1–2	−0.06	−2.00
Age	14.25 ± 1.65	12–17	0.18	−1.12
BMI	19.61 ± 3.44	13.24–37.99	1.05	1.79
Sleeping hours	8.37 ± 1.04	5–12	0.23	0.59
Dietary knowledge				
Choose fruits/vegetables	3.72 ± 0.83	1–5	−1.14	1.21
Eating sugar	2.15 ± 0.62	1–5	1.23	2.81
Eating a variety of food	3.73 ± 0.74	1–5	−1.38	2.15
Diet high in fat	2.11 ± 0.69	1–5	1.18	2.39
Diet of staple food	3.15 ± 0.96	1–5	−0.29	−0.95
Diet of animal products	2.64 ± 0.93	1–5	0.51	−0.82
Reducing fatty meat	3.69 ± 0.82	1–5	−1.26	1.33
Milk and dairy products	4.00 ± 0.54	1–5	−1.87	9.95
Beans and bean products	3.99 ± 0.53	1–5	−1.77	9.92
Preference for activities				
Walking	2.54 ± 0.89	1–5	0.61	0.05
Sports	3.69 ± 1.07	1–5	−0.44	−0.78
Body building	2.86 ± 0.98	1–5	0.49	−0.40
Watching TV	4.05 ± 0.86	1–5	−0.87	0.82
Playing games	3.78 ± 1.09	1–5	−0.52	−0.79
Reading	3.52 ± 0.94	1–5	−0.27	−0.61
Life attitudes				
Praise from parents	2.32 ± 0.77	1–4	0.35	−0.14
Being liked by friends	2.34 ± 0.85	1–4	1.68	10.47
Look fashionable	2.35 ± 0.82	1–4	1.13	6.47
Achieve high scores in school	2.34 ± 0.86	1–4	1.67	10.38

Notes: The amount of missing data varies across variables.

2.2. Instruments

Food preferences. Respondents were asked to describe how much they like ("dislike very much," "dislike," "neutral," "like," "like very much," or "does not eat this food") five kinds of food: (1) fast food (KFC, pizza, hamburgers, etc.); (2) salty snack foods (potato chips, pretzels, French, fries, etc.); (3) fruits and vegetables, and (4) soft drinks and sugared fruit drinks. According to Collins and Lanza (2010) [29], Likert-scale responses are often categorized into binary responses in latent class analyses for ease of interpretation. Thus, the responses to each question for food preferences were collapsed into two categories ('like' and 'dislike'). Specifically, responses of both "like very much" and "like" were grouped into one category of "like," whereas responses of "dislike very much," "dislike," "neutral," or "does not eat this food" were grouped into the other category of "dislike." This approach is consistent with the research practice in previous research (e.g., Hardigan & Sangasubana [30]).

Background variables. Data on social economic status (SES) and other demographic variables were collected from the participants. For the present study, we focused on the following variables: gender, age, education, residence (urban rural rural), BMI, and hours of sleep per day. For gender, male was coded as 1 and female was coded as 2. Age was calculated by subtracting the year of birth from the time of interviewing. Education was classified into five categories ranging from primary school to college. Hours of sleeping was measured by a single item asking for the total hours spent on sleeping in daytime and at night. The BMI was derived from self-reported weight and height [31]. As suggested by Cole, et al. [32], BMI z-score is the optimal measure of adiposity on a single occasion (i.e., not longitudinal change), and so we used the BMI z-score calculated via the R package childsds [33].

Nutrition knowledge. Respondents' knowledge of nutrition was measured by nine items on 5-point Likert scale. The instruction asked the respondents about the degree to which they would agree with each of the nine statements. Some example items were: "choosing a diet with a lot of fresh fruits and vegetables is good for one's health," "choosing a diet with a lot of staple foods 'rice and rice products and wheat and wheat products' is not good for one's health,", and "consuming a lot of animal products daily (fish, poultry, eggs and lean meat) is good for one's health."

Preference for activities. Six items were used to measure participants' preference for activities. Response options ranged from 1 (dislike very much) to 5 (like very much). Listed activities include walking/Tai Chi, sports (ping pong, badminton, tennis, soccer, basketball, volleyball), body building, watching TV, playing computer/video games/surfing the internet, and reading.

Social attitudes. Four items were used to assess the respondents' social attitudes on a 1–4 Likert scale. Participants were asked of the degree to which they care about the following: (a) being praised by their parents, (b) being liked by friends, (c) looking fashionable, and d) achieving high scores in school.

Sleeping. One item was used to measure an adolescent's sleeping duration. The item reads as "including daytime and nighttime, how many hours do you typically spend on sleeping each day?"

2.3. Data Analysis

Latent class analysis (LCA) is a technique often used for identifying "latent" (i.e., unobserved) subgroups of individuals with distinct patterns of responses [34]. Previous studies have shown the advantages of using LCA to identify distinct patterns of food preferences. Specifically, the technique allows researchers to identify different "classes" (i.e., groups) of individuals, with members within the same group being relatively similar and those across groups being relatively dissimilar in food preferences. Once these "latent classes" are statistically identified, it is possible to examine the unique characteristics of each class [35]. Furthermore, identifying subgroups via LCA is especially useful for designing prevention/treatment programs targeting specific groups with higher level of health risk [36].

Latent class analysis was conducted using Mplus version 8.3 [37] with the robust maximum likelihood estimator (MLR). A large number of starting values (500 random sets of start values with 100 best solutions retained) were used to explore the true highest log likelihood value [38]. Comparing models with 1 to 5 profiles, we searched for the optimal number of latent profiles through the following fit indicators: Akaike Information Criterion (AIC), Bayesian Information Criterion (BIC), Sample Size Adjusted BIC (SABIC), Bootstrapped Likelihood Ratio Test (BLRT), Lo-Mendell-Rubin Adjusted Likelihood Ratio Test (LMRT), and Entropy. Generally speaking, lower values of the AIC, BIC, and SABIC suggest a better model fit, whereas higher values of entropy suggest better quality of classification. The two indices of LMRT and BLRT w employed to compare the discrepancy between two models (k classes versus k-1 classes), with statistical significance suggesting that the model with k-1 classes is preferable. However, these fit indices should not be treated as iron rules for comparing models; rather, researchers should take into consideration practical interpretability and theoretical implications in the model-selection process [39,40].

After identifying the optimal number of classes in the sample, we explored the characteristics of the profiles by adding covariates into the LCA model, in light of the recommended three-step approach [41]. The number of predictors was also controlled for all the steps of the statistical procedure. Specifically, conducting multinomial logistic regressions, we investigated the predictive power of multiple variables (demographic variables, personal knowledge of nutrition, preference for activities, and one's social attitudes) for the class memberships. Furthermore, we examined whether adolescents in different classes would differ in BMI and in hours of sleeping. For the very small amount of missing values, we used the list-wise deletion method to handle the missing data, as the percentage of missing values on major variables was generally less than 2%, which could be considered inconsequential in reference to the general standard of 5% [42].

3. Results

3.1. Latent Class Analysis

The values of the fit indicators for model comparison in LCA are reported in Table 2. Specifically, we listed the model fit information for five different models, ranging from 1 class to 5 class. The LL denotes the likelihood ratio of each model, whereas AIC, BIC, and SABIC serve as fit indices of the models. Typically, the smaller the three aforementioned fit indices, the better model fit. The LMRT and BLMRT were conducted to compare two nested models, with statistical significance suggesting that the compared two models are significantly different from each other. Entropy indicates the accuracy of classification, with a larger value indicating higher classification accuracy. The mixing ratio represents the proportion of each latent class in the population. The results showed that the values of the AIC, BIC, and SABIC deceased with the number of latent classes increasing from 1 to 4 incrementally. However, with the number of classes increasing from 4 to 5, values of these indices did not decrease anymore. Furthermore, in terms of BLRT, the p value for the 5-class model was greater than 0.05 (i.e., non-significant), indicating that the 5 class model was not better than the 4 class model. The p values of the LRT showed the 4-class model was better than the models with a smaller number of classes. The values of Entropy, ranging from 0.67 to 0.86, also supported the superiority of the 4-class model over the alternative ones.

Table 2. Fit indices and class proportions for the 1 to 5 class models.

Classes	LL	AIC	BIC	SABIC	LMRT p-Value	BLRT p-Value	Entropy	Mixing Ratio
1	−1987.80	3985.60	4008.04	3992.17	-	-	-	-
2	−1853.49	3728.98	3778.35	3743.42	<0.001	<0.001	0.67	0.45/0.55
3	−1793.25	3620.50	3696.79	3642.82	<0.001	<0.001	0.74	0.46/0.16/0.38
4	−1765.63	3577.25	3680.47	3607.44	<0.001	<0.001	0.84	0.37/0.08/0.20/0.35
5	−1761.94	3581.89	3712.03	3619.96	<0.05	>0.05	0.86	0.34/0.38/0.03/0.07/0.18

Notes: LL = the Log Likelihood; AIC = the Akaike Information Criterion; BIC = the Bayesian Information Criterion; SABIC = the Sample-Size Adjusted BIC; LMRT = the Lo-Mendell-Rubin Adjusted Likelihood Ratio Test.

3.2. Characteristics of Latent Classes

Figure 1 and Table 3 show the patterns of scores on food preference items for each identified class. Specifically, presented in Table 3 are the probabilities of endorsing each item by the respondents classified into a particular class. Figure 1 presents the profiles of each class for the 4 class solution. Class 1, accounting for 19.69% of the sample, was labeled *avoiding vegetables*, because participants in this class showed strong preferences for all types of food except vegetables. Class 2, accounting for 37.09% of the sample, was labeled *varied diet*, as participants in this class were characterized by strong preferences for all five types of food. Class 3, accounting for 7.56% of the sample, was labeled *low appetite*, as participants in this class showed weak preferences for all five types of foods or drinks. Class 4, accounting for 35.66% of the sample, was labeled *healthy diet*, because participants in this class had strong preferences for healthy food types (i.e., fruits and vegetables) but weak preferences for unhealthy food types (i.e., fast food, salty snack food, and soft drinks).

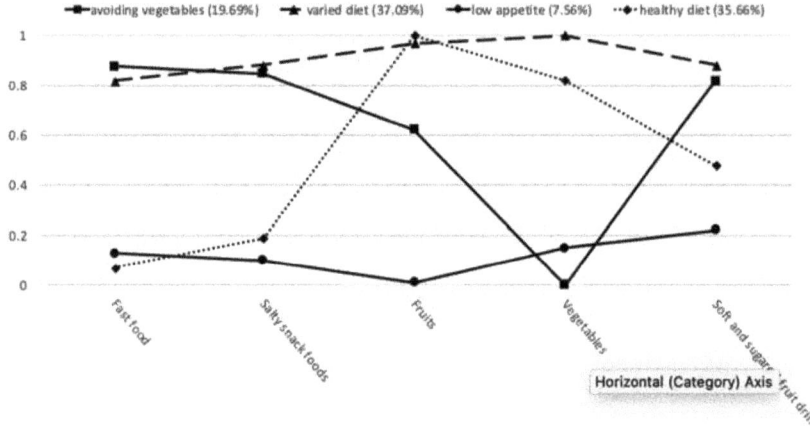

Figure 1. Description of the patterns of food preferences. x-axis = indicators of food preferences (i.e., fast food, salty snack, fruits, vegetables, soft drinks/sugared fruit drinks); y-axis = probability of a "Like" response to each food preference item conditional on latent status membership.

Table 3. Item response probabilities for the four latent classes (avoiding vegetables, varied diet, low appetite, and healthy diet).

Types of Food	Four Latent Classes of Food Preferences			
	Avoiding Vegetables	Varied Diet	Low Appetite	Healthy Diet
	19.69%	37.09%	7.56%	35.66%
	(n = 131)	(n = 254)	(n = 50)	(n = 222)
	Mean ± S.E.	Mean ± S.E.	Mean ± S.E.	Mean ± S.E.
Fast food	0.88 ± 0.05	0.82 ± 0.04	0.13 ± 0.07	0.07 ± 0.04
Salty snack food	0.85 ± 0.04	0.88 ± 0.04	0.10 ± 0.08	0.19 ± 0.05
Fruits	0.62 ± 0.05	0.97 ± 0.01	0.01 ± 0.39	1.00 ± 0.00
Vegetables	0.00 ± 0.00	1.00 ± 0.00	0.15 ± 0.06	0.82 ± 0.07
Soft/sugared fruit drinks	0.82 ± 0.04	0.88 ± 0.03	0.22 ± 0.08	0.48 ± 0.05

3.3. Predictors of Latent Class Membership

To explore how different variables were related to class membership, we used multinomial logistic regression as follow-up analysis to LCA, and examined how different sets of variables could be predictive of the membership in one of the four latent classes. Because multiple post-hoc group comparisons of LCA could lead to inflated overall Type I error rate, we used Bonferroni method for better control of Type I error. To balance statistical power and the Type I error control, we set the overall significance level at 0.10. Thus, the Bonferroni-corrected significance level under each of six comparisons, as shown in Table 4, was set at $\alpha = 0.10/6 \approx 0.02$.

Table 4. Multinomial logistic regression predicting latent class membership as a function of predictors.

	Low Appetite versus Varied Diet			Avoiding Vegetables versus Varied Diet			Healthy Diet versus Varied Diet			Avoiding Vegetables versus Low Appetite			Healthy Diet versus Low Appetite			Healthy Diet versus Avoiding Vegetables		
	B	SE	OR	B	SE	OR	B	SE	OR	B	SE	OR	B	SE	OR	B	SE	OR
Gender	−0.64 *	0.35	0.52	−0.39	0.24	0.68	0.08	0.22	1.09	0.26	0.39	1.29	0.72	0.35	2.06	0.47	0.25	1.59
Residence	−0.01	0.34	0.99	−0.29	0.24	0.75	0.19	0.22	1.21	−0.28	0.37	0.76	0.20	0.34	1.22	0.48 *	0.25	1.62
Education	0.49	0.22	1.64	−0.02	0.16	0.98	0.28 *	0.14	1.32	−0.51 *	0.24	0.59	−0.22	0.22	0.80	0.29	0.16	1.34
Age	0.21 *	0.10	1.24	−0.05	0.08	0.95	0.09	0.07	1.09	−0.27 *	0.11	0.77	−0.13	0.10	0.88	0.14	0.08	1.15
Nutrition knowledge																		
Fruits/vegetables	−0.33 *	0.19	0.72	−0.08	0.14	0.92	0.01	0.14	1.00	0.24	0.21	1.28	0.33	0.20	1.39	0.08	0.15	1.09
Eating sugar	0.52 *	0.27	1.69	0.38 *	0.19	1.47	−0.21	0.19	0.82	−0.14	0.29	0.87	−0.73 **	0.27	0.48	−0.59 **	0.21	0.56
Eating variety	−0.47 *	0.22	0.63	−0.23	0.16	0.80	−0.06	0.16	0.94	0.24	0.23	1.27	0.41 *	0.21	1.51	0.17	0.16	1.18
Diet high in fat	0.30	0.24	1.36	−0.12	0.17	0.89	−0.28	0.16	0.76	−0.43	0.26	0.65	−0.58 *	0.24	0.56	−0.16	0.18	0.86
Staple food	−0.08	0.18	0.93	−0.04	0.13	0.96	0.04	0.12	1.04	0.03	0.20	1.03	0.19	0.18	1.13	0.09	0.14	1.09
Animal products	0.21	0.17	1.23	0.05	0.13	1.05	−0.28 *	0.13	0.75	−0.15	0.18	0.85	−0.49 **	0.17	0.61	−0.34 *	0.14	0.71
Reducing fatty meat	−0.35 *	0.19	0.70	−0.04	0.16	0.96	−0.06	0.14	0.94	0.32	0.22	1.37	0.29	0.18	1.34	−0.02	0.16	0.98
Milk and dairy products	−0.71 *	0.28	0.49	−0.15	0.22	0.86	−0.19	0.24	0.82	0.56 *	0.26	1.74	0.51 *	0.27	1.67	−0.04	0.22	0.96
Beans and bean products	−0.67 *	0.29	0.51	−0.40 *	0.23	0.67	−0.18	0.24	0.84	0.27	0.28	1.31	0.49	0.30	1.64	0.22	0.23	1.25
Physical activities																		
Walking	−0.28	0.20	0.76	−0.34 *	0.14	0.71	−0.11	0.13	0.90	−0.06	0.22	0.94	0.17	0.20	1.19	0.24	0.15	1.27
Sports	−0.35 *	0.16	0.71	−0.05	0.11	0.95	−0.01	0.10	0.99	0.29	0.18	1.34	0.34 *	0.16	1.41	0.05	0.12	1.05
Body building	−0.39	0.21	0.68	−0.09	0.12	0.92	−0.10	0.12	0.90	0.30	0.23	1.35	0.28	0.21	1.33	−0.02	0.13	0.98
Watching TV	−0.90 ***	0.19	0.41	−0.09	0.16	0.91	−0.67 ***	0.16	0.51	0.80 ***	0.20	2.24	0.23	0.17	1.25	−0.56 ***	0.16	0.56
Playing games	−0.39 *	0.17	0.68	0.38 **	0.14	1.46	−0.26 *	0.10	0.77	0.77 ***	0.21	2.16	0.13	0.17	1.14	−0.64 ***	0.14	0.53
Reading	−0.56 **	0.18	0.57	−0.16	0.13	0.86	0.17	0.13	1.19	0.41 *	0.18	1.51	0.74 ***	0.17	2.09	0.33 *	0.13	1.39
Social attitudes																		
Praise from parents	−0.97 **	0.30	0.38	−0.30 *	0.15	0.74	−0.47 **	0.16	0.63	0.67 *	0.31	1.96	0.50	0.29	1.65	−0.17	0.16	0.84
Being liked by friends	−0.95 **	0.30	0.39	−0.29 *	0.14	0.74	−0.42 *	0.19	0.66	0.66 *	0.31	1.93	0.53	0.29	1.70	−0.13	0.17	0.88
Look fashionable	−0.89 **	0.29	0.41	−0.33 *	0.15	0.72	−0.55 **	0.16	0.58	0.56	0.30	1.74	0.34	0.29	1.40	−0.22	0.16	0.80
Achieve high scores in school	−0.96 **	0.32	0.38	−0.30 *	0.14	0.74	−0.42 *	0.19	0.66	0.66 *	0.33	1.93	0.54	0.31	1.72	−0.12	0.17	0.89

Notes: parents care—about parents' praise; friends—care about being liked by friends; fashionable—like being fashionable; school—care about performance in school; SE: approximate standard error; OR = odds ratio; * $p < 0.02$, ** $p < 0.01$, *** $p < 0.001$.

Food preference and demographic variables. Among the background variables, compared to boys, girls were less likely to be in the class of *low appetite* ($OR = 0.52, p < 0.02$). Rural participants were more likely to be in the class of *healthy diet* than urban participants ($OR = 1.62, p < 0.02$). The higher the education, the less likely one would be in the class of *avoiding vegetables*. Compared to younger ones, older adolescents showed a higher likelihood of being in the class of *low appetite* ($OR = 1.24, p < 0.02$) and lower likelihood of being in the class of *avoiding vegetables* ($OR = 0.77, p < 0.02$).

Food preference and nutrition knowledge. Out of the 12 variables for nutrition knowledge, nine factors showed statistically significant predictive effects on adolescents' food preferences. Those believing that eating fruits and vegetables are good for health were less likely to be in the class of *low appetite* than others. Those favoring eating sugar had a high likelihood to be in the classes of *low appetite* or *avoiding vegetables* ($OR = 1.47 \sim 1.69, p < 0.02$), but low likelihood to be in the class of *healthy diet* ($OR = 0.48 \sim 0.56, p < 0.01$). Those who favor dairy food or milk were less likely to be in the class of *low appetite* ($OR = 0.49, p < 0.02$), but were more likely to be in the class of *avoiding vegetables* ($OR = 1.74, p < 0.02$) or *healthy diet* ($OR = 1.67, p < 0.02$). Those who favor animal products were less likely to be in the class of *healthy diet* ($OR = 0.61 \sim 0.75, p < 0.02$). Results also showed that those favoring beans were less likely to be in the classes of *low appetite* ($OR = 0.51, p < 0.02$) or *avoiding vegetables* ($OR = 0.67, p < 0.02$) than in the class of *varied diet*.

Food preference and activity preference. Walking was associated with lower likelihood to be in the class of *avoiding vegetables* ($OR = 0.71, p < 0.02$), whereas sports was associated with lower likelihood of being in the class of *low appetite* ($OR = 0.71, p < 0.02$) but higher likelihood of being in the class of *healthy diet* ($OR = 1.41, p < 0.02$). Body building did not emerge as a significant predictor of any latent class. Watching TV was predictive of lower likelihood of being in the classes of *low appetite* ($OR = 0.41, p < 0.001$) and *healthy diet* ($OR = 0.51, p < 0.001$), but predictive of higher likelihood of being in the class of *avoiding vegetables* ($OR = 2.24, p < 0.001$). The effect of playing games showed a pattern similar to that of watching TV. Interestingly, preference for reading predicted lower likelihood of being in the class of *low appetite* ($OR = 0.57, p < 0.01$) but higher likelihood of being in the classes of *heathy diet* ($OR = 2.09, p < 0.001$) and *avoiding vegetables* ($OR = 1.51, p < 0.02$).

Food preference and social attitudes. High social attitudes (i.e., caring about parents' compliments, friends' likes, being fashionable, and school performance), in general, predicted higher likelihood of being in the class of *varied diet* than in the classes of *low appetite* ($OR = 0.38 \sim 0.41, p < 0.01$), *avoiding vegetables* ($OR = 0.72 \sim 0.74, p < 0.02$), and *healthy diet* ($OR = 0.58 \sim 0.66, p < 0.02$). But, between classes of *avoiding vegetables* and *low appetite*, higher social attitudes signified higher probability of belonging to the former group ($OR = 0.93 \sim 0.96, p < 0.02$).

3.4. Latent Class Membership, BMI and Sleeping Hours

The results showed no statistically significant differences of BMI z-scores among the four latent classes. Interestingly, there was significant difference of sleeping hours among the classes ($\chi^2(3) = 8.35, p = 0.039$). Specifically, adolescents in *healthy diet* group ($M = 8.47, SE = 0.07$) reported longer hours of sleeping than those in *low appetite* group ($M = 8.10, SE = 0.14, \chi^2(1) = 6.12, p < 0.01$) and those in *avoiding vegetables* group ($M = 8.24, SE = 0.09, \chi^2(1) = 4.34, p = 0.037$). Although adolescents in *healthy diet* group ($M = 8.33, SE = 0.07$) reported longer sleeping hours than those in *low appetite* and *avoiding vegetables* groups, the differences were not statistically significant.

4. Discussion

The present study used a national dataset from China and explored adolescents' food preferences and factors related to such preferences. To our knowledge, our study is the first one using the approach of latent class analysis (LCA) to study Chinese adolescents' food preferences. This method has proven to be very useful to identify latent groups, and it provides a novel perspective on prevention and treatment. At the theoretical level, our study contributes to the differentiation between food preference and actual food consumption. Food preferences should be conceptualized as an attitude-related construct instead of a behavior such as actual food consumptions. In this regard, in spite of the studies focusing on the patterns of food consumptions among Chinese adolescents (e.g., [11]), our study is significantly different due to the fact of its focus on food preferences, which have been shown to be related to eating behaviors and psychological well-being We identified four types of food preferences: *avoiding vegetables*, *varied diet*, *low appetite*, and *healthy diet*. Adolescents in the classes of *varied diet* and *healthy diet* accounted for more than 70% of the total respondents. It seems that vegetables and fruits were the major types of food that distinguished respondents' food preferences. Soft drink and fast food, however, were favored options by a large proportion of adolescents.

5. Significant Findings and Implications

Our study found that demographic variables played a significant role in predicting adolescents' food preferences. Girls were more likely to be in the class of *healthy diet* than boys. Although the present study was conducted in the Chinese cultural/social context, the findings echoed those of prior studies conducted in western cultural/social contexts. For example, Caine-Bish and Scheule [43] surveyed American children and reported that food preferences differed across gender. Furthermore, the gender difference varied among elementary, middle, and high school students. Their findings revealed that boys preferred meat, fish, and poultry food, whereas girls preferred fruits and vegetables. Considering the consistency of gender difference in food preference across cultures, practitioners may take into account the role of gender while designing dietary interventions for Chinese adolescents.

One interesting finding speaks to the impact of residence status. In China, people's residence is roughly classified into two types: urban residence vs. rural residence. Urban residents rarely have resources for farming or growing crops or vegetables. In contrast, rural residents are more likely to have access to rich supplies of vegetables. Such a difference may explain why adolescents of rural residence were more likely to be in the class of *healthy diet*, but less likely to be in the class of *avoiding vegetables* than those of urban residence. It is plausible that those growing up in rural regions had easy access to vegetables and formed the habit of eating vegetables over time. As prior studies have shown [44], accessibility of food is a significant predictor of food preference. Thus, health education and promotion programs in China should take into consideration the differences between urban and rural residence.

Regarding the impact of nutrition knowledge, an interesting finding is that nutrition knowledge appears to influence one's food preferences. More specifically, our results showed that one's nutrition knowledge about sugar, animal products, and dairy food was predictive of his/her food preferences. Research has shown that nutrition knowledge is closely related to food intake, especially for healthy eating. Therefore, improving nutrition knowledge could be a target for health education campaigns for promoting healthy eating [45]. On this note, school-based nutrition education for Chinese adolescents could play an important role in promoting healthy eating.

As for the relationship between activity preference and food preferences, the finding about watching TV was in line with prior findings that heavy TV watching may increase children's preferences for unhealthy foods (e.g., high carbohydrate and high fat foods) [46,47]. Not surprisingly, the amount of computer-game playing also emerged to be a significant predictor of food preferences. Past research has shown that both watching TV and playing computer games increased adolescents' cravings for unhealthy snacks and drinks [48]. Our finding speaks to the common nature of the two media activities, which are sedentary and addictive [49,50]. A bit puzzling is the relationship between reading and food preferences, with reading being associated with higher likelihood of being in the class of *healthy diet* as opposed to the classes of *low appetite* or *avoiding vegetables*. One plausible explanation is that those enjoying reading might have learned more about nutrition and healthy dietary practice.

The linkage between social attitudes and food preferences may attest to cultural/social influences. Interestingly, we found that those who cared about parents'/friends' views and one's own social images were more likely to be in the class of *varied diet*, as opposed to be in the other three classes. It is likely that those with higher scores of social attitudes are adaptable to different life contexts, and hence more readily acceptable to varying food choices.

Our study did not reveal any significant differences in BMI z-scores among the four classes of individuals. This finding, however, is in line with some previous studies showing that food preferences were not related, or only marginally related, to BMI [3,51]. Food preferences could be related to nutrition status, but not necessarily to BMI [52].

Finally, the study revealed that adolescents with a high variety of food consumption (i.e., *varied diet*) or healthy food consumption (i.e., *healthy diet*) had longer sleeping hours than those with a low variety of food consumption (i.e., *low appetite*) or unhealthy food consumption (i.e., *avoiding vegetables*). Past research has provided empirical evidence on the linkage between sleep duration and dietary behaviors [53]. For example, Franckle et al. [54] reported that insufficient sleep among children and adolescents was linked to unhealthy dietary behaviors (e.g., decreased vegetables consumption). Future dietary interventions among Chinese adolescents may consider incorporating strategies for improving adolescents' sleep duration.

6. Limitations and Future Directions

The present study has several limitations. First, although we used a national sample of adolescents, the sample size may not be large enough to generalize the findings to the general adolescent population. Second, the measurement of food preferences and nutrition knowledge may not be satisfying due to the small number of items; thus, we highly encourage future researchers to conduct similar studies by using more standardized and well-established instruments (e.g., the General Nutrition Knowledge Questionnaire [55], the Adult Eating Behaviour Questionnaire [56,57]). In reality, there is a much larger variety of food that adolescents consume in their daily lives. Future research should consider more comprehensive instrument(s) to assess food preference. Third, social factors could be much broader, relating to family, community, and cultural contexts. The current study only assessed participants' general attitudes toward parents, friends, and school. Future studies should consider the multidimensional nature of social environment and explore more potential factors in this regard. Adolescence is a vital stage in one's formation of outlooks about life and the world. It would be important to understand what habits and preferences for food will carry over into adulthood and have a lasting impact. Research has shown that adolescents' food preference is related to their general health and well-being. Researchers, if possible, should look at the potential consequences, both proximal and distal, of different food preferences.

7. Conclusions

Our study identified four different types of food preferences among Chinese adolescents, with each presenting its own unique characteristics. We further revealed that various factors (e.g., gender, residence, and nutrition knowledge) were closely related to the types of food preferences. Future dietary interventions (e.g., school-based nutrition education) should target specific groups of Chinese adolescents with attributes known to be associated with low vegetable or high fast food consumption.

Author Contributions: S.S. participated in the study design, performed the statistical analyses, and drafted the manuscript. J.H. led the study design, led the results interpretation, and helped draft the manuscript. X.F. helped draft the manuscript.

Funding: This research received no external funding.

Conflicts of Interest: The authors declare no conflicts of interest.

References

1. Skinner, J.; Carruth, B.R.; Moran, J., III; Houck, K.; Schmidhammer, J.; Reed, A.; Coletta, F.; Cotter, R.; Ott, D. Toddlers' food preferences: Concordance with family members' preferences. *J. Nutr. Educ.* **1998**, *30*, 17–22. [CrossRef]
2. Manios, Y.; Moschonis, G.; Grammatikaki, E.; Mavrogianni, C.; van den Heuvel, E.; Bos, R.; Singh-Povel, C. Food group and micronutrient intake adequacy among children, adults and elderly women in Greece. *Nutrients* **2015**, *7*, 1841–1858. [CrossRef] [PubMed]
3. Davis, C.; Patte, K.; Levitan, R.; Reid, C.; Tweed, S.; Curtis, C. From motivation to behaviour: A model of reward sensitivity, overeating, and food preferences in the risk profile for obesity. *Appetite* **2007**, *48*, 12–19. [CrossRef] [PubMed]
4. Duffy, V.B.; Lanier, S.A.; Hutchins, H.L.; Pescatello, L.S.; Johnson, M.K.; Bartoshuk, L.M. Food preference questionnaire as a screening tool for assessing dietary risk of cardiovascular disease within health risk appraisals. *J. Am. Diet. Assoc.* **2007**, *107*, 237–245. [CrossRef] [PubMed]
5. Umesawa, M.; Iso, H.; Fujino, Y.; Kikuchi, S.; Tamakoshi, A. Salty food preference and intake and risk of gastric cancer: The JACC study. *J. Epidemiol.* **2016**, *26*, 92–97. [CrossRef]
6. Zhang, J.; Wang, H.; Wang, Z.; Du, W.; Su, C.; Zhang, J.; Jiang, H.; Jia, X.; Huang, F.; Ouyang, Y. Prevalence and stabilizing trends in overweight and obesity among children and adolescents in China, 2011–2015. *BMC Public Health* **2018**, *18*, 571. [CrossRef] [PubMed]
7. Lee, Y.-H.; Shelley, M.; Liu, C.-T.; Chang, Y.-C. Assessing the association of food preferences and self-reported psychological well-being among middle-aged and older adults in contemporary China-results from the China Health and Nutrition Survey. *Int. J. Environ. Res. Public Health* **2018**, *15*, 463. [CrossRef]
8. Hu, F.; Liu, Y.; Willett, W. Preventing chronic diseases by promoting healthy diet and lifestyle: Public policy implications for China. *Obes. Rev.* **2011**, *12*, 552–559. [CrossRef]
9. Zickgraf, H.F.; Schepps, K. Fruit and vegetable intake and dietary variety in adult picky eaters. *Food Qual. Prefer.* **2016**, *54*, 39–50. [CrossRef]
10. Birch, L.L. Preschool children's food preferences and consumption patterns. *J. Nutr. Educ.* **1979**, *11*, 189–192. [CrossRef]
11. Zhen, S.; Ma, Y.; Zhao, Z.; Yang, X.; Wen, D. Dietary pattern is associated with obesity in Chinese children and adolescents: Data from China Health and Nutrition Survey (CHNS). *Nutr. J.* **2018**, *17*, 68. [CrossRef]
12. Savage, J.S.; Fisher, J.O.; Birch, L.L. Parental influence on eating behavior: Conception to adolescence. *J. Law Med. Ethics* **2007**, *35*, 22–34. [CrossRef]
13. Pearson, N.; Griffiths, P.; Biddle, S.J.; Johnston, J.P.; Haycraft, E. Individual, behavioural and home environmental factors associated with eating behaviours in young adolescents. *Appetite* **2017**, *112*, 35–43. [CrossRef]
14. Story, M.; Resnick, M.D. Adolescents' views on food and nutrition. *J. Nutr. Educ.* **1986**, *18*, 188–192. [CrossRef]
15. Verstraeten, R.; Leroy, J.L.; Pieniak, Z.; Ochoa-Avilès, A.; Holdsworth, M.; Verbeke, W.; Maes, L.; Kolsteren, P. Individual and environmental factors influencing adolescents' dietary behavior in low-and middle-income settings. *PLoS ONE* **2016**, *11*, e0157744. [CrossRef] [PubMed]
16. Choi, J.E.; Ainsworth, B.E. Associations of food consumption, serum vitamins and metabolic syndrome risk with physical activity level in middle-aged adults: The National Health and Nutrition Examination Survey (NHANES) 2005–2006. *Public Health Nutr.* **2016**, *19*, 1674–1683. [CrossRef] [PubMed]
17. Fussner, L.M.; Luebbe, A.M.; Smith, A.R. Social reward and social punishment sensitivity in relation to dietary restraint and binge/purge symptoms. *Appetite* **2018**, *127*, 386–392. [CrossRef] [PubMed]
18. De Ridder, D.; Kroese, F.; Evers, C.; Adriaanse, M.; Gillebaart, M. Healthy diet: Health impact, prevalence, correlates, and interventions. *Psychol. Health* **2017**, *32*, 907–941. [CrossRef]
19. Coleman, J.C. *The Nature of Adolescence*; Routledge: London, UK, 2011.
20. Das, J.K.; Salam, R.A.; Thornburg, K.L.; Prentice, A.M.; Campisi, S.; Lassi, Z.S.; Koletzko, B.; Bhutta, Z.A. Nutrition in adolescents: Physiology, metabolism, and nutritional needs. *Ann. N. Y. Acad. Sci.* **2017**, *1393*, 21–33. [CrossRef]

21. Movassagh, E.Z.; Baxter-Jones, A.D.; Kontulainen, S.; Whiting, S.; Szafron, M.; Vatanparast, H. Vegetarian-style dietary pattern during adolescence has long-term positive impact on bone from adolescence to young adulthood: A longitudinal study. *Nutr. J.* **2018**, *17*, 36. [CrossRef] [PubMed]
22. Laska, M.N.; Murray, D.M.; Lytle, L.A.; Harnack, L.J. Longitudinal associations between key dietary behaviors and weight gain over time: Transitions through the adolescent years. *Obesity* **2012**, *20*, 118–125. [CrossRef] [PubMed]
23. Peuhkuri, K.; Sihvola, N.; Korpela, R. Diet promotes sleep duration and quality. *Nutr. Res.* **2012**, *32*, 309–319. [CrossRef] [PubMed]
24. St-Onge, M.-P.; Mikic, A.; Pietrolungo, C.E. Effects of diet on sleep quality. *Adv. Nutr.* **2016**, *7*, 938–949. [CrossRef] [PubMed]
25. Frank, S.; Gonzalez, K.; Lee-Ang, L.; Young, M.C.; Tamez, M.; Mattei, J. Diet and sleep physiology: Public health and clinical implications. *Front. Neurol.* **2017**, *8*, 393. [CrossRef] [PubMed]
26. Ma, G. Food, eating behavior, and culture in Chinese society. *J. Ethn. Foods* **2015**, *2*, 195–199. [CrossRef]
27. Deng, S. Adolescents' food preferences in china: Do household living arrangements matter? *Soc. Work Health Care* **2011**, *50*, 625–638. [CrossRef] [PubMed]
28. Shi, Z.; Lien, N.; Kumar, B.N.; Holmboe-Ottesen, G. Socio-demographic differences in food habits and preferences of school adolescents in Jiangsu Province, China. *Eur. J. Clin. Nutr.* **2005**, *59*, 1439. [CrossRef] [PubMed]
29. Collins, L.M.; Lanza, S.T. *Latent Class and Latent Transition Analysis: With Applications in the Social, Behavioral, and Health Sciences*; John Wiley & Sons: Hoboken, NJ, USA, 2009; Volume 718.
30. Hardigan, P.C.; Sangasubana, N. A latent class analysis of job satisfaction and turnover among practicing pharmacists. *Res. Soc. Adm. Pharm.* **2010**, *6*, 32–38. [CrossRef]
31. He, J.; Cai, Z.; Fan, X. Accuracy of using self-reported data to screen children and adolescents for overweight and obesity status: A diagnostic meta-analysis. *Obes. Res. Clin. Pract.* **2017**, *11*, 257–267. [CrossRef]
32. Cole, T.J.; Faith, M.S.; Pietrobelli, A.; Heo, M. What is the best measure of adiposity change in growing children: BMI, BMI%, BMI z-score or BMI centile? *Eur. J. Clin. Nutr.* **2005**, *59*, 419. [CrossRef]
33. Vogel, M. *Childsds: Data and Methods Around Reference Values in Pediatrics*; R Package Version 0.6; Springer: New York, NY, USA, 2017.
34. Lanza, S.T.; Collins, L.M.; Lemmon, D.R.; Schafer, J.L. PROC LCA: A SAS procedure for latent class analysis. *Struct. Equ. Model. A Multidiscip. J.* **2007**, *14*, 671–694. [CrossRef]
35. Séménou, M.; Courcoux, P.; Cardinal, M.; Nicod, H.; Ouisse, A. Preference study using a latent class approach. Analysis of European preferences for smoked salmon. *Food Qual. Prefer.* **2007**, *18*, 720–728. [CrossRef]
36. Lanza, S.T.; Rhoades, B.L. Latent class analysis: An alternative perspective on subgroup analysis in prevention and treatment. *Prev. Sci.* **2013**, *14*, 157–168. [CrossRef] [PubMed]
37. Muthén, L.K.; Muthén, B.O. *Mplus User's Guide*, 7th ed.; Muthén & Muthén: Los Angeles, CA, USA, 1998.
38. Geiser, C. *Data Analysis with Mplus*; Guilford Press: New York, NY, USA, 2012.
39. He, J.; Fan, X. Latent Class Analysis. *Encycl. Personal. Individ. Differ.* **2018**, *1*, 1–4.
40. Marsh, H.W.; Lüdtke, O.; Trautwein, U.; Morin, A.J. Classical latent profile analysis of academic self-concept dimensions: Synergy of person-and variable-centered approaches to theoretical models of self-concept. *Struct. Equ. Model. A Multidiscip. J.* **2009**, *16*, 191–225. [CrossRef]
41. Asparouhov, T.; Muthén, B. Auxiliary variables in mixture modeling: Three-step approaches using M plus. *Struct. Equ. Model. A Multidiscip. J.* **2014**, *21*, 329–341. [CrossRef]
42. Schafer, J.L. Multiple imputation: A primer. *Stat. Methods Med Res.* **1999**, *8*, 3–15. [CrossRef]
43. Caine-Bish, N.L.; Scheule, B. Gender differences in food preferences of school-aged children and adolescents. *J. Sch. Health* **2009**, *79*, 532–540. [CrossRef]
44. Birch, L.L. Development of food preferences. *Annu. Rev. Nutr.* **1999**, *19*, 41–62. [CrossRef]
45. Wardle, J.; Parmenter, K.; Waller, J. Nutrition knowledge and food intake. *Appetite* **2000**, *34*, 269–275. [CrossRef]
46. Boyland, E.J.; Harrold, J.A.; Kirkham, T.C.; Corker, C.; Cuddy, J.; Evans, D.; Dovey, T.M.; Lawton, C.L.; Blundell, J.E.; Halford, J.C. Food commercials increase preference for energy-dense foods, particularly in children who watch more television. *Pediatrics* **2011**, *128*, e93–e100. [CrossRef] [PubMed]

47. Boyland, E.J.; Halford, J.C. Television advertising and branding. Effects on eating behaviour and food preferences in children. *Appetite* **2013**, *62*, 236–241. [CrossRef] [PubMed]
48. Borgogna, N.; Lockhart, G.; Grenard, J.L.; Barrett, T.; Shiffman, S.; Reynolds, K.D. Ecological momentary assessment of urban adolescents' technology use and cravings for unhealthy snacks and drinks: Differences by ethnicity and sex. *J. Acad. Nutr. Diet.* **2015**, *115*, 759–766. [CrossRef] [PubMed]
49. Chaput, J.-P.; Visby, T.; Nyby, S.; Klingenberg, L.; Gregersen, N.T.; Tremblay, A.; Astrup, A.; Sjödin, A. Video game playing increases food intake in adolescents: A randomized crossover study. *Am. J. Clin. Nutr.* **2011**, *93*, 1196–1203. [CrossRef] [PubMed]
50. Thivel, D.; Tremblay, M.S.; Chaput, J.-P. Modern sedentary behaviors favor energy consumption in children and adolescents. *Curr. Obes. Rep.* **2013**, *2*, 50–57. [CrossRef]
51. Jones, A.; Pearce, M.; Adamson, A.; Gateshead Millennium Study Core Team. Food knowledge, attitudes and preferences and BMI in children: The Gateshead Millennium Study. *Proc. Nutr. Soc.* **2010**, *69*, e496. [CrossRef]
52. Maitre, I.; Van Wymelbeke, V.; Amand, M.; Vigneau, E.; Issanchou, S.; Sulmont-Rossé, C. Food pickiness in the elderly: Relationship with dependency and malnutrition. *Food Qual. Prefer.* **2014**, *32*, 145–151. [CrossRef]
53. Lundahl, A.; Nelson, T.D. Sleep and food intake: A multisystem review of mechanisms in children and adults. *J. Health Psychol.* **2015**, *20*, 794–805. [CrossRef]
54. Franckle, R.L.; Falbe, J.; Gortmaker, S.; Ganter, C.; Taveras, E.M.; Land, T.; Davison, K.K. Insufficient sleep among elementary and middle school students is linked with elevated soda consumption and other unhealthy dietary behaviors. *Prev. Med.* **2015**, *74*, 36–41. [CrossRef]
55. Parmenter, K.; Wardle, J. Development of a general nutrition knowledge questionnaire for adults. *Eur. J. Clin. Nutr.* **1999**, *53*, 298. [CrossRef]
56. Hunot, C.; Fildes, A.; Croker, H.; Llewellyn, C.H.; Wardle, J.; Beeken, R.J. Appetitive traits and relationships with BMI in adults: Development of the Adult Eating Behaviour Questionnaire. *Appetite* **2016**, *105*, 356–363. [CrossRef] [PubMed]
57. He, J.; Sun, S.; Zickgraf, H.F.; Ellis, J.M.; Fan, X. Assessing Appetitive Traits Among Chinese Young Adults Using the Adult Eating Behavior Questionnaire: Factor Structure, Gender Invariance and Latent Mean Differences, and Associations With BMI. *Assessment* **2019**, 1073191119864642. [CrossRef] [PubMed]

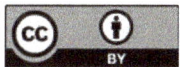

© 2019 by the authors. Licensee MDPI, Basel, Switzerland. This article is an open access article distributed under the terms and conditions of the Creative Commons Attribution (CC BY) license (http://creativecommons.org/licenses/by/4.0/).

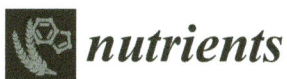

Article

Intake of Sugar-Sweetened Beverages in Adolescents from Troms, Norway—The Tromsø Study: *Fit Futures*

Guri Skeie [1,*], Vårin Sandvær [1,2] and Guri Grimnes [3,4]

1. Department of Community Medicine, UiT the Arctic University of Norway, N-9037 Tromsø, Norway; vsand@hotmail.com
2. Nordland Fylkeskommune, Seksjon for Folkehelse, N-8048 Bodø, Norway
3. Division of Internal Medicine, University Hospital of North Norway, N-9038 Tromsø, Norway; guri.grimnes@unn.no
4. Tromsø Endocrine Research Group, Department of Clinical Medicine, UiT the Arctic University of Norway, N-9037 Tromsø, Norway
* Correspondence: Guri.Skeie@uit.no; Tel.: +47-7764-6594

Received: 1 November 2018; Accepted: 17 January 2019; Published: 22 January 2019

Abstract: High intake of sugar-sweetened beverages (SSB) has been associated with weight gain and chronic disease. The objective of this paper was to study the intake of SSB and characteristics associated with SSB intake in adolescents from Troms, Norway. We present results from a cross-sectional analysis from the Tromsø Study: *Fit Futures*, with 426 female and 444 male students aged 15–17 years (93% participation rate). Descriptive statistics and logistic regression analyses were performed. Among females, 31.8% drank at least one glass of SSB per day on average, compared to 61.0% among males. The adjusted OR (odds ratio) of daily SSB drinking for males vs. females was 3.74 (95% CI (confidence interval) 2.68–5.22). Other dietary habits such as eating snacks, drinking artificially sweetened beverages, fruit juice, and seldom eating breakfast were associated with higher odds for daily SSB drinking, as was daily snuffing. Weight class was not associated with daily SSB drinking. Students in vocational studies, particularly males tended to be more likely to be daily SSB drinkers. The prevalence of participants who on average were daily drinkers was higher than in national studies. We have identified several possible targets for interventions. Clustering of unhealthy behaviours and tendencies to socioeconomic differences are of particular concern.

Keywords: adolescent; dietary behaviour; nutrition; Norway; sugar-sweetened beverages

---

1. Introduction

High intake of sugar-sweetened beverages (SSB) [1] has been associated with several health outcomes. Estimates from the Global Burden of Disease collaboration suggest that worldwide, 184,000 deaths per year are attributable to SSB consumption, mainly due to type 2 diabetes ($n = 133,000$), but also due to cardio-vascular diseases, and cancer [2]. A recent review on diabetes type 2 suggests a 13% higher incidence per serving per day, after adjustment for adiposity [3]. High sugar intake leads to dental decay [4], and SSB is one of the major sugar sources in many demographic groups, including Norwegian youths [5,6]. High SSB intake has also been associated with dental erosion, weight gain, and obesity, although the evidence is not unequivocal [7–9]. While it is the high sugar content that is associated with dental caries, the dental erosion is due to acidity [4,7], and therefore, replacement of SSB with light or artificially sweetened beverages might be beneficial for caries, but not have much effect on erosions. Dental caries has been the most common chronic disease of childhood [10], and damage to the permanent teeth due to caries or erosion, cannot be reverted.

The intake of SSB has been high in Norway, and the authorities have taken initiatives to reduce the intake [11,12]. In the period this study is covering, the aim was to reduce the number of daily consumers of SSB with 20% [13]. Over time, the trend in SSB intake among Norwegian children and adolescents has changed: Nationally representative cross-sectional studies performed in 1989–2001 as part of the international Health Behaviour in Among School-aged Children (HBSC) study, showed both a clear increase in frequency of intake of SSB and an increase in daily users over time [14]. More recently, from the 2005/06 survey, the reported intake has been lower, though not with a continuous decreasing trend [11,15]. In 2014, 11% of the males and 5% of the females drank SSB daily [16]. Another study comparing cross-sectional data from 11–13-year-old children before and after initiatives to reduce SSB consumption showed that the intake of lemonade and regular soft drinks, decreased, the intake of diet soft drinks increased, while juice consumption increased in males, and decreased in females [12].

A higher intake or frequency of intake, of SSB among males [12,15,17,18] and those with lower socio-economic status [12,17] is commonly reported, but in the HBSC study, there was no socio-economic difference in SSB consumption [11]. Some have questioned whether the association between SSB intake and type 2 diabetes is due to the sugar content of the SSB or related lifestyle factors such as other dietary practices, or (lack of) physical activity [19]. Intake of SSB has been associated with lifestyle factors such as physical activity and smoking [18]. Finally, consumption of SSB has been associated with parental modelling and regulation [20–22]. Earlier studies have suggested both poorer dietary habits among adolescents in Northern Norway [23], and found higher prevalence of dental caries as compared to southern parts of the country [24,25]. Our aim was to assess the proportion of daily consumers of SSB in 15–17-year-old adolescents from Troms, Norway, and their characteristics.

2. Material and Methods

The Tromsø study: *Fit Futures* is a population based longitudinal study with repeated measures of various indicators of lifestyle and health among adolescents [26]. The current paper is a cross-sectional analysis from the first survey in 2010–11, where all 1st grade students from all the eight upper secondary schools in Tromsø and Balsfjord municipalities were invited to participate. The catchment area includes both urban and rural populations. In 2010, 1301 students were enrolled as 1st year upper secondary school students, but 70 persons quit before *Fit Futures* 1 was conducted. Furthermore 114 students were sick or not reached for other reasons, leaving 1117 students who were invited to participate [26]. From those invited, 1038 students attended the study, giving a 93% participation rate.

Students were given time off from school and transported to the Clinical Research Unit of the University Hospital of North Norway, where trained personnel performed anthropometrical measurements, took blood samples, performed physical examinations, and conducted clinical interviews. The students completed self-administered digital questionnaires on a variety of health and lifestyle topics in addition to those detailed below. Information regarding school study programme was collected from school records. The Tromsø study: *Fit Futures* has been described in more detail elsewhere [26].

The age of the participants ranged between 15 and 28. Adolescents following a typical Norwegian educational progress are between the ages of 15–17 at 1st year of upper secondary school, and therefore students 18 years and older were excluded from the analyses ($n = 77$). Exclusions were also made for those missing data on variables used in the main analyses ($n = 95$), which therefore included 870 students, 426 females and 444 males.

The Norwegian Data Protection Authorities and the Regional Committee for Medical and Health Research Ethics have approved the *Fit Futures* study (ref no 2009/1282 and 2012/1904). The study was conducted in accordance with the Declaration of Helsinki. All participants in *Fit Futures* signed an informed consent declaration. For students under the age of 16 additional written consent was provided by their guardians.

2.1. Dietary Variables

The questionnaire assessed consumption frequency of 14 different foods/food-groups and 10 different beverages. The questions on diet can be found in supplementary file 1. Questions regarding beverages had the response categories "seldom/never", "1–6 glasses per week", "1 glass per day", "2–3 glasses per day" and "4 glasses or more per day". The replies to the two questions on sugar-sweetened carbonated and non-carbonated soft drinks were summed based on the category midpoints (e.g., if they answered 2–3 glasses per day on both questions, it would be counted as 5 glasses per day). A binary variable was constructed, distinguishing between those who, on average, drank SSB daily and not. Similarly, the two questions on light/artificially sweetened carbonated and non-carbonated beverages were combined into one, as were the four questions on milk/yoghurt. The new variables were categorized in order to avoid low cell counts.

For fruits and vegetables (two questions), the categories were "seldom/never", "1–3 times per month", "1–3 times per week", "4–6 times per week", "1–2 times per day", "3–4 times per day" and "5 times per day". These variables were combined into one variable for number of fruits and vegetables eaten per day. This variable was not normally distributed, and therefore recoded into a categorical variable with four categories, based on the distribution. The variables for sweets (e.g., chocolate and drops) and sweet and savoury snacks (e.g., potato crisps, cakes, cookies, buns) had the same categories as the fruit and vegetables, except "every day" was the highest frequency. Again, categories were combined on a-variable-to-variable basis in order to avoid low cell counts.

We assessed frequency of eating breakfast, dinner (the main hot meal), and lunch. As Norwegian students are not served meals at school, those who do not bring their lunch from home (usually sandwiches) often buy something to eat at some nearby store/kiosk, or possibly a canteen. Therefore, bringing lunch from home could be a marker of a healthier diet, or stronger parental control. For breakfast and dinner, the response categories were "every day", 4–6 days a week", "1–3 days a week" and "seldom/never". For lunch brought to school, categories were "every school day", "3–4 days a week" "1–2 days a week", and "seldom/never". Breakfast and lunch were recoded into three categories covering seldom/never, most days, and every (school) day. Dinner was recoded into every day/not every day.

2.2. Other Variables

Study program was classified as general studies (including sports and physical education studies) and vocational studies. We combined the information about physical activity from two questions: First, the students indicated whether or not they were doing sports or physical activity (such as skateboarding, soccer, dancing or running) outside school hours. Then, weekly sports/physical activity outside school hours was assessed with the original categories: "none", "about 30 min", "about 30–90 min", "about 2–3 h", "about 4–6 h", "7 h or more". Those who on the first question indicated no activity were combined with the lowest group on the second question and coded none. The next three categories for weekly activity outside school hours were coded as up to three h a week, and the last two as 4 h or more.

Students were asked about average time spent in front of computers, TV, DVD or similar outside of school hours, differentiating between school days and weekend days. Categories were the same as for physical activity, except for the highest categories: "about 7–9 h" or "10 h or more". School days and weekend days were weighted 5/7 and 2/7 respectively and combined into one variable. The variable daily screen time was split into categories of "<2 h", "2–3.99 h" and "≥4 h" per day.

Students were asked about smoking and snuff (or snus, a form of smokeless tobacco, a moist powder tobacco placed under the upper lip) habits, with response categories "no, never", "sometimes" or "daily". Due to few daily smokers, they were combined with occasional smokers. Students were asked how often they drank alcohol, with options "never", "once per month or less", "2–4 times per month", "2–3 times per week" or "4 times or more per week". The highest categories had few responders and were combined into the category "2 times per month or more".

A question on who the students lived with (some form of family guardian, friends or alone) was used to differentiate between those who had moved out of home and not. Students answering that they lived both with parents and had moved out of home ($n = 7$) were assumed to be commuters and were therefore included in the group that had moved out of home. Only two students answered living in an institution (and having moved out of home). They were still included in the group living at home, as it is likely that an institution would have an adult in charge of the food environment.

BMI was calculated as weight in kg divided by the square of height in meters (kg/m^2) and Cole and Lobstein's revised gender- and age-specific cut-offs [27] were used for classification of BMI categories. Due to few thin and obese students, these groups were merged with the categories normal weight and overweight, respectively.

Students were asked about parents' educational level. The categories "primary school" and "upper secondary school" were combined due to few responders. Furthermore, this variable differentiated between higher education for less and more than four years. The category "do not know" was combined with "missing". Since around 25% of the students did not know or did not answer the questions on mother's and father's education, the variables were only used for additional analyses, and not introduced in the main statistical model.

2.3. Statistical Analyses

Descriptive and analytic statistical analyses were performed using SAS version 9.4 (SAS Institute Inc., Cary, NC, USA). Two-sided p-values < 0.05 were considered statistically significant. As the variables included in the analyses were categorical, unadjusted analyses were performed using contingency tables with chi-square tests, with the percentage of students that on average reported daily drinking of SSB as outcome. Data from all participants were used to calculate the percentage daily drinkers, but the numbers for non-daily drinkers have been suppressed for increased legibility. Adjusted analyses of characteristics associated with daily drinking of SSB were performed using logistic regression. We considered health related characteristics (smoking, using snuff, drinking alcohol, physical activity, screen time, body mass index), school programme, whether the student lived with parents/guardians, dietary variables (fruits and vegetables, sweets, snacks, beverages other than SSB, and meals eaten) as potential covariates. As there was a large difference in SSB drinking between sexes, both unadjusted and adjusted analyses were performed for each sex separately. However, in order to compare the results obtained between sexes, the adjusted logistic regression model was constructed by including independent variables which were associated with daily drinking of SSB ($p < 0.25$) in the unadjusted analyses of the total sample, weighted for sex. Variables were manually excluded until only significant covariates remained in the model. An additional model was constructed including also sex, mother's and father's education, in order to estimate the effect of sex, and study socio-economic differences from an additional perspective. Father's education was not a significant covariate and was not included in the final analyses. To assess potential sex differences in the associations, we fitted interaction terms with sex, and re-ran the regression analyses for each covariate.

No indication of multicollinearity was observed when evaluating the variance inflation factor. Hosmer and Lemeshow's goodness-of-fit test was used to evaluate overall fit of the regression models. To evaluate how much of the variance in daily drinking of SSB the model explained, pseudo R^2 (Nagelkerke/Cragg and Uhler's) was assessed.

3. Results

The mean age of the participants was 16.1 year (Table 1). While most females were in general study programs (61.7%), most males had chosen vocational studies (55.0%). Most students lived with their parents/guardian (females 85.9% and males 87.8%). More males (61.3%) than females (32.2%) reported drinking SSB on average every day ($p < 0.001$). Females tended to drink water more frequently than males, while males tended to drink milk more often than females. About half of the students had breakfast daily, and about one-third brought lunch to school every school day, females slightly more often than males. Almost 60% of the females and 73% of the males had dinner daily.

Table 1. Characteristics [1] of the participants in the Tromsø study: *Fit Futures*.

	Females (*n* = 426)	Males (*n* = 444)
Age, years	16.1	16.1
Living with parent(s)	85.9	87.8
Mother's education		
Elementary or secondary school	34.3	32.0
College/university < 4 years	19.0	16.4
College/university 4 years or more	23.5	22.3
Unknown/missing	23.2	29.3
Father's education		
Elementary or secondary school	38.7	39.0
College/university < 4 years	13.4	13.5
College/university 4 years or more	18.8	18.2
Unknown/missing	29.1	29.3
General study programme (including sports)	61.7	45.1
Drink sugar-sweetened beverages daily	32.2	61.3
Servings of fruits and vegetables, daily		
Less than 0.6	22.8	34.7
0.6–1.3	18.1	22.3
1.4–2.3	26.3	22.1
More than 2.3	32.8	20.9
Consume chocolate/sweets at least weekly	70.2	68.5
Consume sweet or savoury snacks at least weekly	64.3	68.0
Light/artificially sweetened beverages, daily		
None	40.6	43.9
0.5 glass	32.6	26.6
1 glass or more	26.8	29.5
Fruit juice, daily		
0.5 glass or less	65.5	63.7
1 glass	19.2	21.4
2.5 glasses or more	15.3	14.9
Milk, daily [2]		
1 glass or less	42.7	40.6
1.5–2.5 glass	31.5	26.1
2.5 glasses or more	25.8	33.3
Water, daily		
1 glass or less	18.3	31.1
2–3 glasses	34.5	33.8
4 or more glasses	47.2	35.1
Breakfast		
Seldom/never	15.0	12.2
1–3 days per week	35.2	35.3
Every day	49.8	52.5
Bring lunch for school		
Seldom/never	23.0	34.9
1–6 days/week	43.4	39.0
Every school day	33.6	26.1
Dinner daily	58.5	73.4
Overweight/obese	19.3	23.7

Table 1. Cont.

	Females (n = 426)	Males (n = 444)
Screen time, daily [3]		
<2 h	26.3	14.0
2–3.99 h	38.7	38.3
4 h or more	35.0	47.7
Physical activity outside school hours, weekly		
Not active	30.0	33.3
3 h or less	30.3	26.6
4 h or more	39.7	40.1
Smoking daily or occasionally	20.0	23.4
Use of snuff		
Never	67.1	60.4
Occasionally	14.3	12.8
Daily	18.6	26.8
Alcohol drinking		
Never	23.5	32.7
Once per month or less often	46.9	37.1
Twice per month or more often	29.6	30.2

[1] Mean age, otherwise percentage distributions. [2] Sum of four different milk types (different fat content) and yoghurt. Includes both plain and fermented milk. [3] Weighted mean of weekends and weekdays.

The prevalence of overweight/obesity was high, 19.3% in females and 23.7% in males (Table 1). A larger proportion of males than females was in the group with the highest screen time (47.7% vs. 35.0%). Regarding physical activity outside school hours, the distribution in females and males seemed to be similar. While 20.0% of females and 23.4% of males smoked occasionally or daily, 32.9% of females and 39.6% of males used snuff occasionally or daily. The proportion of students reporting never drinking alcohol was quite low (females 23.5%, males 32.7%).

More than 50% of the females and males drank carbonated SSB 1–6 times a week, but more males than females drank them daily (Figure 1a). Non-carbonated SSB was drunk less frequently than carbonated SSB, and the majority reported drinking them seldom/never, though males also consumed these beverages more often than females (Figure 1b).

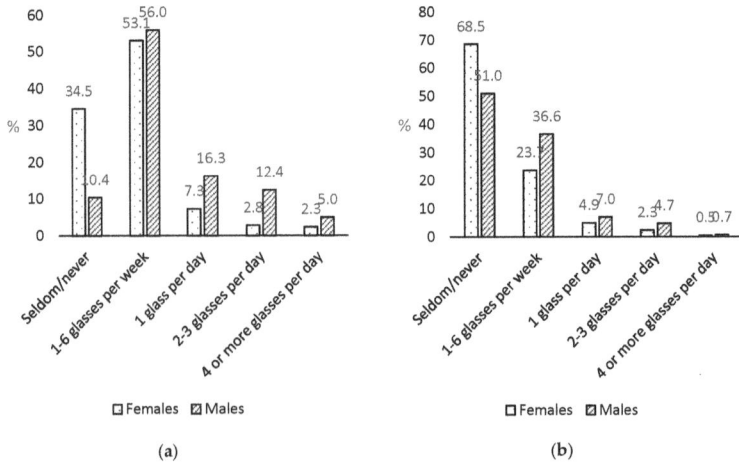

Figure 1. Intake of (a) carbonated sugar-sweetened beverages (SSB); and (b) non-carbonated SSB, by sex.

In univariate analyses, living with parents/guardians was not associated with daily SSB drinking, neither in females nor in males (Table 2). Almost 70% of males in vocational studies were daily drinkers, compared to half of the males in general studies. In females the corresponding percentages were slightly less than 50 in vocational studies and just above 20 in general studies ($p < 0.001$ in both sexes).

Table 2. Daily drinkers of sugar-sweetened beverages according to demographic, dietary and lifestyle characteristics, by sex in the Tromsø study: *Fit Futures*.

Characteristic	Females (n = 426) [1]		Males (n = 444) [1]	
	Daily Drinkers % (n [2])	*p*-Value [3]	Daily Drinkers % (n [2])	*p*-Value [3]
Living with parent(s)		0.63		0.84
Yes	32.6 (119/365)		61.4 (239/389)	
No	29.5 (18/61)		60.0 (33/55)	
School programme		<0.0001		0.0003
Vocational	46.6 (76/163)		68.9 (168/244)	
General (including sports)	23.2 (61/263)		52.0 (104/200)	
Servings of fruits and vegetables, daily		0.008		0.05
Less than 0.6	40.2 (39/97)		69.5 (107/154)	
0.6–1.3	42.9 (33/77)		60.6 (60/99)	
1.4–2.3	24.1 (27/112)		53.1 (52/98)	
More than 2.3	27.1 (38/140)		57.0 (53/93)	
Consumption of chocolate/sweets		0.007		0.007
Not weekly	22.8 (29/127)		52.1 (73/140)	
Weekly	36.1 (108/299)		65.5 (199/304)	
Consumption of sweet or savoury snacks		<0.0001		0.004
Not weekly	18.4 (28/152)		51.4 (73/142)	
Weekly	39.8 (109/274)		65.9 (199/302)	
Light/artificially sweetened beverages, daily		<0.0001		0.003
None	24.3 (42/173)		54.4 (106/195)	
0.5 glass	20.9 (29/139)		56.8 (67/118)	
1 glass or more	57.9 (66/114)		75.6 (99/131)	
Fruit juice, daily		0.0006		0.002
0.5 glass	25.8 (72/279)		55.1 (156/283)	
1 glass	43.9 (36/82)		72.6 (69/95)	
2.5 glasses or more	44.6 (29/65)		71.2 (47/66)	
Milk, daily [4]		0.28		0.10
1 glass or less	34.6 (63/182)		67.2 (121/180)	
1.5–2.5 glass	26.9 (36/134)		56.0 (65/116)	
2.5 glasses or more	34.6 (38/110)		58.1 (86/148)	
Water, daily		0.02		0.0005
1 glass or less	41.0 (32/78)		74.6 (103/138)	
2–3 glasses	36.1 (53/147)		56.0 (84/150)	
4 glasses or more	25.9 (52/201)		54.5 (85/156)	
Breakfast		<0.0001		0.002
Seldom/never	67.2 (43/64)		74.1 (40/54)	
1–6 days/week	31.3 (47/150)		68.2 (107/157)	
Every day	22.2 (47/212)		53.7 (125/233)	

Table 2. Cont.

Characteristic	Females (n = 426) [1]		Males (n = 444) [1]	
	Daily Drinkers % (n [2])	p-Value [3]	Daily Drinkers % (n [2])	p-Value [3]
Bring lunch to school		<0.0001		0.0006
Seldom/never	50.0 (49/98)		68.4 (106/155)	
1–4 days/week	31.4 (58/185)		64.7 (112/173)	
Every school day	21.0 (30/143)		46.6 (54/116)	
Dinner		0.09		0.21
Not daily	36.7 (65/177)		66.1 (78/118)	
Daily	28.9 (72/249)		59.5 (194/326)	
Weight class		0.38		0.59
Thin/normal weight	33.1 (114/344)		62.0 (210/339)	
Overweight/obese	28.1 (23/82)		59.1 (62/105)	
Screen time, daily [5]		0.002		0.24
<2 h	22.3 (25/112)		54.8 (34/62)	
2–3.99 h	29.7 (49/165)		58.8 (100/170)	
4 h or more	42.3 (63/149)		65.1 (138/212)	
Physical activity outside school hours, weekly		0.0001		0.06
Not active	46.9 (60/128)		65.5 (97/148)	
3 h or less	26.4 (34/129)		66.1 (78/118)	
4 h or more	25.4 (43/169)		54.5 (97/178)	
Smoking		< 0.0001		0.005
Never	26.7 (91/341)		57.7 (196/340)	
Occasionally or daily	54.1 (46/85)		73.1 (76/104)	
Use of snuff		< 0.0001		0.001
Never	23.1 (66/286)		54.9 (147/268)	
Occasionally	39.3 (24/61)		63.2 (36/57)	
Daily	59.5 (47/79)		74.8 (89/119)	
Alcohol drinking		0.1		0.02
Never	29.0 (29/100)		52.4 (76/145)	
Once a month or less often	29.0 (58/200)		67.9 (112/165)	
Twice a month or more often	39.7 (50/126)		62.7 (84/134)	

[1] All participants are used to calculate the percentage of daily drinkers, but the numbers for the non-daily drinkers have been suppressed for better legibility. [2] The n is the number of daily drinkers/the total number of participants reporting the given characteristic. [3] Chi-square test. [4] Sum of four different milk types (different fat content) and yoghurt. Includes both plain and fermented milk. [5] Weighted mean of weekends and weekdays.

Among females eating less than 0.6 servings of fruits and vegetables daily, there were 40.2% daily drinkers of SSB, compared to 27.1% among those eating 2.3 servings or more ($p = 0.008$). The corresponding numbers for males were 69.5% and 57.0% ($p = 0.05$). Both among males and females, those who drank a glass or more of light/artificially sweetened beverages or fruit juice daily, also had a higher tendency to drink SSB daily. There were differences in prevalence of daily drinkers of SSB of 20–30 percentage points between the highest and lowest categories of these beverages for both sexes. Similar, but smaller, differences were found for more frequent consumption of sweets and snacks. In both sexes, the higher the intake of water, the lower the percentage of daily SSB drinkers ($p < 0.02$). There was no association between drinking SSB and milk consumption.

Rarely eating breakfast or bringing lunch to school was associated with daily SSB drinking, with 20–40% higher prevalence of daily SSB drinking than among those eating these meals every day (Table 2). No association was found between frequency of having dinner and daily SSB drinking. Weight class (thin/normal vs. overweight/obese) was not associated with daily SSB drinking, neither in females nor males. Those not physically active were more often daily drinkers of SSB than the more active, though the distributions differed between sexes, and the difference was only borderline significant in males. Higher daily screen time was associated with daily SSB drinking in females ($p = 0.002$), but not in males. Smokers and snuff users were more likely to be daily SSB drinkers. Among males, never drinkers of alcohol were less likely to be daily SSB drinkers than more frequent alcohol drinkers, among females, there was no significant association between alcohol drinking and daily SSB drinking in univariate analyses.

In the adjusted model, students in vocational studies had a 59% higher chance of drinking SSB daily compared to those in general studies (only borderline significant for females) (Table 3). Daily drinking of SSB was associated with several dietary variables: eating snacks weekly vs. not (females OR 3.67, 95%CI 2.03–6.64, males OR 2.03, 95% CI 1.29–3.19), drinking light/artificially sweetened beverages (>1 glass daily vs never—females OR 4.05, 95%CI 2.22–7.36, males OR 2.20, 95% CI 1.30–3.72). The same was seen for fruit juice, those drinking a glass or more daily had an odds ratio of daily SSB drinking of 2 or more, compared to never drinkers (significant for both sexes). Not eating breakfast was associated with higher odds of daily drinking of SSB compared to eating everyday (females OR 4.03, 95% CI 1.88–8.63, males OR 2.02, 95% CI 0.97–4.22). Other health behaviours were also associated with daily SSB drinking: A significant association with daily snuffing (females OR 4.93, 95% CI 2.40–10.14, males OR 2.18, 95% CI 1.14–4.16), and the same tendency, although not statistically significant, was seen for daily/occasional smoking. Never drinkers of alcohol had a higher OR of daily SSB drinking than those drinking alcohol twice a month or more often, at least in females (females OR 2.59, 95% CI 1.19–5.66, males OR 1.60, 95% CI 0.84–3.03). Water consumption was no longer a significant covariate. The adjusted model explained 40.8% of the variation in daily drinking of sugar-sweetened beverages for females and 20.6% for males. However, there was no interaction with sex (all p-values for interaction >0.08).

Table 3. Characteristics Associated with being a daily drinker of sugar-sweetened beverages in the Tromsø study: *Fit Futures*.

	Females (n = 426)		Males (n = 444)	
Characteristic	OR	95% CI	OR	95% CI
School programme				
General	Ref		Ref	
Vocational	1.59	(0.94–2.68)	1.59	(1.03–2.46)
Consumption of sweet or savoury snacks				
Not weekly	Ref		Ref	
Weekly	3.67	(2.03–6.64)	2.03	(1.29–3.19)
Light/artificially sweetened beverages, daily				
None	Ref		Ref	
0.5 glass	0.77	(0.41–1.46)	0.99	(0.60–1.64)
1 glass or more	4.05	(2.22–7.36)	2.20	(1.30–3.72)
Fruit juice, daily				
0.5 glass or less	Ref		Ref	
1 glass	2.12	(1.13–3.95)	2.82	(1.62–4.92)
2.5 glasses or more	2.34	(1.18–4.64)	2.13	(1.13–4.03)
Breakfast				
Every day	Ref		Ref	
1–6 days/week	1.19	(0.68–2.08)	1.68	(1.04–2.70)
Seldom/never	4.03	(1.88–8.63)	2.02	(0.97–4.22)

Table 3. *Cont.*

Characteristic	Females (n = 426) OR	95% CI	Males (n = 444) OR	95% CI
Smoking				
Never	Ref		Ref	
Occasionally or daily	1.92	(0.98–3.76)	1.59	(0.84–2.99)
Use of snuff				
Never	Ref		Ref	
Occasionally	2.35	(1.12–4.91)	1.14	(0.56–2.30)
Daily	4.93	(2.40–10.14)	2.18	(1.14–4.16)
Alcohol drinking				
Twice a month or more often	Ref		Ref	
Once a month or less often	1.39	(0.76–2.54)	2.00	(1.13–3.53)
Never	2.59	(1.19–5.66)	1.60	(0.84–3.03)

Mutually adjusted logistic regression analyses. Ref = reference category, OR = odds ratio, CI = confidence interval.

In the model including sex and mother's education, males had 3.74 times higher odds of being daily SSB drinkers compared to females (95% CI 2.68–5.22) (Figure 2). Compared to students with mothers with the longest education, those with mothers with short (OR 1.74, 95% CI 1.11–2.72) or medium length of education (OR 2.06, 95% CI 1.24–3.43), had higher odds of being daily SSB drinkers. Else the results were similar to the main model, with OR estimates between what was found for females and males, but estimates for smoking and alcohol were stabilized. This model explained 37.6% of the variation in daily SSB drinking. There was no interaction with sex, (all *p*-values for interaction >0.12).

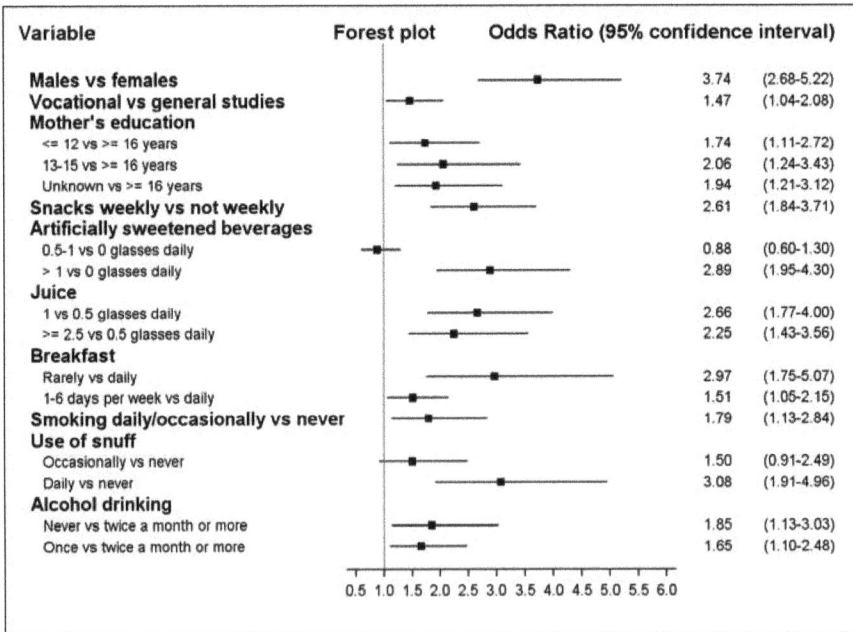

Figure 2. Odds for being a daily drinker of sugar-sweetened beverages in the Tromsø study: *Fit Futures*. Mutually adjusted model including sex and mother's education, n = 870.

4. Discussion

We found high prevalence of daily SSB drinking in this group of adolescents from Northern Norway. Socio-economic factors (study programme, mother's education), sex, diet (snacks, breakfast), other drinking habits (light/artificially sweetened beverages, fruit juice), and health-related habits (smoking, snuffing, alcohol drinking) all contributed to explaining the variation in daily SSB drinking. The model explained more of the variation in daily SSB drinking in females than in males.

In our study, there were more than twice as many daily drinkers as in the edition of HBSC that took place in the same period and age group, 61% of the males and 32% of the females vs. 25 and 11% [11,15]. We included two questions (carbonated and non-carbonated SSB) rather than one, but it is not likely that this, and differences in response categories, explains the difference in prevalence, but rather that there are differences in intake between the two studies. The HBSC study included a lower number of students from the Northern region, but they used a cluster sampling to ensure a nationally representative sample [11], how this might have influenced the results is uncertain. A previous study from Northern Norway found that among boys, as many as 52.3% of eighth graders and 74.0% of tenth graders were daily drinkers of carbonated SSB, corresponding numbers for girls were 42.1% and 46.8% [23]. In addition, 48.9% of the boys and 45.0% of the girls drank other soft drinks ("squash") daily. That survey took place five years before our study. As we found that 61% of the males and 32% of the females were daily drinkers (of carbonated and non-carbonated SSB combined), this might support the decreasing trend in SSB intake seen over time in the HBSC study [11]. However, the number of daily drinkers still is higher than what is reported in national studies and studies from other parts of Norway. Some of this difference can be explained by differences in age groups and questions included in the different studies, but not all. While our questions covered more than HBSC, we did not include energy/sports drinks, so our prevalence estimates could still be underestimated. Our participants represented urban and rural adolescents in Northern Norway. We excluded some students due to age, and some due to missing variables, but with an exceptionally high participation rate, we still think that the results are representative for adolescents in the region.

Conflicting results exists concerning the stability of SSB consumption. The Oslo Youth survey found moderate to high stability of soft drink consumption from age 15 to 25, but low stability from age 15 to 33 [18]. The FVMM study on the other hand observed a decrease in SSB consumption, and an increase in consumption of artificially sweetened beverages from age 11 to 26 [28]. Hence, continued monitoring of our participants would be interesting in order to gain more knowledge about the stability of the SSB intake.

Higher or more frequent intake in boys than in girls has been reported in several studies [17,29–32]. However, some of the other results were surprising; we did not see associations with BMI, sedentary behaviour, or physical activity in the final models. A lack of association between BMI and consumption of SSB has also been reported in other studies [29]. One study found no association in cross-sectional analyses, but higher BMI in SSB consumers in longitudinal analyses [30]. The same study found associations both cross-sectionally and longitudinally for percentage body fat. A review on confectionery consumption and overweight/obesity found that in cross-sectional studies, obese and overweight children had lower confectionary intakes than normal weight children [33]. In addition, they reported no association in longitudinal studies. Our study is a cross-sectional study, so no causal inferences can be drawn. It is possible that those with high BMI underreport their SSB consumption, or actually reduce their consumption in order to lose weight [29]. Alternatively, BMI might not be the best measure of body fatness, or this could be a true association. Spending much time on sedentary activities could also mean spending much time on homework, and need not be only a negative feature.

One could assume that more frequent consumption of one drink would be mirrored by lower/less frequent consumption of other drinks, but daily drinking of SSB was associated with higher consumption of juice. The picture was more mixed for artificially sweetened soft drinks, however, daily drinkers were more frequently never consumers of alcohol, at least among females. In the univariate analyses, there was less SSB consumption among those that drank water more frequently. This association was not significant in the adjusted analyses. Replacing SSB with water would be the healthiest option, but interventions have only produced medium size increases in water consumption [6]. Longitudinal analyses of stability and change across the spectrum of beverages would provide interesting complimentary data. Those rarely eating breakfast had a very high odds for daily SSB-drinking. For this group, availability of healthy options in schools might be an issue.

A recent publication with data from the Nordic countries in the HBSC study found no socioeconomic differences in SSB drinking, as measured by the family affluence scale [11], however, our study suggested that both own educational choice and mother's education were associated with daily SSB drinking, in line with other studies [12,17,20,28–30,32,34]. To the best of our knowledge, this is the first Norwegian study to look at school programme, an indicator of the students own socioeconomic status, in association with SSB consumption. If longitudinal studies can confirm that school programme is a predictor of SSB consumption, targeted interventions in vocational school programmes might be an important avenue for further reducing the SSB consumption. Not living with parents did not influence SSB drinking, but the group was small, so no strong conclusions can be drawn.

The HELENA study assessed the beverage consumption among European adolescents in eight countries [31]. SSB was the second most frequently consumed beverage, after only water, and 55% of the 15–17.5 year olds reported drinking SSB (including sports drinks) during the two days the study covered, compared with our 61% daily drinkers among males and 32% among females. In half the countries studied, SSB were the largest contributor to energy intake among all beverages.

SSB are major contributors to sugar intake in Norwegian adolescents [35], and dietary patterns characterized by high sugar and fat content have been associated with adiposity later in adolescence [36]. The current national plan of action for a better diet aims at halving the number of 15-year-olds that drink SSB 5 times a week or more often [37]. Continued monitoring, and interventions targeting SSB consumption in general, and in males, students in vocational programmes and Northern Norway in particular are warranted, in order to accomplish that goal. Reviews have suggested that education programmes and changes in school environment (restricted access) will reduce intake, but also that substitution of SSB with low sugar/artificially sweetened beverages will reduce sugar and energy intake [38,39]. This is in line with children's own opinions [40]. Restricting access at home and ensuring good parental modelling is another possible avenue [20,22,38,40]. A recent review showed only small decreases in SSB consumption in adolescents after interventions [6], specific analyses on most successful intervention settings could not be done in adolescents, but for children, home-based interventions and modelling/demonstrating the behaviour seemed to improve intervention effects.

This study has several strengths, a fairly large, population-based sample, a very high participation rate, and assessment of a range of covariates that might confound analyses of SSB intake and health. The sample was homogenous with respect to age, and included both rural and urban participants. Taken together, this suggests that our results are representative for adolescents in Northern Norway. Separate questions were asked for both carbonated and non-carbonated SSB, as this better captures the range of products that can be grouped as SSB [41].

The study also has several limitations. The questions about SSB used in this study have not been used in other studies in adolescents and, in general, most of the studies cited here have used different definitions or response categories, hampering comparisons between studies. For instance, not all studies distinguish between carbonated and non-carbonated SSB, and many do not include sports drinks (and neither did ours). Not including sports drinks/energy drinks in the definition probably means that frequency of intake reported here is underestimated. Lack of comparability is a recognized problem, and a recent review has suggested methods that should be used in future studies [41].

The most frequently reported intake category in our study was wide (1–6 glasses per week), and created possibilities for misclassification when combining the data for carbonated and non-carbonated SSB into one variable. Some studies distinguish weekday and weekend consumption, as this may differ considerably [17], but we did not have that information. Consequently, some of the participants we labelled "daily SSB drinkers" might have consumed larger amounts of SSB on one or two days, rather than one (or more) glass daily. The total amount of sugar and energy ingested will be the same, independent of how the consumption is distributed, but the length of time the teeth are exposed will affect dental caries risk.

Furthermore, the food/drink questions have not been validated. A review on validity of food frequency questionnaires used in adolescents showed that not assessing portion size, shorter time span, medium length, and administration directly to the adolescent, not via a parent gave the best validity [42]. Our questionnaire did not specify the time-span for the food questions, but the other factors were fulfilled. Our study only included participants from Northern Norway, and the results might not be representative for the rest of the country.

As cutting down on sugar intake has been official policy during the last years, and initiatives have been taken to reduce consumption of SSB [13], social desirability bias, i.e., underreporting consumption of products the health authorities discourage, could be an issue. Given the high consumption reported, this seems less likely, but it cannot be ruled out. Although the sample was relatively large, the skewed distribution of some of the variables led to large uncertainty in some of the estimates. The study was cross-sectional, so it is not possible to make causal inferences. For some reason, the variables explained the variation in SSB intake in females better than in males. We lacked information regarding, e.g., individual choices vs. family or peer influence, and availability, or money to purchase SSB [20,21,34,40]. Perhaps such variables are more important for males' food choices than females'. Females reach puberty earlier and have a stronger body focus, and possibly also health focus than males [43,44], this may explain some of the sex differences we found.

5. Conclusions

In conclusion, particularly males are frequent drinkers of SSB, despite efforts at reducing consumption in recent years. In both males and females, higher prevalence of daily drinking was found than in a national survey. Our study has identified several factors associated with daily SSB drinking, many of them are other unhealthy lifestyle choices, and are important to adjust for in analyses of SSB intake and health. If these associations are confirmed using stronger study designs, these factors could be targeted together in future comprehensive intervention studies. The higher consumption of SSB in vocational studies is of particular concern, suggesting that socio-economic differences in diet start early.

Supplementary Materials: The following are available online at http://www.mdpi.com/2072-6643/11/2/211/s1, Supplementary File 1: Dietary questions used in the Tromsø study: *Fit Futures 1*.

Author Contributions: Conceptualization: G.S. and V.S.; data curation: V.S. and G.G.; formal analysis: G.S.; funding acquisition: G.G.; investigation: G.G.; methodology: G.S.; project administration: G.S. and G.G.; resources: G.G.; supervision: G.S.; writing—original draft: G.S., V.S., and G.G.; writing—review and editing: G.S., V.S., and G.G.

Funding: The Tromsø study: *Fit Futures 1* was set up with contributions from Helse Nord Infrastrukturmidler, UNN Forskningsposten, Helsefak UiT, Troms fylkeskommune, Odd Berg medisinske forskningsfond, Sparebankens gavefond, Simon Fougner Hartmanns Familiefond, and Eckbos legat. The funding bodies had no role in the design, analysis, or interpretation of this paper. The publication charges for this paper have been funded by a grant from the publication fund of UiT The Arctic University of Norway.

Acknowledgments: We wish to thank all the adolescents who participated in the Tromsø study: *Fit Futures 1*. Also, we want to thank everyone who contributed to setting up the Tromsø study: *Fit Futures*, and to the data collection, particularly the Clinical Research Department at the University Hospital of North Norway.

Conflicts of Interest: The authors declare no conflict of interest.

Abbreviations

BMI	Body mass index (kg/m^2)
CI	Confidence interval
HBSC	Health Behaviour among School Children study
OR	Odds ratio
SSB	Sugar-sweetened beverages

References

1. Division of Nutrition, Physical Activity, and Obesity; National Center for Chronic Disease Prevention and Health Promotion. Get the Facts: Sugar-Sweetened Beverages and Consumption. Available online: https://www.cdc.gov/nutrition/data-statistics/sugar-sweetened-beverages-intake.html (accessed on 8 January 2018).
2. Singh, G.M.; Micha, R.; Khatibzadeh, S.; Lim, S.; Ezzati, M.; Mozaffarian, D. Estimated Global, Regional, and National Disease Burdens Related to Sugar-Sweetened Beverage Consumption in 2010. *Circulation* **2015**, *132*, 639–666. [CrossRef] [PubMed]
3. Imamura, F.; O'Connor, L.; Ye, Z.; Mursu, J.; Hayashino, Y.; Bhupathiraju, S.N.; Forouhi, N.G. Consumption of sugar sweetened beverages, artificially sweetened beverages, and fruit juice and incidence of type 2 diabetes: Systematic review, meta-analysis, and estimation of population attributable fraction. *Br. J. Sports Med.* **2016**, *50*, 496–504. [CrossRef] [PubMed]
4. Moynihan, P.J.; Kelly, S.A. Effect on caries of restricting sugars intake: Systematic review to inform WHO guidelines. *J. Dent. Res.* **2014**, *93*, 8–18. [CrossRef] [PubMed]
5. Andersen, L.F.; Overby, N.; Lillegaard, I.T. Intake of fruit and vegetables among Norwegian children and adolescents. *Tidsskrift for den Norske Laegeforening Tidsskrift for Praktisk Medicin ny Raekke* **2004**, *124*, 1396–1398.
6. Vargas-Garcia, E.J.; Evans, C.E.L.; Prestwich, A.; Sykes-Muskett, B.J.; Hooson, J.; Cade, J.E. Interventions to reduce consumption of sugar-sweetened beverages or increase water intake: Evidence from a systematic review and meta-analysis. *Obes. Rev.* **2017**, *18*, 1350–1363. [CrossRef] [PubMed]
7. Lussi, A.; Jaeggi, T.; Zero, D. The role of diet in the aetiology of dental erosion. *Caries Res.* **2004**, *38* (Suppl. 1), 34–44. [CrossRef] [PubMed]
8. Trumbo, P.R.; Rivers, C.R. Systematic review of the evidence for an association between sugar-sweetened beverage consumption and risk of obesity. *Nutr. Rev.* **2014**, *72*, 566–574. [CrossRef] [PubMed]
9. Malik, V.S.; Pan, A.; Willett, W.C.; Hu, F.B. Sugar-sweetened beverages and weight gain in children and adults: A systematic review and meta-analysis. *Am. J. Clin. Nutr.* **2013**, *98*, 1084–1102. [CrossRef]
10. Marshall, T.A.; Levy, S.M.; Broffitt, B.; Warren, J.J.; Eichenberger-Gilmore, J.M.; Burns, T.L.; Stumbo, P.J. Dental caries and beverage consumption in young children. *Pediatrics* **2003**, *112*, e184–e191. [CrossRef]
11. Fismen, A.S.; Smith, O.R.; Torsheim, T.; Rasmussen, M.; Pedersen Pagh, T.; Augustine, L.; Ojala, K.; Samdal, O. Trends in Food Habits and Their Relation to Socioeconomic Status among Nordic Adolescents 2001/2002–2009/2010. *PLoS ONE* **2016**, *11*, e0148541. [CrossRef]
12. Stea, T.H.; Overby, N.C.; Klepp, K.I.; Bere, E. Changes in beverage consumption in Norwegian children from 2001 to 2008. *Public Health Nutr.* **2012**, *15*, 379–385. [CrossRef] [PubMed]
13. Ministry of health and Care Services. *Norwegian Action Plan on Nutrition (2007–2011)—Recipe for a Healthier Diet*; Norwegian Ministries: Oslo, Norway, 2007.
14. Åstrøm, A.N.; Klepp, K.I.; Samdal, O. Konsum av sukret mineralvann og søtsaker blant norske skoleelever: Sterk økning fra 1989 til 2001. *Nor Tannlegeforen Tid* **2004**, *114*, 816–821.
15. Samdal, O.; Bye, H.H.; Torsheim, T.; Birkeland, M.S.; Diseth, Å.R.; Fismen, A.-S.; Haug, E.; Leversen, I.; Wold, B. *Sosial Ulikhet i Helse og Læring Blant Barn og Unge. Resultater fra den Landsrepresentative Spørreskjemaundersøkelsen "Helsevaner Blant Skoleelever. En WHO-Undersøkelse i Flere Land"*; HEMIL-Senteret, Universitetet i Bergen: Bergen, Norway, 2012.
16. Samdal, O.; Mathisen, F.; Torsheim, T.; Diseth, Å.; Fismen, A.-S.; Larsen, T.; Wold, B.; Årdal, E. *Helse og Trivsel Blant Barn og Unge. Resultater fra den Landsrepresentative Spørreundersøkelsen «Helsevaner Blant Skoleelever. En WHO-Undersøkelse i Flere Land»*; HEMIL-Senteret, Universitetet i Bergen: Bergen, Norway, 2016.

17. Bjelland, M.; Lien, N.; Grydeland, M.; Bergh, I.H.; Anderssen, S.A.; Ommundsen, Y.; Klepp, K.I.; Andersen, L.F. Intakes and perceived home availability of sugar-sweetened beverages, fruit and vegetables as reported by mothers, fathers and adolescents in the HEIA (HEalth In Adolescents) study. *Public Health Nutr.* **2011**, *14*, 2156–2165. [CrossRef] [PubMed]
18. Kvaavik, E.; Andersen, L.F.; Klepp, K.I. The stability of soft drinks intake from adolescence to adult age and the association between long-term consumption of soft drinks and lifestyle factors and body weight. *Public Health Nutr.* **2005**, *8*, 149–157. [CrossRef]
19. Greenwood, D.C.; Threapleton, D.E.; Evans, C.E.L.; Cleghorn, C.L.; Nykjaer, C.; Woodhead, C.; Burley, V.J. Association between sugar-sweetened and artificially sweetened soft drinks and type 2 diabetes: Systematic review and dose–response meta-analysis of prospective studies. *Br. J. Nutr.* **2014**, *112*, 725–734. [CrossRef] [PubMed]
20. Gebremariam, M.K.; Lien, N.; Torheim, L.E.; Andersen, L.F.; Melbye, E.L.; Glavin, K.; Hausken, S.E.; Sleddens, E.F.; Bjelland, M. Perceived rules and accessibility: Measurement and mediating role in the association between parental education and vegetable and soft drink intake. *Nutr. J.* **2016**, *15*, 76. [CrossRef] [PubMed]
21. Gebremariam, M.K.; Henjum, S.; Terragni, L.; Torheim, L.E. Correlates of fruit, vegetable, soft drink, and snack intake among adolescents: The ESSENS study. *Food Nutr. Res.* **2016**, *60*, 32512. [CrossRef]
22. Melbye, E.L.; Bergh, I.H.; Hausken, S.E.S.; Sleddens, E.F.C.; Glavin, K.; Lien, N.; Bjelland, M. Adolescent impulsivity and soft drink consumption: The role of parental regulation. *Appetite* **2016**, *96*, 432–442. [CrossRef]
23. Øvrebø, E.M. Food habits of school pupils in Tromsø, Norway, in the transition from 13 to 15 years of age. *Int. J. Consum. Stud.* **2011**, *35*, 520–528. [CrossRef]
24. Statistics Norway. Dental Status by Age, 18-Year Olds. Available online: https://www.ssb.no/statistikkbanken/SelectVarVal/saveselections.asp (accessed on 19 November 2015).
25. Mulic, A.; Fredriksen, O.; Jacobsen, I.D.; Tveit, A.B.; Espelid, I.; Crossner, C.G. Dental erosion: Prevalence and severity among 16-year-old adolescents in Troms, Norway. *Eur. J. Paediatr. Dent.* **2016**, *17*, 197–201.
26. Winther, A.; Dennison, E.; Ahmed, L.A.; Furberg, A.S.; Grimnes, G.; Jorde, R.; Gjesdal, C.G.; Emaus, N. The Tromso Study: Fit Futures: A study of Norwegian adolescents' lifestyle and bone health. *Arch. Osteoporos.* **2014**, *9*, 185. [CrossRef] [PubMed]
27. Cole, T.J.; Lobstein, T. Extended international (IOTF) body mass index cut-offs for thinness, overweight and obesity. *Pediatr. Obes.* **2012**, *7*, 284–294. [CrossRef] [PubMed]
28. Bolt-Evensen, K.; Vik, F.N.; Stea, T.H.; Klepp, K.I.; Bere, E. Consumption of sugar-sweetened beverages and artificially sweetened beverages from childhood to adulthood in relation to socioeconomic status—15 years follow-up in Norway. *Int. J. Behav. Nutr. Phys. Act.* **2018**, *15*, 8. [CrossRef] [PubMed]
29. Park, S.; Blanck, H.M.; Sherry, B.; Brener, N.; O'Toole, T. Factors Associated with Sugar-Sweetened Beverage Intake among United States High School Students. *J. Nutr.* **2012**, *142*, 306–312. [CrossRef] [PubMed]
30. Laverty, A.A.; Magee, L.; Monteiro, C.A.; Saxena, S.; Millett, C. Sugar and artificially sweetened beverage consumption and adiposity changes: National longitudinal study. *Int. J. Behav. Nutr. Phys. Act.* **2015**, *12*, 137. [CrossRef] [PubMed]
31. Duffey, K.J.; Huybrechts, I.; Mouratidou, T.; Libuda, L.; Kersting, M.; De Vriendt, T.; Gottrand, F.; Widhalm, K.; Dallongeville, J.; Hallstrom, L.; et al. Beverage consumption among European adolescents in the HELENA study. *Eur. J. Clin. Nutr.* **2012**, *66*, 244–252. [CrossRef] [PubMed]
32. Vereecken, C.A.; Inchley, J.; Subramanian, S.V.; Hublet, A.; Maes, L. The relative influence of individual and contextual socio-economic status on consumption of fruit and soft drinks among adolescents in Europe. *Eur. J. Public Health* **2005**, *15*, 224–232. [CrossRef]
33. Gasser, C.E.; Mensah, F.K.; Russell, M.; Dunn, S.E.; Wake, M. Confectionery consumption and overweight, obesity, and related outcomes in children and adolescents: A systematic review and meta-analysis. *Am. J. Clin. Nutr.* **2016**, *103*, 1344–1356. [CrossRef]
34. Nordnes, E.T.; Melbye, E.L.; Pedersen, I.; Bjelland, M. Hva Betyr Kjønn, Foreldres Utdanningsnivå og Foreldrepraksis for Ungdommers Inntak av Ulike Typer Drikke? Master's Thesis, Norwegian University of Life Sciences, Ås, Norway, 2016; pp. 6–12.
35. Hansen, L.B.; Myhre, J.B.; Johansen, A.M.W.; Paulsen, M.M.; Andersen, L.F. *UNGKOST 3. Landsomfattende Kostholdsundersøkelse Blant Elever i 4.—og 8. Klasse i Norge, 2015*; Folkehelseinstituttet: Oslo, Norway, 2016.

36. Ambrosini, G.L.; Johns, D.J.; Northstone, K.; Emmett, P.M.; Jebb, S.A. Free Sugars and Total Fat Are Important Characteristics of a Dietary Pattern Associated with Adiposity across Childhood and Adolescence. *J. Nutr.* **2016**, *146*, 778–784. [CrossRef]
37. Ministries. *Norwegian Action Plan for a Better Diet (2017–2021)*; Ministries: Oslo, Norway, 2017.
38. Avery, A.; Bostock, L.; McCullough, F. A systematic review investigating interventions that can help reduce consumption of sugar-sweetened beverages in children leading to changes in body fatness. *J. Hum. Nutr. Diet.* **2015**, *28* (Suppl. 1), 52–64. [CrossRef]
39. Grieger, J.A.; Wycherley, T.P.; Johnson, B.J.; Golley, R.K. Discrete strategies to reduce intake of discretionary food choices: A scoping review. *Int. J. Behav. Nutr. Phys. Act.* **2016**, *13*, 57. [CrossRef] [PubMed]
40. Battram, D.S.; Piche, L.; Beynon, C.; Kurtz, J.; He, M. Sugar-Sweetened Beverages: Children's Perceptions, Factors of Influence, and Suggestions for Reducing Intake. *J. Nutr. Educ. Behav.* **2016**, *48*, 27–34. [CrossRef] [PubMed]
41. Riordan, F.; Ryan, K.; Perry, I.J.; Schulze, M.B.; Andersen, L.F.; Geelen, A.; Van't Veer, P.; Eussen, S.; van Dongen, M.; Wijckmans-Duysens, N.; et al. A systematic review of methods to assess intake of sugar-sweetened beverages among healthy European adults and children: A DEDIPAC (DEterminants of DIet and Physical Activity) study. *Public Health Nutr.* **2017**, *20*, 578–597. [CrossRef] [PubMed]
42. Kolodziejczyk, J.K.; Merchant, G.; Norman, G.J. Reliability and validity of child/adolescent food frequency questionnaires that assess foods and/or food groups. *J. Pediatr. Gastroenterol. Nutr.* **2012**, *55*, 4–13. [CrossRef] [PubMed]
43. Abreu, A.P.; Kaiser, U.B. Pubertal development and regulation. *Lancet Diabetes Endocrinol.* **2016**, *4*, 254–264. [CrossRef]
44. Kantanista, A.; Osinski, W.; Borowiec, J.; Tomczak, M.; Krol-Zielinska, M. Body image, BMI, and physical activity in girls and boys aged 14–16 years. *Body Image* **2015**, *15*, 40–43. [CrossRef] [PubMed]

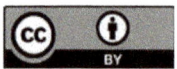

© 2019 by the authors. Licensee MDPI, Basel, Switzerland. This article is an open access article distributed under the terms and conditions of the Creative Commons Attribution (CC BY) license (http://creativecommons.org/licenses/by/4.0/).

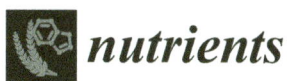

Article

Nutritional Behaviors of Polish Adolescents: Results of the Wise Nutrition—Healthy Generation Project

Joanna Myszkowska-Ryciak [1,*], Anna Harton [1], Ewa Lange [1], Wacław Laskowski [2] and Danuta Gajewska [1]

1. Department of Dietetics, Faculty of Human Nutrition and Consumer Sciences, Warsaw University of Life Sciences (WULS), 159C Nowoursynowska Str, 02-776 Warsaw, Poland
2. Department of Organization and Consumption Economics, Faculty of Human Nutrition and Consumer Sciences, Warsaw University of Life Sciences (WULS), 159C Nowoursynowska Str, 02-776 Warsaw, Poland
* Correspondence: joanna_myszkowska_ryciak@sggw.pl; Tel.: +48-22-593-7022; Fax: +48-22-593-7018

Received: 9 June 2019; Accepted: 11 July 2019; Published: 13 July 2019

Abstract: Background: Recognition of the dominant dietary behaviors with respect to gender and specific age groups can be helpful in the development of targeted and effective nutritional education. The purpose of the study was to analyze the prevalence of the selected eating behaviors (favorable: Consuming breakfasts, fruit, vegetables, milk and milk beverages, whole grain bread and fish; adverse: Regular consumption of sweets, sugared soft drinks and fast-foods) among Polish adolescents. Methods: Data on the nutritional behaviors were collected using a questionnaire. Body mass status was assessed based on weight and height measurements. Results: 14,044 students aged 13–19 years old from 207 schools participated in the study. Significant differences were found in the nutritional behaviors depending on age, gender and nutritional status. Favorable nutritional behaviors corresponded with each other, the same relationship was observed for adverse behaviors. The frequency of the majority of healthy eating behaviors decreased with age, whereas the incidence of adverse dietary behaviors increased with age. Underweight adolescents more often consumed sugared soft drinks, sweets and fast food compared to their peers with normal and excessive body mass. Conclusions: A significant proportion of adolescents showed unhealthy nutritional behaviors. Showing changes in the incidence of nutritional behaviors depending on age, gender and body weight status, we provide data that can inform the development of dietary interventions tailored to promote specific food groups among adolescents on different stages of development to improve their diet quality.

Keywords: nutrition; nutritional behavior; diet quality; adolescents

---

1. Introduction

The health of children and adolescents is dependent upon food intake that provides sufficient energy and nutrients to promote optimal physical, cognitive and social growth and development [1–3]. However, in practice, the implementation of proper nutrition recommendations in these population groups is extremely difficult due to the existing barriers, e.g., availability of healthy food, inadequate nutritional knowledge of caregivers and children and personal food preferences [4–7]. A great body of the literature indicates the low overall diet quality in children and adolescents, both in terms of the amounts (deficits or excesses) of food/nutrients, and the selection of food groups/food products. One in four Polish 17–18 years old female adolescents did not eat breakfast regularly, and nearly half of them consumed fish only one time per month [8]. Almost 35% of schoolchildren and adolescents aged 9–13 years from rural parts of Poland regularly ate sweets, and 46% failed to consume vegetables and fruit at least once a day [9]. These inadequacies in the assortment and quantities of food products result in an incorrect supply of energy and nutrients. The average European adolescents' diet is too high in saturated fatty acids and sodium, whereas too low in monounsaturated fatty acids, vitamin D, folate and iodine [10]. In Poland a significant increasing trend in calcium intake in teenagers aged 11–15 years was noted in the last 20 years, but the observed values are still lower than the recommendations [11]. In the US nearly 40% of total energy consumed by two- to 18-year-olds came in the form of empty calories (including 365 kcal from added sugars) [12]. Poor quality of the diet in early life may impair growth and development rate, and also increases the risk of some diet-related diseases (e.g., obesity, type 2 diabetes mellitus, cardiovascular disease and osteoporosis) in the future [3,13].

Although correct nutrition is important throughout the life span, it is possible to distinguish particularly critical periods, i.e., the first 2–3 years [3] and the period of puberty [14,15]. Dramatic physical growth and development during puberty significantly increases requirements for energy, protein, and also others nutrients compared to late childhood. Biological changes related to puberty might significantly affect psychosocial development. Rapid changes in body size, shape and composition in girls might lead to poor body image experience and development of eating disorders [16]. At this age, girls may experience nutritional behaviors leading to weight loss, e.g., alternative diets promoted in the media. Nevertheless, a delay in biological development might lower self-esteem and increase the risk of eating disorders among male teenagers [17]. As young teens are highly influenced by a peer group, then the desire to conform may also affect nutritional behaviors and food intake. Moreover, food choices can be used by adolescents as a way to express their independence from families and parents. At this age, young people may prefer to eat fast-food meals in a peer group instead of meals at home with their families. During middle adolescence (15–17 years) importance of peer groups even raising, and their influence regarding individual food choices peaks. Finally, in the late stage of adolescence (18–21 years) the influence of peer groups decreases, whereas an ability to comprehend how current health behaviors may affect the long-term health status significantly increases [18], which in turn can enhance the effectiveness of nutritional education.

Although nutritional knowledge does not always translate into proper nutritional behavior [19], some data indicate the association between nutritional knowledge and the diet quality among adolescents [20]. Joulaei et al. (2018) observed that an increase in functional nutrition literacy was associated with lower sugar intake and better energy balance among boys and higher dairy intake among girls. Therefore, recognition of the dominant dietary behaviors with respect to gender and specific age groups can be helpful in the development of targeted and effective nutritional education.

In Poland, there are many studies on nutritional behaviors of adolescents [8,9,11], but their limitation is the small number of participants and the lack of representativeness in their selection. The only study involving a large, representative group of Polish adolescents is the health behavior in school-aged children (HBSC) [21], conducted for over 30 years, now in more than 40 countries, including Poland. The HBSC study does not allow us to assess nutritional behaviors of older adolescents, because it covers only the group of 11-, 13- and 15-year-old boys and girls. In Poland there is no research including the wide age range of respondents with all periods of adolescence at the same time and with the same methodology. Therefore, the purpose of the present study was to analyze the frequency of occurrence of the behaviors important in terms of overall diet quality amongst Polish adolescents. The frequency of occurrence of nutritional behaviors was analyzed in the age categories with regard to gender and taking into account the criteria of the weight status.

2. Materials and Methods

2.1. General Information

The presented study is a part of the research and education program Wise nutrition—healthy generation granted by The Coca-Cola Foundation, and addressed to the secondary and upper secondary school youth, their parents and teachers. The main objective of the program was to educate the secondary and upper secondary school students regarding the importance of healthy nutrition and physical activity in the prevention of the diet-related diseases. The research part of the project included assessing the selected dietary behaviors and parameters related to physical activity of the students and performing anthropometric measurements to assess their nutritional status. Those with diagnosed abnormal body mass were invited to the dietary counseling program (two individual meetings with a dietician). The diagram presenting the overall activities within the project is provided in the supplementary materials (Figure S1). Participation in the project was voluntary and totally free of charge for all participants (schools, students and parents). All educational and research activities were carried out in schools participating in the program by trained dieticians. After receiving patronages from the government educational institutions and local authorities, written invitations were sent to all secondary and upper secondary schools in Poland. Nearly 14,000 educational institutions listed in the electronic register of schools of the Minister for National Education were invited to participate. Finally, 2058 schools attended by nearly 450,000 students joined the project in 2013–2015.

This paper focused on the results concerning nutritional behaviors of students (Figure S1). The program was carried out following the standards required by the Helsinki Declaration, and the protocol was approved by the Scientific Committee of the Polish Society of Dietetics. School directors provided written informed consent to participate in the study. Parents were provided with a detailed fact sheet describing the program and had to give written informed consent if they wanted their child to participate. All students over 16 years of age were asked to give their written informed consent to participate in the study.

2.2. Study Participants

To examine the selected nutritional behaviors and nutritional status of Polish teenagers, participants were recruited from schools participating in the project. To ensure a representative selection of students, these schools were randomly selected using the stratified sampling method from all of the 2058 enrolled institutions. The sampling was stratified by province and location (large, medium, small city and countryside), as well as the type of school (secondary and upper secondary). Secondary schools (called "gimnazjum" in Poland) are compulsory for all adolescents aged 13–16 years, and are located close to the students' place of residence. Upper secondary schools (high schools, technical schools and basic vocational schools) include, depending on the type, youth from 16 to 20 years of age. As in the case of secondary schools, students typically live with their families and commute to school. Within the selected schools, as the next step, students were randomly selected from the class registry. Exclusion criteria included: Diagnosed disease that required the use of a special diet, pregnancy or lactation in girls or lack of written consent. All the personal data of participants were fully anonymized. The schools, and consequently, students came from all over Poland, therefore the research was of a nationwide character. In total, 207 schools of the 2058 institutions were enrolled (~10%), and finally 14,044 students participated in the study, including 7553 (53.8%) girls and 6491 (46.2%) boys. The age categories for the studied group were adopted in accordance with the HBSC methodology [21].

2.3. Anthropometric Measurements

The assessment of the body weight status of the examined individuals was based on anthropometric measurements (body weight and height) conducted by a trained dietitian. All the measurements were carried out with the equipment provided by The Polish Society of Dietetics: Digital floor scales (TANITA HD-380 BK, Tanita Corporation, Tokyo, Japan) and a steel measuring tape (0–200 cm). All dieticians conducting the measurements were specially trained and followed the same procedures according to Anthropometry Procedures Manual by National Health and Nutrition Examination Survey (NHANES) [22] to minimize bias. The school was obliged to provide a room suitable for the measurements.

Weight of the individuals was measured twice to the nearest 0.1 kg, and the mean value was recorded. Measurements were conducted on individuals dressed in basic clothes (e.g., underwear, trousers/skirt and t-shirt) and without shoes. From the final result 0.5 kg was subtracted (predicted weight of the basic clothes).

For height measurements individuals stood on a flat surface in an upright position with their back against the wall, and the heels together and toes apart (without shoes and socks). They were asked to stand as tall as possible with the head in the Frankfort horizontal plane [22]. The height measurement was conducted twice to the nearest 0.1 cm, and the mean value was recorded.

Based on the body height and weight data, body mass index (BMI) value was calculated. BMI was calculated as body weight in kilograms divided by the square of height in meters. Depending on the age of the subjects different criteria for assessing the body weight status were used. For individuals aged 13–18 years old, calculated BMI value was plotted on gender BMI centile charts for age (with an accuracy of one month) [23]. The percentile value was read from percentile grids and the body mass status was assessed according to the International Obesity Task Force (IOTF) criteria (underweight <5 percentile, normal weight 5–85 percentile, overweight >85 and ≤95 percentile, obese >95 percentile) [24]. For students above the age of 18 years old, the standard World Health Organization (WHO) body mass index criteria were applied: Underweight for BMI <18.5 kg/m^2, normal body weight for BMI between 18.5 and 24.9 kg/m^2, overweight between 25 and 29.9 kg/m^2 and obesity ≥30 kg/m^2 [25].

2.4. Analysis of Nutritional Behaviors

Data on the selected nutritional behaviors were collected prior to the anthropometric measurements and dietary counseling. The paper questionnaire containing questions about the selected nutritional practices, physical activity and self-esteem satisfaction (data not included in this article) was carried out in individuals by a dietitian. This provided the opportunity to clarify possible doubts or ask additional questions. After its completion the questionnaire was collected by a dietician. Due to the large sample group and direct methods of data acquisition, it was decided that the questionnaire has to be short, and must contain questions about the critical determinants of teenagers diet quality. Taking into account the health behavior in school-aged children (HBSC) questionnaire (developed for 11, 13 and 15 year olds) concerning nutritional behaviors [26], and available data on nutritional characteristics of the Polish youth population [21], nine questions were finally formulated with the possibility of answering "yes" or "no". The first six questions concerned favorable aspects of the nutritional behaviors, while the last three questions referred to the adverse nutritional practices. Healthy nutritional behaviors included: (1) Regular consumption of breakfast before leaving for school, (2) daily consumption of at least one serving of fresh fruit and (3) daily consumption of at least two servings of vegetables (recommended diet quality indicators adapted from HBSC questionnaire [26]. Additionally, taking into account the importance for the overall diet quality and the low consumption in the Polish population [21,27], the three extra questions were added: (4) Daily consumption of milk and/or milk fermented beverages (as the main source of calcium in the diet), (5) daily consumption of whole grains (as the main source of complex carbohydrates and dietary fiber) and (6) consumption of fish at least once week (as the main source of docosahexaenoic acid (DHA), eicosapentaenoic acid (EPA), vitamin D and iodine in the diet). On the other hand, negative dietary determinants (unfavorable nutritional practices increasing the share of free sugars, saturated fat and trans fatty acids in the diet) were considered as: Drinking sugared soft drinks (soda and other carbonated soft drinks) several times during the week, eating sweets more than once a day (adapted from HBSC), and consuming fast food more than twice a week. Prior to the main study, a pilot study ($n = 50$) was conducted to examine whether the questions were understandable to the respondents. The questionnaire was validated: Repeatability was verified by determining the correlation coefficient between the results obtained in the same group ($n = 50$, age 13–19 years old) twice; correlation coefficients for individual questions were on average 0.76 (95% CI = 0.71–0.83) and ranged from 0.18 to 0.96.

2.5. Statistical Analysis

Statistical data processing was performed using Statistica version 13.1 (Copyright©StatSoft, Inc, 1984–2014, Cracow, Poland). Data were analyzed in the total group, according to age, gender and body weight status. Statistical significances for nominal (categorical) variables were determined using the

Pearson's chi-square test. Additionally, contingency coefficient Cramér's V was used to indicate the strength of association between categorical variables. Quantitative data was tested for normality of distribution; in the case of its absence the Mann–Whitney test was used for comparisons of independent groups. The correspondence analysis was used to study the relationship between dietary behaviors. The differences were considered significant at $p \leq 0.05$.

3. Results

The total sample group consisted of 14,044 students, including 7553 girls and 6491 boys. The detailed characteristics of the group in terms of age distribution, sex and the body mass index are presented in Table 1. Data on examined dietary behaviors are presented in Table 2. All data are expressed as number values and in percentages.

3.1. Characteristics of the Study Group

The characteristics of the study population in terms of age distribution and the body mass index (BMI) in the whole group and separately for girls and boys are presented in Table 1. The predominant group was students aged 17 (followed by 18 and 16 olds in girls, and 16 and 18 olds in boys), while the smallest groups were students aged 13 and 19 between both sex groups. There were significant differences in the average BMI between girls and boys in the total group and in the case of all age categories except the 13 year olds.

Table 1. Age and body mass index (BMI) distribution of the individuals: In the total group and divided by gender.

Age (years)	Total Group			Girls			Boys			p-Value
	N	%	BMI mean ± SD	N	%	BMI mean ± SD	N	%	BMI mean ± SD	
13	1270	9.0	20.1 ± 3.66	670	8.9	19.9 ± 3.55	600	9.2	20.3 ± 3.78	0.0854
14	1876	13.4	20.5 ± 3.48	1004	13.3	20.3 ± 3.41	872	13.4	20.6 ± 3.54	0.0414 [1]
15	2011	14.3	20.8 ± 3.37	1040	13.8	20.6 ± 3.17	971	15.0	21.0 ± 3.56	0.0485 [1]
16	2386	17.0	21.3 ± 3.31	1257	16.6	21.1 ± 3.08	1129	17.4	21.6 ± 3.54	0.0024 [1]
17	2781	19.8	21.8 ± 3.48	1538	20.4	21.3 ± 3.30	1243	19.2	22.3 ± 3.61	0.0000 [1]
18	2551	18.2	21.9 ± 3.41	1436	19.0	21.3 ± 3.16	1115	17.2	22.7 ± 3.56	0.0000 [1]
19	1169	8.3	22.2 ± 3.61	608	8.1	21.7 ± 3.68	561	8.6	22.6 ± 3.48	0.0000 [1]
All age groups	14044	100.0	21.3 ± 3.51	7553	53.8	20.9 ± 3.33	6491	46.2	21.7 ± 3.68	0.0000 [1]

[1] Significant differences in average BMI between girls and boys for age categories and for the total (all age groups), the Mann–Whitney test.

3.2. Characteristics of Nutritional Behaviors

Figure 1 presents the relationship between the examined nutritional behaviors in the whole group. Based on the correspondence analysis, it is possible to indicate the connections between the analyzed nutritional behaviors. Beneficial nutritional behaviors such as consuming breakfast, fruit, vegetables, whole-grain bread, milk or milk beverages and fish were linked together. In opposite, unfavorable eating behaviors such as skipping breakfast, low consumption of milk products, fruits, vegetables, fish and whole-grain bread were related. Behaviors such as fast food, sweets and sugared soft drinks consumption were linked together and corresponded more to the adverse nutritional behaviors.

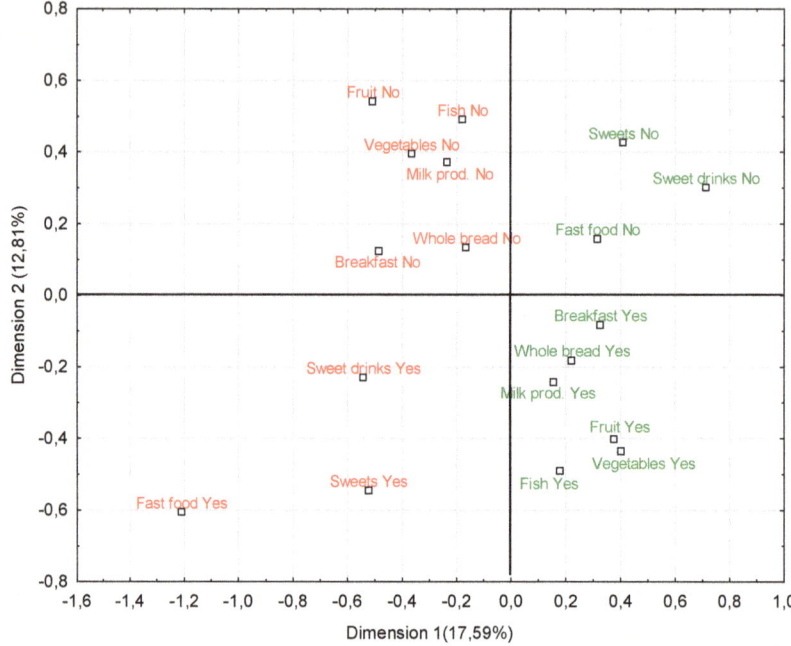

Figure 1. The results of the analysis of correspondence of all examined variables (nutritional behaviors) in the total group. Behaviors beneficial to the overall diet quality are marked in green; unfavorable behaviors are marked in red.

The frequencies of examined nutritional behaviors in the total group, and for girls and boys separately are presented in Table 2.

Breakfast was regularly consumed by seven out of 10–13 year olds but only by half of 19 year olds. There was a statistically significant (but small) effect of age in the total group, and separately for girls and boys. Boys were more likely to eat breakfast in comparison to girls, and differences were particularly noticeable in the younger age groups. The frequency of eating at least one serving of fruit per day also decreased with age. A statistically significant (but small) effect in the total group, and separately for girls, and boys was noted. Girls were more likely to include fresh fruits to the daily diet in comparison to boys. There was a significant effect of age on the consumption of vegetables in the total group. Half of the 13-year-olds consumed at least two servings of vegetables a day, but the frequency of consumption decreased to 43% for the group of 19-year-olds. Similarly, the influence of age was observed in the group of girls, and boys. Girls consumed at least two servings of vegetables daily more often than boys in all age groups, except for 18-year-olds. The consumption of milk or milk beverages decreased with age. Significant age effects were observed throughout the total group, and among girls, and boys. In all age groups fewer girls drank milk and fermented milk beverages compared to boys. With age, the proportion of teenagers consuming whole grain bread in everyday diet decreased. However, age effects were not observed for girls, and neither for boys, separately. Considering gender, in all age groups, the greater percentage of girls consumed whole wheat bread in their usual diet. No significant effect of age was observed on fish consumption, neither in the total group, nor in girls, and boys. However, significant gender effects were observed: A greater percentage of boys consumed fish at least one a week in all age groups compared to girls. The effect of age was observed in regards of drinking sugared soft drinks a few times a week, for the whole group, and for both genders. The proportion of adolescents drinking sugared soft drinks increased with age. A higher percentage of boys consumed sugared soft drinks compared to girls in all age categories. Less than half of the students declared consuming sweets more than once a day. No age effects were observed, neither for the whole group, nor for the girls. A small effect of age was found only among boys. On the other hand, a relationship with gender was observed: In all age groups, a higher percentage of girls declared such behavior compared to boys. There was a significant relationship between fast-food consumption and age. The percentage of adolescents consuming fast food more than twice a week increased with age, and an analogous relationship was observed for girls and boys. In all age groups, a higher number of boys declared such nutritional behaviors comparing to girls.

Table 2. Nutritional behaviors of the individuals: In the total group and divided by gender.

Age Category (years)	Total Group		Girls		Boys		p-Value (V Cramer) Girls vs. Boys
	N	%	N	%	N	%	
Having breakfast every day before leaving for school							
All age groups	8400	59.81	4178	55.32	4222	65.05	
13	897	70.63	431	64.33	466	77.67	
14	1222	65.14	595	59.26	627	71.90	
15	1267	63.00	587	56.44	680	70.03	0.0000 [4] (0.10)
16	1405	58.89	682	54.26	723	64.04	
17	1620	58.25	836	54.36	784	63.12	
18	1391	54.53	751	52.30	640	57.40	
19	598	51.15	296	48.68	302	53.83	
p-value	0.0000 [1]		0.0001 [2]		0.0000 [3]		
V Cramer	0.10		0.08		0.14		
Consuming fresh fruit every day (at least one serving)							
All age groups	8071	57.47	4506	59.66	3565	54.93	
13	857	67.48	468	69.85	389	64.83	
14	1242	66.20	686	68.33	556	63.76	
15	1267	63.00	673	64.71	594	61.17	0.0000 [4] (0.05)
16	1322	55.41	746	59.35	576	51.02	
17	1490	53.58	865	56.24	625	50.32	
18	1322	51.82	751	52.30	571	51.21	
19	571	48.85	317	52.14	254	45.28	
p-value	0.0000 [1]		0.0000 [2]		0.0000 [3]		
V Cramer	0.13		0.13		0.13		
Consuming vegetables every day (at least two servings)							
All age groups	6678	47.55	3658	48.43	3019	46.52	
13	662	52.13	372	55.52	290	48.33	
14	1010	53.84	561	55.88	449	51.49	
15	996	49.53	533	51.25	463	47.68	0.0241 [4] (0.02)
16	1130	47.36	614	48.85	516	45.70	
17	1245	44.77	698	45.38	547	43.96	
18	1135	44.51	616	42.90	519	46.56	
19	500	42.77	264	43.42	236	42.07	
p-value	0.0000 [1]		0.0000 [2]		0.0061 [3]		
V Cramer	0.0		0.07		0.05		
Drinking milk or milk beverages (yoghurt/kefir/butter milk, etc.) every day							
All age groups	8478	60.38	4172	55.24	4306	66.36	
13	860	67.72	438	65.37	422	70.33	
14	1279	68.18	643	64.04	636	72.94	
15	1305	64.89	610	58.65	695	71.58	0.0000 [4] (0.11)
16	1392	58.34	674	53.62	718	63.60	
17	1583	56.92	780	50.72	803	64.65	
18	1435	56.27	729	50.80	706	63.32	
19	624	53.42	298	49.01	326	58.21	
p-value	0.0000 [1]		0.0000 [2]		0.0000 [3]		
V Cramer	0.10		0.11		0.09		

Table 2. Cont.

Age Category (years)	Total Group		Girls		Boys		p-Value (V Cramer) Girls vs. Boys
	N	%	N	%	N	%	
Consuming whole-grained bread every day							
All age groups	5962	42.46	3302	43.72	2659	40.97	
13	556	43.78	297	44.33	259	43.17	
14	809	43.12	447	44.52	362	41.51	
15	871	43.33	467	44.95	404	41.61	0.0010 [4] (0.03)
16	1065	44.64	578	45.98	487	43.14	
17	1198	43.08	679	44.15	519	41.71	
18	1020	39.98	598	41.64	422	37.85	
19	443	37.90	236	38.82	207	36.90	
p-value V Cramer	0.0007 [1] 0.04		p = 0.0566		p = 0.0548		
Consuming fish at least once a week							
All age groups	7023	50.02	3412	45.19	3610	55.63	
13	662	52.13	341	50.90	321	53.50	
14	965	51.44	463	46.12	502	57.57	
15	1021	50.80	469	45.10	552	56.91	0.0000 [4] (0.1)
16	1188	49.81	564	44.90	624	55.27	
17	1330	47.84	673	43.79	657	52.82	
18	1260	49.39	626	43.59	634	56.86	
19	597	51.07	276	45.39	321	57.22	
p-value V Cramer	0.1057		0.0640		0.2130		
Drinking sugared soft drinks few times a week							
All age groups	7977	56.80	3764	49.83	4212	64.90	
13	650	51.18	305	45.52	345	57.50	
14	1069	56.98	512	51.00	557	63.88	
15	1202	59.77	540	51.92	662	68.18	0.0000 [4] (0.15)
16	1374	57.59	633	50.36	741	65.63	
17	1546	55.59	719	46.75	827	66.51	
18	1441	56.49	720	50.14	721	64.66	
19	695	59.45	335	55.10	360	64.17	
p-value V Cramer	0.0000 [1] 0.05		0.0026 [2] 0.05		0.0019 [3] 0.06		
Consuming sweets more than once a day							
All age groups	6156	43.84	3428	45.39	2727	42.02	
13	548	43.15	311	46.42	237	39.50	
14	840	44.78	465	46.31	375	43.00	
15	926	46.05	486	46.73	440	45.31	0.0000 [4] (0.03)
16	1065	44.65	573	45.62	492	43.58	
17	1216	43.73	690	44.86	526	42.27	
18	1068	41.87	628	43.73	440	39.46	
19	493	42.17	275	45.23	218	38.86	
p-value V Cramer	p = 0.0912		p = 0.7863		0.0480 [3] 0.04		
Consuming fast food (e.g., chips, burgers etc.) more than two times a week							
All age groups	2906	20.70	1360	18.01	1545	23.81	
13	206	16.22	99	14.78	107	17.83	
14	314	16.74	145	14.54	168	19.27	
15	385	19.14	170	16.35	215	22.14	0.0000 [4] (0.07)
16	513	21.50	226	17.98	287	25.42	
17	622	22.37	299	19.44	323	25.93	
18	590	23.14	295	20.54	295	26.48	
19	276	23.63	125	20.56	151	26.96	
p-value V Cramer	0.0000 [1] 0.06		0.0002 [2] 0.06		0.0000 [3] 0.07		

[1] Significant differences in the examined nutritional behaviors between age categories in the total group; [2] significant differences in the examined nutritional behaviors between age categories in girls; [3] significant differences in the examined nutritional behaviors between age categories in boys; [4] significant differences in the examined nutritional behaviors between girls and boys, the chi^2 Pearson test.

The data on the prevalence of examined nutritional behaviors depending on the nutritional status (underweight, normal body mass, overweight and obesity) are presented in Table 3.

Table 3. Nutritional behaviors of the individuals depending on body weight status: In the total group and divided by gender.

BMI Category	Total Group		Girls		Boys	
	N	%	N	%	N	%
Having breakfast every day before leaving for school						
Underweight	422	59.44	256	55.65	166	66.40
Normal	6567	60.99	3302	56.28	3265	66.62
Overweight	908	55.64	407	52.38	501	58.60
Obesity	502	53.98	212	47.53	290	59.92
p value	0.0000 [1]		0.0012 [2]		0.0000 [3]	
V Cramer	0.05		0.04		0.06	
Consuming fresh fruit every day (at least one serving)						
Underweight	360	50.70	233	50.65	127	50.80
Normal	6108	56.72	3467	59.09	2641	53.89
Overweight	994	60.91	499	64.22	495	57.89
Obesity	606	65.16	305	68.39	301	62.19
p value	0.0000 [1]		0.0000 [2]		0.0006 [3]	
V Cramer	0.06		0.07		0.05	
Consuming vegetables every day (at least two servings)						
Underweight	334	47.04	214	46.52	120	48.00
Normal	5086	47.23	2828	48.20	2258	46.07
Overweight	799	48.99	384	49.42	415	48.59
Obesity	457	49.14	230	51.57	227	46.90
p value	0.4228		0.4139		0.5479	
V Cramer						
Drinking milk or milk beverages (yoghurt / kefir / butter milk, etc.) every day						
Underweight	392	55.21	233	50.65	159	63.60
Normal	6538	60.72	3266	55.68	3272	66.76
Overweight	1000	61.27	429	55.21	571	66.78
Obesity	545	58.67	241	54.04	304	62.94
p value	0.0174 [1]		0.2010		0.2830	
V Cramer	0.03					
Consuming whole-grained bread every day						
Underweight	285	40.14	177	38.48	108	43.20
Normal	4522	42.00	2547	43.42	1975	40.30
Overweight	713	43.69	352	45.30	361	42.22
Obesity	440	47.31	224	50.22	216	44.63
p value	0.0059 [1]		0.0031 [2]		0.1984	
V Cramer	0.03		0.04			
Consuming fish at least once a week						
Underweight	323	45.49	193	41.96	120	52.00
Normal	5356	49.75	2632	44.88	2176	55.59
Overweight	849	52.02	370	47.62	376	56.02
Obesity	493	53.01	216	48.43	207	57.23
p value	0.0071 [1]		0.1157		0.5947	
V Cramer	0.03					
Drinking sugared soft drinks few times a week						
Underweight	435	61.27	260	56.52	175	70.00
Normal	6140	57.02	2943	50.16	3197	65.23
Overweight	901	55.21	361	46.46	540	63.16
Obesity	499	53.66	199	44.62	300	61.98
p value	0.0096 [1]		0.0007 [2]		0.1098	
V Cramer	0.03		0.05			

Table 3. Cont.

BMI Category	Total Group		Girls		Boys	
	N	%	N	%	N	%
	Consuming sweets more than once a day					
Underweight	403	56.76	272	59.13	131	52.40
Normal	4900	45.51	2751	46.89	2149	43.85
Overweight	572	35.05	278	35.78	294	34.39
Obesity	280	30.14	127	28.54	153	31.61
p value	0.0000 [1]		0.0000 [2]		0.0000 [3]	
V Cramer	0.11		0.13		0.09	
	Consuming fast food (e.g., chips, burgers etc.) more than two times a week					
Underweight	187	26.34	115	25.00	72	28.80
Normal	2311	21.46	1090	18.58	1221	24.92
Overweight	274	16.80	105	13.51	169	19.79
Obesity	134	14.41	50	11.21	84	17.36
p value	0.0000 [1]		0.0000 [2]		0.0000 [3]	
V Cramer	0.06		0.07		0.06	

[1] Significant differences in the examined nutritional behaviors in the total group; [2] significant differences in the examined nutritional behaviors between girls; [3] significant differences in the examined nutritional behaviors between boys; the chi^2 Pearson test.

Analyzing the prevalence of selected nutritional behaviors in the whole group of adolescents depending on the body weight status, significant relationships were observed for all eating behaviors except for consuming vegetables. Regular consumption of breakfast was more often declared by adolescents with normal body weight and underweight in total group and both for girls and boys. The percentage of subjects consuming at least one portion of fruit was the smallest in the underweight group, and the largest among the obese adolescents. Consumption of milk and milk beverages was declared by a higher percentage by overweight adolescents, whereas in the smallest percentage by underweight individuals. At the same time, no relationship was observed between this nutritional behavior and the nutritional status separately for girls and boys. The frequency of regular consumption of whole-grain bread increased with the category of body weight in the whole group and in the case of girls. The relationship between fish consumption and the nutritional status was observed only in the whole group. As in the case of bread, the frequency of declared fish consumption increased with the BMI category. In the case of the last three nutritional behaviors: Drinking sweet beverages, eating sweets and fast foods, the incidence of these behaviors decreased with the BMI category, both in the whole group and among girls and boys (with the exception of drinking sweet drinks among boys, where no relation was observed with the body weight status).

4. Discussion

Since adolescence is a time of tremendous biological, psychosocial and cognitive changes, nutrition interventions need to be tailored not only to the developmental stage, but also to the nutritional needs of individuals [18]. Based on dietary recommendation, nutritional behaviors crucial for the overall diet quality of children and adolescents might be determined. The "key" determinants of the healthy diet include eating breakfasts, regular consumption of vegetables, fruits, dairy products, whole grain products, fish, as well as avoiding sugared soft drinks, sweets and fast foods (empty calories) [26,28,29]. Literature data indicate the prevalence of selected nutritional behaviors, as well as typical nutritional errors in children and adolescents at different stages of development [8,30–32]. Hiza et al. [33] and Bandield et al. [33] reported a poorer diet quality in adolescents compared to younger children. In the US students, a decrease in fruit and vegetable consumption and an increase in fast food intake have been reported from childhood and young adolescence to older adolescence [34]. Nevertheless, Lipsky et al. [29] observed a modest improvement in diet quality between 16.5 and 20.5 years of age reflected, among others, in more frequent breakfasts consumption.

Based on the analysis of correspondence, it can be noticed that regardless of age or sex, beneficial (or adverse) nutritional behaviors cluster together. Thus, individuals who, for example, do not consume breakfast, more often show other adverse nutritional behaviors (a low consumption of fruit, vegetables, fish and whole grain bread). A typical breakfast in Poland includes bread or cereals, dairy and/or meat products as well as vegetables and/or fruit. Thus, omitting breakfast may lead to a reduction in the supply of these products in the overall diet. Our results suggest that if one irregularity is found in a teenager's diet, it can be assumed that the overall diet quality is low. Interestingly, consuming (or not consuming) sweets, sugared soft drinks and fast food cluster together, but did not correspond to other determinants of the quality of the diet. It may suggest that such products might be consumed together as a meal (e.g., meal typical for fast-food restaurants). It may also suggest the need for educational activities aimed at these products, regardless of the general education about healthy nutrition.

In our study, the frequency of regular breakfast consumption decreased with age, both among boys and girls. In addition, girls significantly less often declared eating breakfast compared to boys. Our observations are consistent with data from the HBSC study [26] where older children and girls were less likely to eat breakfast every weekday. However, more Polish 13- and 15 years olds declared this beneficial nutritional behavior compared to the average among their European peers [26]. Interestingly, we noted a significant relationship between the regularity of consuming breakfast and the body mass status. Regular breakfast consumption was declared by the highest percentage of students with normal body mass (61%) and the lowest with obesity (54%). It could be hypothesized that skipping breakfasts can be a strategy to reduce the weight of adolescents. However, this hypothesis requires additional research. Fayet-Moore et al. [35] observed a lower prevalence of overweight among breakfast consumers compared to skippers (n = 4487, 2–16 years). Moreover, individuals who eat breakfast had significantly higher intake of calcium and folate, and significantly lower intake of total fat than breakfast skippers, which indicates the important role of breakfast not only in maintaining a healthy body weight but also in the quality of the diet. Our results indicate a strong need to increase education activities promoting the regular breakfast consumption, especially among older girls and students with abnormal body mass status.

Regular fruit and vegetables consumption is linked to many positive health outcomes [36]. The WHO recommends at least 400 g of fruit and vegetables daily, however studies in 10 European countries indicate that the majority of teenagers fail to meet the recommendations [37]. Only 37% of 13-year-olds and 33% 13-year-olds reported eating fruit at least once a day, whereas vegetables were consumed every day or more than once a day by 35% of the 13-year-olds and 33% of the 13-year-olds, respectively (average from 38 countries and regions) [26]. We observed a decrease in the daily fruit and vegetables consumption with age in the total group, and for both genders; in the total group the percentage of teenagers reporting daily fruit consumption decreased from 67% in 13-years-olds to 49% in 19-years-olds. In the case of vegetables, we did not observe a relationship with body weight status, but the frequency of daily fruit consumption was related to the nutritional state. Regular consumption of fruit was most often declared by obese teenagers, and least frequently by underweight adolescents. The fruit, in contrast to vegetables, have a higher energy value, which, with high consumption, may increase the energy value of the diet. In the case of vegetables and fruit there is still a substantial room for improvement in all subgroups, however education should emphasize differences in the caloric value between fruit and vegetables, especially promoting the latter.

Dairy products, especially milk and milk beverages, contribute to a healthy diet by providing energy, protein, and nutrients such as calcium, magnesium and vitamins B_1, B_2 and B_{12} [38]. Regular consumption of at least two servings of dairy products in adolescents resulted in a significant weight loss and a reduction in body fat [39,40]. However, data from HELENA study reported that European adolescents eat less than two-thirds of the recommended amount of milk (and milk products) [37], which reflected in low calcium intake, especially in oldest girls group [10]. We also observed a decrease in the percentage of students declaring daily milk and milk beverages consumption with age. The trend was particularly pronounced among girls: From 56% among 13-year-olds to 43%

in 19-year-olds. We also observed a relationship between milk consumption and nutritional status in total group. In this case regular daily milk consumption most often has been declared by individuals with normal body weight. Based on our findings, nutritional education concerning promotion of milk products should be especially targeted at older girls.

As in the case of vegetables and fruits, consumption of whole grain products is associated with a lower risk of many diet-related diseases, e.g., cardiovascular disease and stroke, hypertension, insulin sensitivity, diabetes mellitus type 2, obesity and some types of cancer [41]. Papanikolaou et al. [42] reported a better diet quality and nutrients intake in US children and adolescents consuming grain food products compared to those consuming no grains. In our study less than half of students consumed whole grains bread every day, and the percentage of those decreased with age. Interestingly, the frequency of whole-grain bread consumption was the highest among adolescents with excessive body mass, especially in girls. This may suggest that although consumption of whole grain bread improves the quality of a diet, it may also contribute to increasing the overall caloric value of the diet.

Regular intake of fish, particularly fatty fish, has positive health outcomes, especially in the long term. It reduces the risk of CHD mortality and ischaemic stroke [43]. Fish consumption in adolescents has been associated with better school achievements and performance in cognitive tests [44]. Handeland et al. [45] observed a small beneficial effect of fatty fish consumption on processing speed in tests of attention conducted in 426 students age 14–15 years old. In our study only half of students consumed fish at least once a week, and no age effect has been observed. However, boys declared consumption of fish more often compared with girls. Additionally, the significant relation has been noted between fish consumption and body weight status: The percentage of fish consumers increased with body mass status (45% in underweight and 53% in obese individuals). However, considering the beneficial role of fish and their low intake, nutritional education should be carried out in all subgroup of adolescents, regardless of age, sex or weight status.

Sugared soft drinks, sweets and fast foods are the sources of empty calories that contribute to a substantial share of the total energy intake in children and adolescents [46]. Intake of soft (sweetened) drinks among adolescents is higher than in other age groups (nearly 20% of 13- and 15-years olds reported their regular daily consumption), and it is associated with a greater risk of weight gain, obesity and chronic diseases and directly affects dental health by providing excessive amounts of sugars [26]. In our study, consumption of sugared soft drinks increased with the age category in total group, and both for boys and girls, but in the same time was the lowest in the case of obese individuals compared to other weight groups (except for boys). Sweetened beverages provide a high-energy amount in liquid form that contributes to increasing the simple-carbohydrate content of the diet and influencing the other nutrients' intake [12,47]. Interestingly, similar relationships were also observed in the case of fast food consumption. While sweets consumption was significantly higher in girls and underweight students, but no effect of age has been noted. The HBSC data also highlighted gender differences in daily sweets intake (27% of 13-years old girls compared to 23% of boys in the same age). Taking into account the prevalence of these adverse behaviors, nutritional education should be directed at all adolescents, but with particular focus on older age groups.

Strengths and Limitations

The strength of the study is the sample size. To our knowledge there is no research on such a scale covering all age categories over a large geographic area. With such a large sample, the advantage is also the way of obtaining data. All questionnaires were filled in by a trained dietician who could explain the respondents' doubts on an ongoing basis. Moreover, all anthropometric data were obtained through measurements conducted also by a dietician, which ensured obtaining reliable results and minimize the bias.

Respondents for our study were recruited from schools participating in the project, which can be a certain limitation. However, the number of schools allowed a random selection of the sample taking into account different types of institutions and their geographic location. The small number of questions with the very limited possibilities of answers in the questionnaire may also be a certain limitation. However, the questions have been developed on the basis of large, international studies on the nutritional behaviors of school-aged children [21,26], and include the most important healthy and unhealthy behaviors concerning nutrition. Additionally, the questionnaire was validated before the main study.

5. Conclusions

By analyzing the differences in nutritional behaviors between age and gender groups, we provide data that can inform the development of dietary interventions tailored to answer the needs of adolescents at different stage of development and to improve the quality of their diet. We observed significant changes in the frequencies of analyzed eating behaviors depending on gender as well as on age. Furthermore, we have shown that the incidence of undesirable eating behavior is higher among underweight adolescents compared to their peers with an excessive body mass. Information on the most frequent nutritional errors on every stage of adolescents might be used to determine the type of educational messages given when counseling this challenging group, e.g., education activities regarding regular breakfast consumption should be intensified in older age groups, as the percentage of young people who eat breakfast decreases with age. On the other hand, education on the adverse effects of consumption of sweets, sugared soft drinks and fast food should be directed not only to adolescents with excessive body weight, but mainly to those underweight, as the consumption of these products is more frequent in this group. Moreover, regardless of age and sex, both favorable and adverse nutritional behaviors corresponded with each other. The present findings can be used both for the development of educational programs and for educational activities carried out by teachers at the school level.

Supplementary Materials: The following are available online at http://www.mdpi.com/2072-6643/11/7/1592/s1, Figure S1: The diagram of the Wise Nutrition—Healthy Generation project.

Author Contributions: Conceptualization, J.M.-R., D.G. and A.H.; methodology D.G., J.M.-R., A.H. and E.L.; investigation, D.G., A.H. and J.M.-R.; data curation, W.L. and A.H.; statistical analysis, W.L. and J.M.-R.; funding acquisition, D.G.; project administration, A.H.; writing—original draft preparation, J.M.-R.; writing—review and editing, all authors.

Funding: This research was funded by The Coca-Cola Foundation, the research and education grant Wise Nutrition—Healthy Generation.

Acknowledgments: The authors want to express their gratitude to Agata Wawrzyniak and Jadwiga Hamułka (Department of Human Nutrition, Faculty of Human Nutrition and Consumer Sciences, WULS, Warsaw, Poland) for their help with development of the questionnaire used in the study, and psychologist Bianca-Beata Kotoro for her professional support during the project. We also want to thank all the dieticians, school directors and teachers involved in the program.

Conflicts of Interest: The authors declare no conflict of interest. The founding sponsor had no role in the design of the study; in the collection, analyses, or interpretation of data; in the writing of the manuscript, and in the decision to publish the results. The preliminary results of nutritional behaviors were presented as an oral poster (Selected aspects of the nutrition style of Polish adolescents participating "Wise Nutrition—Healthy Generation" project. Joanna Myszkowska-Ryciak, Anna Harton, Ewa Lange, Wacław Laskowski, Danuta Gajewska) at the 8th DIETS/EFAD Conference "Health 2020—supporting vulnerable groups", Athens, Greece, 9–12 October 2014.

References

1. Hurley, K.M.; Yousafzai, A.K.; Lopez-Boo, F. Early Child Development and Nutrition: A Review of the Benefits and Challenges of Implementing Integrated Interventions1234. *Adv. Nutr.* **2016**, *7*, 357–363. [CrossRef] [PubMed]
2. World Health Organization. Nutrition for Health and Development (NHD) Sustainable Development and Healthy Environments (SDE) for Health and Development: A Global Agenda for Combating Malnutrition Nutrition. Available online: https://apps.who.int/iris/bitstream/handle/10665/66509/WHO_NHD_00.6.pdf?sequence=1 (accessed on 13 July 2019).

3. Cusick, S.E.; Georgieff, M.K. The Role of Nutrition in Brain Development: The Golden Opportunity of the "First 1000 Days". *J. Pediatr.* **2016**, *175*, 16–21. [CrossRef] [PubMed]
4. United Nations Children's Fund. *Improving Child. Nutrition: The Achievable Imperative for Global Progress*; United Nations Children's Fund (UNICEF): New York, NY, USA, 2013; ISBN 978-92-806-4686-3.
5. Nepper, M.J.; Chai, W. Parents' barriers and strategies to promote healthy eating among school-age children. *Appetite* **2016**, *103*, 157–164. [CrossRef] [PubMed]
6. Downs, S.M.; Farmer, A.; Quintanilha, M.; Berry, T.R.; Mager, D.R.; Willows, N.D.; McCargar, L.J. From Paper to Practice: Barriers to Adopting Nutrition Guidelines in Schools. *J. Nutr. Educ. Behav.* **2012**, *44*, 114–122. [CrossRef] [PubMed]
7. Mozaffarian, D.; Angell, S.Y.; Lang, T.; A Rivera, J. Role of government policy in nutrition—Barriers to and opportunities for healthier eating. *BMJ* **2018**, *361*, k2426. [CrossRef]
8. Przysławski, J.; Stelmach, M.; Grygiel-Górniak, B.; Mardas, M.; Walkowiak, J. Dietary habits and nutritional status of female adolescents from the great poland region. *Pol. J. Food Nutr. Sci.* **2011**, *61*, 73–78. [CrossRef]
9. Kołłątaj, W.; Sygit, K.; Sygit, M.; Karwat, I.D.; Kołłątaj, B. Eating habits of children and adolescents from rural regions depending on gender, education, and economic status of parents. *Ann. Agric. Environ. Med.* **2011**, *18*, 393–397.
10. Diethelm, K.; Huybrechts, I.; Moreno, L.; De Henauw, S.; Manios, Y.; Beghin, L.; Gonza-Gross, M.; Le Donne, C.; Cuenca-Garcı, M.; Castillo, M.J.; et al. Nutrient intake of European adolescents: Results of the HELENA (Healthy Lifestyle in Europe by Nutrition in Adolescence) Study. *Public Health Nutr.* **2014**, *17*, 486–497. [CrossRef]
11. Chwojnowska, Z.; Charzewska, Z.; Jajszczyk, B.; Chabrom, E. Trendy w spożyciu wapnia i witaminy D w dietach młodzieży szkolnej. *Probl. Hig. Epidemiol.* **2010**, *91*, 544–548. (In Polish)
12. Reedy, J.; Krebs-Smith, S.M. Dietary Sources of Energy, Solid Fats, and Added Sugars among Children and Adolescents in the United States. *J. Am. Diet. Assoc.* **2010**, *110*, 1477–1484. [CrossRef]
13. Sebert, S.; Sharkey, D.; Budge, H.; E Symonds, M.; Symonds, M. The early programming of metabolic health: Is epigenetic setting the missing link? *Am. J. Clin. Nutr.* **2011**, *94*, 1953S–1958S. [CrossRef] [PubMed]
14. Das, J.K.; Salam, R.A.; Thornburg, K.L.; Prentice, A.M.; Campisi, S.; Lassi, Z.S.; Koletzko, B.; Bhutta, Z.A. Nutrition in adolescents: Physiology, metabolism, and nutritional needs. *Ann. N. Y. Acad. Sci.* **2017**, *1393*, 21–33. [CrossRef] [PubMed]
15. Das, J.K.; Lassi, Z.S.; Hoodbhoy, Z.; Salam, R.A. Nutrition for the Next Generation: Older Children and Adolescents. *Ann. Nutr. Metab.* **2018**, *72*, 56–64. [CrossRef] [PubMed]
16. Kakhi, S.; McCann, J. Anorexia nervosa: Diagnosis, risk factors and evidence-based treatments. *Prog. Neurol. Psychiatry* **2016**, *20*, 24–29c. [CrossRef]
17. Lavender, J.M.; Brown, T.A.; Murray, S.B. Men, Muscles, and Eating Disorders: An Overview of Traditional and Muscularity-Oriented Disordered Eating. *Curr. Psychiatry Rep.* **2017**, *19*, 32. [CrossRef] [PubMed]
18. Stang, J.; Story, M. (Eds.) *Guidelines for Adolescent Nutrition Services*; University of Minnesota: Minneapolis, MN, USA, 2005.
19. Vaitkeviciute, R.; Ball, L.E.; Harris, N. The relationship between food literacy and dietary intake in adolescents: A systematic review. *Public Health Nutr.* **2015**, *18*, 649–658. [CrossRef] [PubMed]
20. Joulaei, H.; Keshani, P.; Kaveh, M.H. Nutrition literacy as a determinant for diet quality amongst young adolescents: A cross sectional study. *Prog. Nutr.* **2018**, *20*, 455–464. [CrossRef]
21. Mazur, J. Zdrowie i Zachowania Zdrowotne Młodzieży Szkolnej w Polsce na tle Wybranych Uwarunkowań Socjodemograficznych. In *Wyniki badań HBSC 2014*; Instytut Matki i Dziecka: Warszawa, Poland, 2015. (In Polish)
22. National Health and Nutrition Examination Survey (NHANES Anthropometry Procedures Manual. January 2007. Available online: https://www.cdc.gov/nchs/data/nhanes/nhanes_07_08/manual_an.pdf (accessed on 20 March 2019).
23. Kułaga, Z.; Litwin, M.; Tkaczyk, M.; Palczewska, I.; Zajączkowska, M.; Zwolińska, D.; Krynicki, T.; Wasilewska, A.; Moczulska, A.; Morawiec-Knysak, A.; et al. Polish 2010 growth references for school-aged children and adolescents. *Eur. J. Pediatr.* **2011**, *170*, 599–609. [CrossRef]
24. Cole, T.J.; Bellizzi, M.C.; Flegal, K.M.; Dietz, W.H. Establishing a standard definition for child overweight and obesity worldwide: International survey. *BMJ* **2000**, *320*, 1240. [CrossRef]

25. Body Mass Index—BMI. Available online: http://www.euro.who.int/en/health-topics/disease-prevention (accessed on 5 May 2019).
26. Inchley, J.; Currie, D.; Young, T.; Eds. Health Policy for Children and Adolescents, No. 7 Growing up Unequal: Gender and Socioeconomic Differences in Young People's Health and Well-Being. Health Behaviour in School-Aged Children (HBSC) Study: International Report from the 2013/2014 Survey. WHO Regional Office for Europe: Copenhagen, Denmark, 2016. Available online: http://www.euro.who.int/__data/assets/pdf_file/0003/303438/HSBC-No.7-Growing-up-unequal-Full-Report.pdf?ua (accessed on 20 March 2019).
27. Sygnowska, E.; Waśkiewicz, A.; Głuszek, J.; Kwaśniewska, M.; Biela, U.; Kozakiewicz, K.; Zdrojewski, T.; Rywik, S. Spożycie produktów spożywczych przez dorosłą populację polski. Wyniki programu WOBASZ. *Kardiol. Pol.* **2005**, *63*, 649–654. (In Polish)
28. Voortman, T.; Jong, J.C.K.-D.; Geelen, A.; Villamor, E.; A Moll, H.; De Jongste, J.C.; Raat, H.; Hofman, A.; Jaddoe, V.W.; Franco, O.H.; et al. The Development of a Diet Quality Score for Preschool Children and Its Validation and Determinants in the Generation R Study. *J. Nutr.* **2014**, *145*, 306–314. [CrossRef] [PubMed]
29. Lipsky, L.M.; Nansel, T.R.; Haynie, D.L.; Liu, D.; Li, K.; Pratt, C.A.; Iannotti, R.J.; Dempster, K.W.; Simons-Morton, B. Diet quality of US adolescents during the transition to adulthood: Changes and predictors12. *Am. J. Clin. Nutr.* **2017**, *105*, 1424–1432. [CrossRef] [PubMed]
30. De Assumpção, D.; Barros, M.B.D.A.; Fisberg, R.M.; Carandina, L.; Goldbaum, M.; Cesar, C.L. Diet quality among adolescents: A population-based study in Campinas, Brazil. *Brazil. Rev. Bras. Epidemiol.* **2012**, *15*, 605–616. [CrossRef] [PubMed]
31. Kambek, L.; Pitsi, T.; Eha, M.; Gluškova, N. *Dietary Habits of Adolescents in Estonia: Equity and Social Determinants*; World Health Organization: Geneva, Switzerland, 2013.
32. Banfield, E.C.; Liu, Y.; Davis, J.S.; Chang, S.; Frazier-Wood, A.C. Poor Adherence to US Dietary Guidelines for Children and Adolescents in the National Health and Nutrition Examination Survey Population. *J. Acad. Nutr. Diet.* **2016**, *116*, 21–27. [CrossRef] [PubMed]
33. Hiza, H.A.; Casavale, K.O.; Guenther, P.M.; Davis, C.A. Diet Quality of Americans Differs by Age, Sex, Race/Ethnicity, Income, and Education Level. *J. Acad. Nutr. Diet.* **2013**, *113*, 297–306. [CrossRef] [PubMed]
34. Larson, N.I.; Neumark-Sztainer, D.; Hannan, P.J.; Story, M. Trends in adolescent fruit and vegetable consumption, 1999–2004: Project EAT. *Am. J. Prev. Med.* **2007**, *32*, 147–150. [CrossRef] [PubMed]
35. Fayet-Moore, F.; Kim, J.; Sritharan, N.; Petocz, P. Impact of Breakfast Skipping and Breakfast Choice on the Nutrient Intake and Body Mass Index of Australian Children. *Nutrients* **2016**, *8*, 487. [CrossRef] [PubMed]
36. Slavin, J.L.; Lloyd, B. Health Benefits of Fruits and Vegetables1. *Adv. Nutr.* **2012**, *3*, 506–516. [CrossRef] [PubMed]
37. Diethelm, K.; Jankovic, N.; Moreno, L.A.; Huybrechts, I.; De Henauw, S.; De Vriendt, T.; Gonzalez-Gross, M.; Leclercq, C.; Gottrand, F.; Gilbert, C.C.; et al. Food intake of European adolescents in the light of different foodbased dietary guidelines: Results of the HELENA (Healthy Lifestyle in. Europe by Nutrition in Adolescence) Study. *Public Health Nutr.* **2012**, *15*, 386–398. [CrossRef] [PubMed]
38. Pereira, P.C. Milk nutritional composition and its role in human health. *Nutrition* **2014**, *30*, 619–627. [CrossRef] [PubMed]
39. Abreu, S.; Santos, R.; Moreira, C.; Vale, S.; Santos, P.C.; Soares-Miranda, L.; Marques, A.I.; Mota, J.; Moreira, P. Association between dairy product intake and abdominal obesity in Azorean adolescents. *Eur. J. Clin. Nutr.* **2012**, *66*, 830–835. [CrossRef] [PubMed]
40. Abreu, S.; Santos, R.; Moreira, C.; Santos, P.C.; Vale, S.; Soares-Miranda, L.; Mota, J.; Moreira, P. Milk intake is inversely related to body mass index and body fat in girls. *Eur. J. Nucl. Med. Mol. Imaging* **2012**, *171*, 1467–1474. [CrossRef] [PubMed]
41. O'Neil, C.E.; Nicklas, T.A.; Zanovec, M.; Cho, S. Whole grain consumption is associated with diet quality and nutrient intake in adults: The National Health and Nutrition Examination Survey (NHANES) 1999–2004. *J. Am. Diet. Assoc.* **2010**, *110*, 1461–1468. [CrossRef] [PubMed]
42. Papanikolaou, Y.; Jones, J.M.; Fulgoni, V.L. Several grain dietary patterns are associated with better diet quality and improved shortfall nutrient intakes in US children and adolescents: A study focusing on the 2015–2020 Dietary Guidelines for Americans. *Nutr. J.* **2017**, *16*, 266. [CrossRef] [PubMed]
43. Dinter, J.; Bechthold, A.; Boeing, H.; Ellinger, S.; Leschik-Bonnet, E.; Linseisen, J.; Lorkowski, S.; Wolfram, G. Fish intake and prevention of selected nutrition-related diseases. *Ernähr. Umsch.* **2016**, *63*, 148–154.

44. Kim, J.; Winkvist, A.; Åberg, M.A.; Åberg, N.; Sundberg, R.; Torén, K.; Brisman, J. Fish consumption and school grades in Swedish adolescents: A study of the large general population. *Acta Paediatr.* **2010**, *99*, 72–77. [CrossRef] [PubMed]
45. Handeland, K.; Øyen, J.; Skotheim, S.; Graff, I.E.; Baste, V.; Kjellevold, M.; Frøyland, L.; Lie, Ø.; Dahl, L.; Kjell, M. Stormark 3 Fatty fish intake and attention performance in 14–15 year old adolescents: FINS-TEENS a randomized controlled trial. *Nutr. J.* **2017**, *16*, 64. [CrossRef]
46. Poti, J.M.; Slining, M.M.; Popkin, B.M. Where are kids getting their empty calories? Stores, schools, and fast-food restaurants each played an important role in empty calorie intake among US children during 2009-2010. *J. Acad. Nutr. Diet.* **2013**, *114*, 908–917. [CrossRef]
47. Vartanian, L.R.; Schwartz, M.B.; Brownell, K.D. Effects of Soft Drink Consumption on Nutrition and Health: A Systematic Review and Meta-Analysis. *Am. J. Public Heal.* **2007**, *97*, 667–675. [CrossRef]

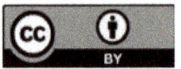

© 2019 by the authors. Licensee MDPI, Basel, Switzerland. This article is an open access article distributed under the terms and conditions of the Creative Commons Attribution (CC BY) license (http://creativecommons.org/licenses/by/4.0/).

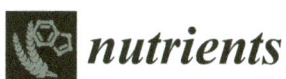

Article

Non-Milk Extrinsic Sugars Intake and Food and Nutrient Consumption Patterns among Adolescents in the UK National Diet and Nutrition Survey, Years 2008–16

Heidi T. Lai [1,2], Jayne Hutchinson [1] and Charlotte E. L. Evans [1,*]

1. Nutritional Epidemiology Group (NEG), School of Food Science and Nutrition, University of Leeds, Leeds LS2 9JT, UK
2. Friedman School of Nutrition Science and Policy, Tufts University, 150 Harrison Ave, Boston, MA 02111, USA
* Correspondence: c.e.l.evans@Leeds.ac.uk; Tel.: +44(0)113-343-3956

Received: 25 April 2019; Accepted: 12 July 2019; Published: 17 July 2019

Abstract: The revised guidelines from the Department of Health (DoH) in the UK state that mean population intakes of free sugars should be below 5% of the total energy (TE) consumption of the British population. However, very few studies have assessed the impact of this recommendation on diet quality in the UK. We explored the dietary patterns and intakes of micronutrients of British adolescents with low intakes of non-milk extrinsic sugars (NMES) (similar to free sugars but not equal, with slight differences in the categorisation of fruit sugars from dried, stewed or canned fruit and smoothies), using the National Diet and Nutrition Survey Rolling Programme, years 1–8 (NDNS RP). The sample included 2587 adolescents aged 11–18 years. Four percent (112) of adolescents reported consuming 5% or lower NMES as a proportion of TE. The odds of being categorised as a low-sugar consumer in adolescents (≤5% TE from NMES) were significantly lower with higher intakes of sweetened drinks, fruit juice, cakes, biscuits, sugar and sweet spreads, chocolate confectionery and sugar confectionery, and significantly higher with higher intakes of pasta and rice, wholemeal and brown bread, and fish. Across the five categories of NMES intakes, micronutrient intakes were lowest for those consuming either ≤5% TE or more than 20% TE from NMES, and optimal for those consuming between 10–15% of energy from NMES. These findings confirm the difficulties of meeting the free sugars recommended intake for adolescents. Care needs to be taken to ensure that an adequate consumption of micronutrients is achieved in those adhering to the revised guidelines on free sugars.

Keywords: free sugars; added sugars; non-milk extrinsic sugars; diet quality; nutrient intake

1. Introduction

The prevalence of obesity is high in the UK [1,2]; nearly 25% of adults are obese and the risk of obesity in adulthood is much higher for those who are obese in childhood or adolescence [3]. The causal factors for obesity are complex and multi-factorial, but many are modifiable through individual and policy action to improve dietary and activity behaviour. As such, the World Health Organization (WHO) recommends that individuals reduce their intakes of fats and sugars and increase their consumption of fruits and vegetables to improve their health [2], which includes limiting the consumption of free sugars in foods and drinks.

There are several factors which suggest that a diet high in non-milk extrinsic sugars (NMES) could result in a poor-quality diet, including excess energy intake, low satiety, poor compensation in terms of energy intake, a less nutritious diet higher in nutrient-poor foods and lower in nutrient-rich foods. NMES are similar to free sugars [4] and was the definition used for recommending sugars intakes before

2015 in the UK. Ultimately, a diet rich in these sugars results in weight gain [5,6]. Based on further evidence from systematic reviews of dietary sugars and body weight [7], and on dental caries [2], the WHO and the Scientific Advisory Committee on Nutrition (SACN) revised the recommendations to restrict added and free sugars intake in 2015. The recommended % total energy (%TE) from free sugars was lowered from 10% TE [8] to 5% TE [9].

To date, no national studies have reported on diet patterns with different categories of NMES intake. Two studies assessed micronutrient adequacy by dietary sugar intake [10,11], but reported no firm basis to describe an optimal intake of added sugars with regard to micronutrient adequacy, given how divergent the reported relationships were between micronutrients and added sugar were across studies. Whilst most studies report either no association between added sugars intakes and dietary adequacy or some deterioration with high intakes, some also describe a curvilinear association with poorer micronutrient status at the lower extremes of added sugars intake [12]. This may be related to low overall food intakes in low-sugars consumers, which could be due to deliberate energy restriction for weight reduction, distorted reporting of all or specific foods, or avoidance of foods which are particularly rich sources of micronutrients.

Whilst it is clearly important to determine the impact of high consumption of free or added sugars, it is equally important to explore associations with micronutrient intakes in individuals adhering to the guidelines on added or free sugars, as significant deviations from the general UK dietary pattern might have been adopted [13]. Our study therefore aimed to examine the potential impact of adherence to the revised guidelines on the intakes of important key foods and nutrients in British adolescents. We quantified existing dietary intakes of major food groups and nutrients in participants of the National Diet and Nutrition Survey Rolling Programme years 1–8, categorised by percentage of energy from NMES.

2. Materials and Methods

2.1. The National Diet and Nutrition Survey Rolling Programme

In the UK, the National Diet and Nutrition Survey Rolling Programme (NDNS RP) provides an authoritative source of information on the nutritional status of the UK population, providing descriptors of food and nutrient intakes, biomarkers of nutritional status and anthropometric indices of over, and underweight. This survey is funded by the Public Health arm of the Department of Health for England (Public Health England) as a means of monitoring diet and nutrient trends and the adequacy of the UK diet. Fieldwork was carried out between 2008 and 2016 to collect dietary and lifestyle information from approximately 1000 participants every year from private households, providing sufficient statistical power to observe differences between dietary intake groups. Further details of the survey and sampling methods were reported elsewhere [14]. Data files from years 1–8 of the NDNS Rolling Programme (2008–2016) were obtained under licence from the UK Data Service.

2.2. Dietary Information

Dietary information was collected using a four-day food diary. The participants were required to complete the diary by reporting portions of food and drink consumed, using household measures over four consecutive days assigned randomly by the interviewer's computer-assisted personal interview (CAPI), beginning on any day of the week. For children aged 11 years, a parent/carer was asked to complete the four-day diary with help from the child as appropriate. Photographs of food portions were included in the diary to aid portion size descriptions and younger children (<16 years) were provided with an age-appropriate version of the Young Person's Food Photograph Atlas [14]. Consumption was expressed as grams per day (g/day). Data on food group consumption and total nutrient intakes averaged over 4 days (and in some cases 3 days) were provided for each adolescent participant.

2.3. Characteristics

Participant characteristics were collected using a CAPI programme and self-completion questionnaires during the interviewer visit in the first stage of the survey. Classification of socio-economic status was undertaken based on occupation, according to the UK National Statistics-Socio-Economic Classification (NS-SEC). Participants were initially divided into eight NS-SEC categories and reclassified into three categories: (1) managerial/professional, (2) intermediate, and (3) routine/manual, in addition to 'unemployed/don't know' or 'missing'. Height and weight were measured, and the mean of three valid measurements were recorded, from which BMI (kg/m^2) was derived. Waist circumference (cm) and waist-to-hip ratio measurements were taken during a consented nurse visit during the second stage of the survey. Waist and hip circumference (cm) was measured, and the mean of three valid measurements were recorded.

2.4. Statistical Analyses

Survey weights from the dataset were applied to account for bias in non-response and probability of selection by age, sex and Government Office Region relative to the total population in the UK, as addressed elsewhere [14–16].

The food groups (Supplementary Table S1) investigated here are similar to previous literature, and a full list can be found in the supplementary tables in the NDNS report [15]. In this study, we focused on foods high in sugar, as well as foods which provide alternative substantial energy from protein, fat, and carbohydrates. Sugar sweetened drinks included carbonated and cordial drinks but not pure fruit juice, milk-based drinks or tea and coffee. A number of different dietary sugar variables were derived from the food diary analysis. In line with the SACN recommendation, NMES as a percent of total energy was the variable used for this analysis (rather than percent of food energy). However, the proposed SACN guidelines refer to 'free sugars' which also include sugars in pure fruit juice and 50% of sugars in fruit purees that are not included in NMES; therefore NMES values are likely to be slightly lower than free sugars levels [13]. Participants were categorised by percentage (%) of total energy from NMES into 5 groups ($\leq$5%, >5–10%, >10–15%, >15–20%, >20%) with means reported. Wald tests were carried out to determine statistically significant differences in mean characteristics, such as anthropometric measures, between the NMES consumption categories. Chi-square tests were used to determine differences in categorical variables, such as smoking, between NMES consumption groups reported as percentages and 95% confident intervals (CI) in table 1.

Energy, food and nutrient intakes (excluding supplements) by the %NMES category were reported as means (g/day and mg/day or μg/day) and 99% confidence intervals (CI). Wald tests were carried out to determine statistically significant differences in intake between the % NMES categories. Patterns of food consumption were visualised using a radar chart. Logistic regression was undertaken to determine the odds (99% CI) of being classified as a low NMES consumer ($\leq$5% NMES) compared with any other NMES category with increasing food intake by typical portions (g/day). This was adjusted by age and gender. Sensitivity analyses excluded 6.5% of participants, who were dieting (n = 152). We also adjusted for those who reported dieting. When dieters were excluded, only 94 individuals remained in the lowest NMES group for the sensitivity analyses. The proportion of adolescents consuming less than the Lower Reference Nutrient Intake (LRNI) for vitamins A, C, B12, riboflavin, and folate, and the minerals iron, calcium, magnesium, potassium, zinc and iodine was reported as a % and 99% CI by category of %NMES consumption, and a graph of the % was produced. Stata version 14.1 was used for all statistical analyses and statistical significance was determined using $p \leq 0.01$ due to multiple testing.

The extent of under-reporting was explored using estimates of the basal metabolic rate derived from standard Harris–Benedict equations [17] multiplied by a very low physical activity level (PAL) of 1.2 [18]. This value was used to reflect an implausible level of energy intake reported from the 4-day survey diary. However, under-reporting using even this conservative approach was so pervasive and generated such high numbers of potential under-reporters that their exclusion would render the analysis unfeasible. Accordingly, no individuals were excluded on the basis of under-reporting.

2.5. Research Ethics

Ethical approval for the NDNS RP had already been obtained from the Oxfordshire A Research Ethics Committee. The letters of approval for the original submission and subsequent substantial amendments, together with the approved documents, were sent to all the Local Research Ethics Committees (LRECs) covering the areas where the fieldwork was conducted. No further approval was required.

3. Results

The analysis was carried out on 2587 adolescents aged 11 to 18 years. Their mean intake of NMES in grams was 72 g/day (95% CI 70 to 74), and as a percentage of total energy intake, this was 14.9% (95% CI 14.5 to 15.2). They were categorised by level of % total energy from NMES consumption, as described in the methods, and 4% ($n = 112$) of the sample consumed ≤5% NMES, and therefore met the recommended level of intake. This category consumed a mean of 13 g of NMES. The category with the highest number of participants (34%) consumed 10–15% of energy from NMES with an average daily intake of 60 g/day of NMES. The highest NMES consumption group, with intakes greater than 20% of total energy, included almost a fifth of the sample (18%), with an average daily intake of 122 g/day of NMES.

Few statistically significant differences in participant characteristics between the categories of NMES consumption were observed (see Table 1) but individuals from ethnic minorities were more likely to be in the lowest NMES consumption group. Although more females and obese individuals tended to be in this group, differences were not statistically significant. The proportion of adolescent participants within each NMES intake category with implausible recorded energy intakes was consistently high across all categories, but was markedly greater in the lowest NMES consumers at 79%, compared with 49% in the highest consumers.

Table 1. Characteristics of adolescents aged 11 to 18 years in the National Diet and Nutrition Survey Y1-8 by category of non-milk extrinsic sugar consumption as a percentage of total energy after the application of Y1-8 survey weights (n = 2587).

Variables *	N	TOTAL	Quantiles of Non-Milk Extrinsic Sugars Consumption (% of Total Energy/Day)					Wald/Chi² p-Value
			≤5	>5-10	>10-15	>15-20	>20	
No. of participants, n (%)	2587	-	112 (4%)	470 (17%)	795 (34%)	699 (27%)	511 (18%)	-
Age, years	2587	15 (14, 15)	15 (14, 15)	14 (14, 15)	15 (14, 15)	15 (14, 15)	15 (14, 15)	0.33
Female, %	2587	49 (46, 51)	55 (43, 67)	50 (44, 56)	51 (47, 55)	46 (41, 50)	47 (41, 52)	0.37
Body Mass Index, kg/m²	2493	22 (21, 22)	24 (23, 25)	22 (21, 22)	22 (21, 22)	22 (21, 22)	22 (21, 22)	0.29
Normal weight, %	1620	66 (63, 69)	51 (38, 64)	66 (59, 71)	64 (60, 69)	69 (64, 73)	69 (64, 75)	
Overweight, %	349	13 (12, 15)	15 (8, 26)	12 (9, 16)	14 (11, 17)	14 (11, 18)	12 (9, 17)	0.09
Obese, %	524	21 (18, 23)	34 (24, 47)	23 (18, 28)	22 (18, 26)	17 (14, 21)	18 (14, 23)	
Waist circumference, cm	1870	76 (75, 76)	81 (77, 85)	75 (74, 77)	76 (74, 77)	75 (74, 76)	75 (73, 77)	0.10
Waist-to-hip ratio	1869	0.81 (0.80, 0.81)	0.82 (0.80, 0.85)	0.81 (0.80, 0.82)	0.80 (0.80, 0.81)	0.81 (0.80, 0.81)	0.80 (0.79, 0.81)	0.42
Dieting	2586	7 (5, 8)	21 (13, 33)	7 (4, 10)	6 (4, 9)	7 (5, 10)	3 (2, 6)	<0.01
Achieving 5-a-day F & V	2587	8 (7, 10)	7 (3, 18)	10 (7, 15)	9 (7, 12)	8 (6, 11)	6 (4, 9)	0.33
Under-reporters †	2587	55 (52, 57)	79 (68, 88)	65 (59, 71)	54 (49, 58)	49 (44, 54)	49 (43, 54)	<0.01
Have longstanding illness	2587	16 (14, 18)	21 (12, 33)	15 (11, 21)	15 (12, 18)	19 (15, 23)	13 (9, 17)	0.18
Socio-economic status of parent								
Professional/Managerial, %	1032	42 (40, 45)	39 (27, 52)	44 (38, 50)	41 (36, 45)	45 (40, 50)	39 (34, 45)	
Intermediate, %	552	23 (21, 25)	19 (11, 30)	22 (17, 27)	24 (20, 28)	24 (20, 29)	23 (18, 28)	0.53
Routine/Manual, %	875	35 (32, 37)	42 (30, 55)	34 (29, 40)	35 (31, 40)	31 (26, 36)	38 (33, 44)	
Ethnic groups								
White, %	2309	83 (81, 85)	69 (54, 80)	79 (72, 84)	81 (77, 85)	88 (84, 92)	86 (80, 90)	<0.01
Non-white, %	276	17 (15, 19)	31 (20, 46)	21 (16, 28)	19 (15, 23)	12 (8, 16)	14 (10, 20)	
Total Energy (TE), kcal/day	2587	1761 (1734, 1788)	1390 (1258, 1523)	1593 (1542, 1644)	1778 (1735, 1821)	1830 (1777, 1884)	1872 (1800, 1944)	<0.01
Non-milk extrinsic sugars (NMES)	2587	72 (70, 74)	13 (12, 15)	34 (33, 35)	60 (58, 62)	85 (82, 88)	122 (116, 127)	<0.01
NMES, % of TE	2587	14.9 (14.5, 15.2)	3.5 (3.2, 3.8)	8.0 (7.8, 8.2)	12.6 (12.5, 12.8)	17.4 (17.2, 17.5)	24.5 (24.0, 25.1)	<0.01

* Variables expressed as mean (95% CI) for continuous variables, percentage (95% CI) for categorical variables, unless otherwise stated. † % with EI:BMR < 1.2, BMR calculated using Harris-Benedict equations.

3.1. Foods

Differences in mean intake (g/day) of selected foods by category of sugars consumption (% energy) are displayed in Table 2. There was a general trend across the categories for pasta and rice, wholemeal bread and high fibre breakfast cereals to be eaten in larger quantities in the lower NMES categories. Conversely, consumption of biscuits, cakes, and ice-cream was higher with each increase in the NMES category; however, no significant difference was observed for pudding intake. Confectionery, sugars and sweet spreads increased with increasing added sugars across the categories. Sweetened soft drinks, fruit juices and beer consistently increased over all the NMES categories, but low-calorie drinks did not show a clear trend across the categories. Non-low-calorie soft drinks consumption was particularly high in the highest NMES category, with a daily mean intake of about 500mls in the highest category compared with 12 mL in the lowest. The highest intakes of cheese, yogurt and other dairy desserts were found in the middle groups of NMES intake. The intake of savoury snacks, such as crisps, increased over increasing sugars categories. The intake of disaggregated total fish and vegetables generally decreased across increasing sugars categories.

Table 2. Food group intakes (g/day) of adolescents aged 11 to 18 years in the National Diet and Nutrition Survey Y1-8 by category of non-milk extrinsic sugar (NMES) consumption as a percentage of total energy after the application of Y1-8 survey weights, expressed as mean (99% CI).

Variables	Total	Consumers n (%)	Quantiles of Non-Milk Extrinsic Sugars Consumption (% of Total Energy/Day)				
			≤5	>5-10	>10-15	>15-20	>20
No. of participants, n (%)	2587 (100%)		112 (4%)	470 (17%)	795 (34%)	699 (27%)	511 (18%)
Food Groups							
Carbohydrate rich foods							
Pasta, rice and other cereals ***	104 (98, 110)	2265 (90%)	130 (93, 167)	119 (103, 135)	107 (96, 117)	99 (87, 110)	88 (75, 101)
White bread	56 (53, 59)	2274 (87%)	44 (29, 58)	58 (50, 65)	56 (50, 62)	60 (54, 66)	52 (45, 58)
Wholemeal, brown, granary, wheatgerm bread ***	21 (19, 23)	1153 (46%)	34 (19,49)	26 (19, 33)	25 (20, 29)	16 (13, 20)	14 (10, 18)
High fibre breakfast cereals **	13 (12, 15)	963 (37%)	20 (7, 34)	14 (9, 19)	16 (12, 19)	12 (9, 15)	9 (6, 12)
Other breakfast cereals	10 (9, 11)	1146 (46%)	8 (3, 12)	10 (7, 12)	10 (8, 12)	11 (9, 13)	11 (8, 14)
Biscuits ***	17 (16, 19)	1697 (67%)	7 (4, 11)	15 (12, 18)	17 (15, 20)	19 (17, 22)	20 (14, 26)
Buns, cakes, pastries and fruit pies ***	20 (18, 22)	1352 (53%)	3 (1, 4)	12 (9, 14)	21 (17, 23)	23 (19, 27)	25 (19, 31)
Puddings	11 (9, 13)	579 (24%)	7 (1, 12)	8 (4, 12)	11 (8, 14)	12 (9, 15)	11 (7, 16)
Dairy products							
Milk	132 (122, 142)	2137 (81%)	147 (57, 237)	141 (114, 167)	138 (120, 155)	131 (111, 151)	112 (92, 132)
Cheese ***	11 (10, 12)	1486 (60%)	8 (5, 12)	13 (10, 15)	13 (11, 14)	10 (8, 12)	8 (6, 10)
Yogurt, fromage frais and other dairy desserts **	20 (18, 22)	933 (37%)	10 (3, 17)	19 (14, 25)	22 (17, 27)	22 (18, 26)	17 (13, 22)
Ice cream ***	9 (7, 10)	698 (26%)	2 (−1, 5)	5 (3, 7)	9 (6, 12)	10 (8, 13)	11 (8, 14)
Egg and egg dishes	12 (11, 15)	896 (36%)	21 (6, 37)	14 (10, 18)	14 (10, 17)	10 (8, 13)	12 (8, 15)
Total fat spreads	8 (7, 8)	2103 (80%)	9 (6, 11)	8 (7, 9)	8 (7, 9)	8 (7, 9)	7 (5, 8)
Potato and potato products							
Chips, fried roast potatoes and potato dishes	50 (47, 53)	2022 (78%)	42 (22, 61)	43 (36, 50)	53 (47, 59)	52 (47, 57)	51 (44, 59)
Other potatoes, potato salads and dishes	31 (28, 34)	1474 (54%)	34 (17, 52)	32 (25, 38)	34 (29, 39)	31 (26, 35)	25 (20, 30)
Crisps and savoury snacks **	13 (12, 13)	1775 (69%)	10 (4, 15)	11 (9, 13)	12 (10, 13)	14 (12, 16)	13 (11, 16)
Sugar, preserves and confectionery							
Sugars, preservatives and sweet spreads ***	7 (6, 7)	1553 (61%)	2 (0, 3)	4 (3, 5)	6 (5, 8)	8 (7, 10)	9 (7, 11)
Sugar confectionery ***	7 (6, 8)	848 (33%)	1 (0, 1)	2 (1, 3)	4 (3, 5)	8 (6, 10)	15 (12, 19)
Chocolate confectionery ***	12 (11, 13)	1498 (56%)	3 (1, 4)	6 (5, 8)	10 (9, 12)	15 (12, 17)	18 (14, 21)
Beverages							
Fruit juice ***	78 (69, 87)	1218 (49%)	7 (1, 13)	31 (23, 39)	68 (57, 80)	99 (82, 117)	125 (91, 160)
Soft drinks, not low calorie ***	230 (213, 247)	1957 (75%)	12 (2, 21)	65 (52, 78)	164 (143, 185)	280 (251, 308)	484 (432, 535)
Soft drinks, low calorie **	184 (165, 202)	1454 (54%)	183 (71, 294)	225 (179, 271)	199 (162, 237)	160 (131, 189)	151 (114, 189)
Beer, lager, cider and perry ***	31 (19, 42)	2408 (93%)	4 (−3, 11)	16 (−1, 34)	30 (13, 47)	29 (10, 49)	52 (18, 98)
Disaggregated Food Groups †							
Total Fruit	59 (54, 63)	2169 (83%)	53 (30, 75)	69 (54, 83)	61 (53, 69)	55 (47, 63)	51 (40, 62)
Total vegetables ***	112 (107, 117)	2570 (95%)	115 (92, 138)	119 (107, 138)	121 (113, 130)	110 (101, 119)	89 (80, 98)
Total meat	97 (93, 101)	2500 (96%)	99 (72, 125)	97 (87, 106)	99 (92, 106)	98 (91, 105)	91 (83, 99)
Total fish ***	12 (11, 14)	1214 (50%)	18 (10, 25)	16 (10, 22)	12 (10, 15)	11 (9, 13)	8 (6, 11)

*** = $p < 0.001$, ** = $p < 0.01$, significant difference across NMES groups using wald test. † Disaggregated food groups include estimated portions of foods that are in composite dishes in order to provide a more complete estimate of intake at the individual food level.

Differences by category of NMES for the selected drinks and foods are also displayed in radial graphs for ease of interpretation (Figures 1 and 2, respectively). Participants in the higher categories of NMES consumption had high intakes of full-sugar soft drinks, which was highest in the highest NMES category and lowest in the lowest NMES category. The remaining drinks such as milk, fruit juice and low-calorie soft drinks varied little by NMES category. The participants in the higher NMES categories had particularly high intakes of biscuits, cakes and both sugar and chocolate confectionery. There was less variation between the categories of NMES for puddings, yogurt and other dairy desserts, breakfast cereals, ice-cream and sugars and sweet spreads. Mean intakes by weight were highest for cakes, chocolate confectionery, and yogurts.

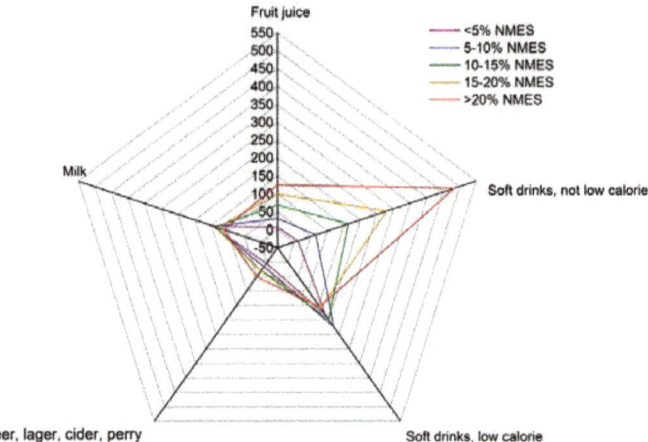

Figure 1. Consumption of alcoholic and non-alcoholic beverages (g/day) by adolescents in the National Diet and Nutrition Survey aged 11 to 18 years, by category of non-extrinsic milk sugar after the application of survey weights.

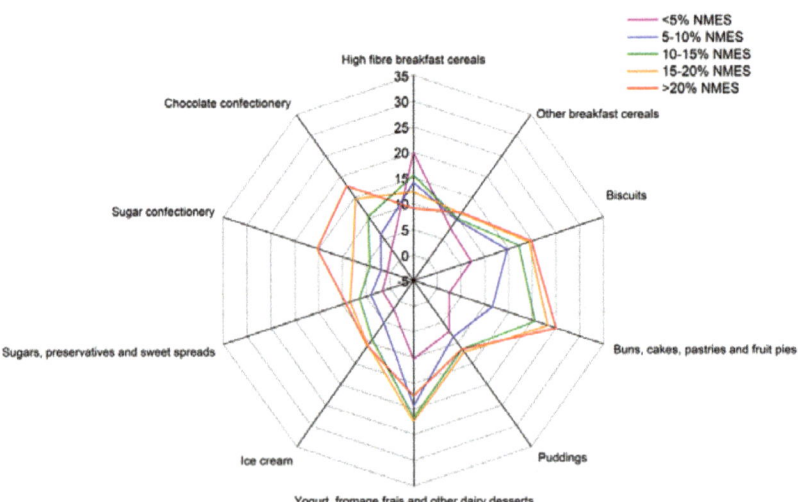

Figure 2. Consumption of sweet foods (g/day) from adolescents aged 11 to 18 years in the National Diet and Nutrition Survey, by category of non-extrinsic milk sugar after the application of survey weights.

The odds of being categorised as a low-sugars consumer (≤5% NMES) varied by food type. The age- and gender-adjusted results are provided in Figure 3. The odds of an adolescent being categorised as a low-sugars consumer compared with any of the other NMES categories were significantly lower with greater consumption of biscuits, cakes, sugar and sweet spreads, confectionery, fruit juice and full-sugar soft drinks. The odds of being categorised as a low-sugars consumer were significantly higher with higher intakes of wholemeal and brown bread. Similar findings were reported when dieters were excluded or adjusted for, although on exclusion of dieters, the odds were also significantly lower in relation to greater consumption of ice-cream and significantly higher with greater consumption of eggs, but not significant for wholemeal bread (see Supplementary Table S2).

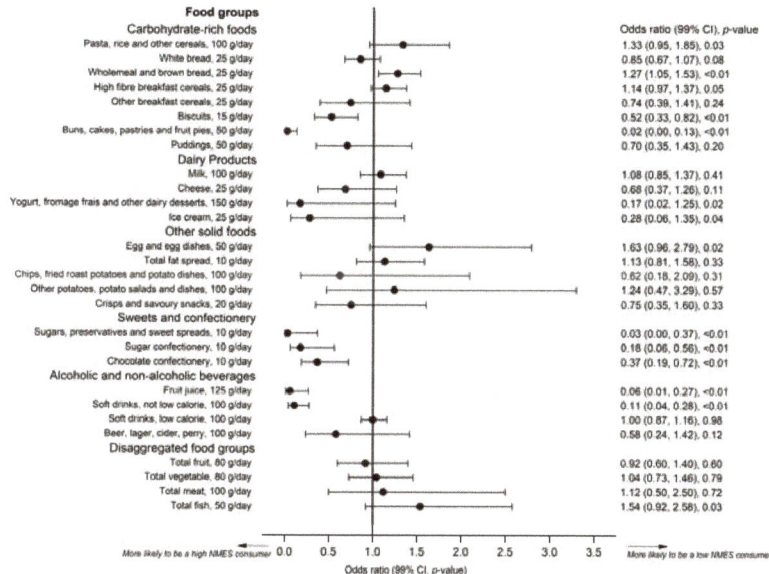

Figure 3. The odds (99% CI, p-value) of adolescents aged 11 to 18 years being categorised as consuming <10% NMES of total energy with increasing consumption of various foods by portion (g/day) in the National Diet and Nutrition Survey.

3.2. Nutrients

Energy and nutrient intakes by category of percentage of energy from NMES are reported in Table 3. Energy intakes (both food-derived and total) were consistently lowest in participants reporting the smallest intakes of NMES, increasing with increasing NMES intake. Protein and dietary fibre were lowest in the highest NMES group, and fibre was consistently low across all the NMES intake categories. Intakes of energy from total fat and total carbohydrate were reciprocally associated with higher carbohydrate and lower fat intakes in the highest NMES consumers. Intakes of alcohol were low, as might be expected, but were equivalent to about 2 units per week on average in the highest NMES consumers.

Table 3. Daily mean (99% CI) nutrient intakes of adolescents aged 11 to 18 years in the National Diet and Nutrition Survey Y1-8 by percentage of non-milk extrinsic sugars consumption of total energy (n = 2587) after the application of survey weights.

Variables	Total	Quantiles of Non-Milk Extrinsic Sugars Consumption (% of Total Energy/Day)					p-Value
		≤5	>5–10	>10–15	>15–20	>20	
No. of participants, n	2587 (100%)	112 (4%)	470 (17%)	795 (34%)	699 (27%)	511 (18%)	
Macronutrients							
Total Energy (TE), kcal/day	1761 (1726, 1797)	1390 (1216, 1565)	1593 (1526, 1661)	1778 (1721, 1835)	1830 (1760, 1901)	1872 (1777, 1967)	<0.01
Food Energy (FE), kcal/day	1750 (1714, 1785)	1389 (1215, 1563)	1585 (1519, 1652)	1765 (1709, 1822)	1820 (1750, 1890)	1855 (1761, 1949)	<0.01
Total Energy (TE), kJ/day	7417 (7268, 7569)	5854 (5120, 6588)	6707 (6425, 6988)	7485 (7247, 7723)	7708 (7412, 8002)	7890 (7490, 8290)	<0.01
Food Energy (FE), kJ/day	7369 (7221, 7516)	5847 (5114, 6581)	6672 (6393, 6950)	7432 (7195, 7668)	7664 (7370, 7958)	7821 (7426, 8216)	<0.01
Protein (g)	66 (64, 67)	66 (54, 78)	68 (64, 71)	68 (66, 71)	65 (63, 68)	60 (57, 63)	<0.01
Fat, % of TE	34 (33, 34)	35 (33, 37)	35 (34, 36)	35 (34, 35)	33 (33, 34)	31 (30, 32)	<0.01
CHO, % of TE	51 (50, 51)	46 (44, 48)	48 (47, 48)	49 (49, 50)	52 (51, 52)	56 (55, 56)	<0.01
Total sugars	101 (98, 104)	38 (32, 45)	64 (61, 68)	91 (87, 94)	114 (111, 119)	149 (140, 156)	<0.01
Total sugars, % of TE	21 (21, 22)	10 (9, 12)	15 (15 16)	19 (19, 20)	24 (23, 24)	30 (29, 31)	<0.01
Non-milk extrinsic sugars (NMES)	72 (69, 74)	13 (11, 15)	34 (32, 35)	60 (58, 62)	85 (81, 88)	122 (115, 128)	<0.01
NMES, % of TE	15 (15, 15)	4 (3, 4)	8 (8, 8)	13 (12, 13)	17 (17, 18)	25 (24, 25)	<0.01
AOAC fibre (g)	16 (15, 16)	15 (13, 17)	16 (15, 17)	17 (16, 17)	16 (15, 16)	14 (13, 15)	<0.01
Non-starch polysaccharides (NSP) (g)	12 (12, 12)	11 (10, 13)	12 (11, 13)	12 (12, 13)	12 (11, 12)	10 (9, 11)	<0.01
Alcohol (g)	1.7 (1.2, 2.1)	0.2 (−0.1, 0.5)	1.2 (0.2, 2.0)	1.8 (0.8, 2.8)	1.5 (0.7, 2.2)	2.4 (0.8, 3.9)	<0.01
Micronutrients							
Vitamin A, μg/day	624 (590, 680)	495 (376, 614)	653 (548, 759)	634 (588, 682)	624 (557, 690)	610 (537, 683)	0.07
Thiamin, mg/day	1.4 (1.4, 1.4)	1.3 (1.1, 1.5)	1.4 (1.3, 1.4)	1.5 (1.4, 1.5)	1.4 (1.4, 1.5)	1.3 (1.3, 1.4)	0.01
Riboflavin, mg/day	1.4 (1.4, 1.5)	1.3 (0.9, 1.6)	1.4 (1.3, 1.5)	1.5 (1.4, 1.5)	1.4 (1.4, 1.5)	1.4 (1.3, 1.5)	0.30
Niacin equivalents, mg/day	32 (31, 33)	31 (26, 36)	32 (30, 34)	33 (32, 34)	32 (30, 33)	31 (29, 33)	0.40
Vitamin B6, mg/day	1.9 (1.8, 1.9)	1.6 (1.3, 1.9)	1.7 (1.6, 1.9)	1.8 (1.7, 1.9)	1.9 (1.8, 2.0)	2.1 (1.8, 2.4)	<0.01
Vitamin B12, μg/day	4.2 (4.0, 4.4)	4.0 (3.0, 5.0)	4.4 (4.0, 4.7)	4.3 (4.0, 4.6)	4.1 (3.8, 4.4)	4.1 (3.7, 4.5)	0.37
Folate, μg/day	205 (200, 211)	181 (153, 209)	201 (186, 216)	214 (196, 220)	208 (197, 220)	194 (181, 206)	<0.01
Vitamin C, mg/day	80 (76, 83)	51 (40, 63)	61 (55, 68)	78 (72, 84)	84 (78, 90)	99 (88, 111)	<0.01
Vitamin D, μg/day	2.2 (2.1, 2.3)	2.1 (1.7, 2.5)	2.2 (2.1, 2.4)	2.3 (2.1, 2.5)	2.1 (2.0, 2.2)	1.9 (1.7, 2.2)	<0.01
Vitamin E, mg/day	8.8 (8.5, 9.1)	7.7 (6.8, 8.5)	8.5 (8.0, 9.0)	9.3 (8.8, 9.7)	8.9 (8.5, 9.3)	8.3 (7.7, 8.9)	<0.01
Iron, mg/day	9.5 (9.3, 9.7)	8.3 (6.9, 9.6)	9.3 (8.9, 9.7)	9.9 (9.5, 10.2)	9.6 (9.2, 10.0)	9.0 (8.4, 9.5)	<0.01
Calcium, mg/day	782 (758, 805)	664 (525, 804)	774 (722, 826)	812 (772, 853)	788 (746, 830)	750 (693, 808)	0.03
Magnesium, mg/day	210 (205, 214)	189 (162, 216)	207 (195, 219)	217 (209, 225)	211 (203, 219)	201 (190, 211)	<0.01
Potassium, mg/day	2305 (2255, 2355)	2024 (1710, 2339)	2211 (2098, 2324)	2391 (2300, 2484)	2355 (2265, 2445)	2224 (2105, 2344)	<0.01
Zinc, mg/day	7.3 (7.2, 7.5)	7.2 (6.0, 8.3)	7.7 (7.2, 8.2)	7.7 (7.4, 8.0)	7.2 (6.9, 7.5)	6.6 (6.2, 7.0)	<0.01
Iodine, mg/day	124 (119, 129)	105 (80, 130)	128 (115, 140)	130 (119, 141)	122 (114, 130)	118 (108, 129)	0.07
Sodium, mg/day	2114 (2063, 2164)	1898 (1631, 2165)	2052 (1944, 2161)	2185 (2096, 2274)	2150 (2049, 2250)	2038 (1908, 2168)	0.01

TE = total energy, FE= Food energy, AOAC = Association of Official Analytical Chemists.

In terms of water-soluble vitamins, intakes of riboflavin, niacin equivalents and B12 tended not to vary greatly by NMES intake category. However, the highest folate, zinc, magnesium, calcium, iron, vitamin E, Vitamin D, iodine, potassium and sodium intakes were consumed in the middle NMES consumer group (>10–15%), whilst vitamin C intakes increased with increasing NMES consumption. All micronutrient intakes were lower in the lowest NMES intake group (meeting recommended NMES levels) compared with those in the intermediate categories (5–10% and 10–15% of energy categories). The results were similar, albeit slightly attenuated when dieters were excluded (see Table S3 and Figure S1).

Table 4 shows the percentage of adolescents consuming less that the LRNI (very low micronutrient consumers who are likely to be deficient if usual intake is below this level) for micronutrients by category of percentage energy from NMES. Generally, for the nutrients of concern, there was evidence of a U-shaped relationship between the percentage of energy from NMES and the proportion of each category reporting less than the LRNI for vitamins A, riboflavin and folate and also for the minerals calcium iron, magnesium, potassium, zinc and iodine (see Figure 4). Those consuming between 10–15% of energy from NMES had the smallest proportion of individuals consuming below the LRNI for most micronutrients. The lowest and highest NMES consumer categories had the greatest percentage of individuals consuming less than the LRNI. For example, 44% in the lowest NMES intake category, and 33% in the highest category did not consume more than the LRNI for iron, compared with 25% to 30% of participants in the middle NMES categories. 20% or more of participants with the lowest NMES intakes reported consuming less than the LRNI for vitamin A, riboflavin, iron, calcium, magnesium, potassium, zinc and iodine.

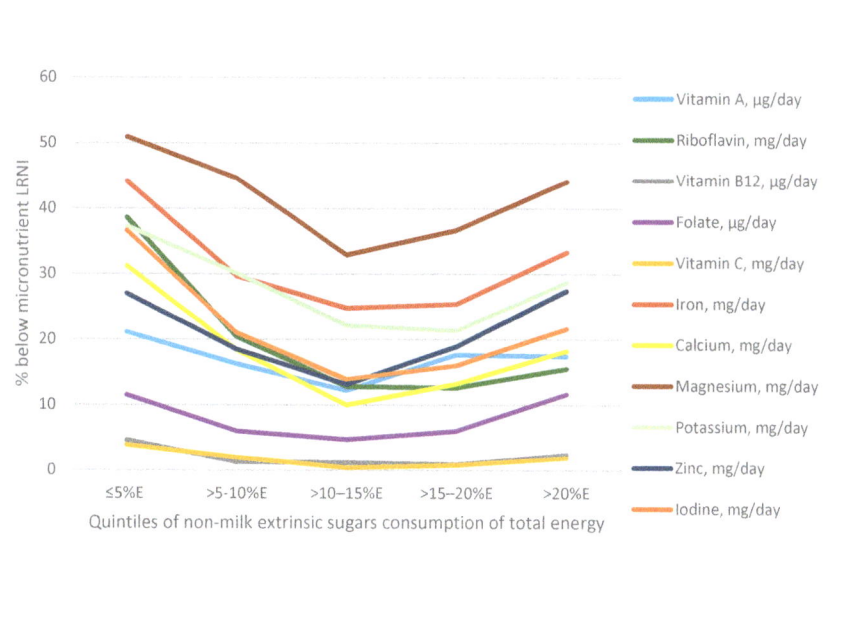

Figure 4. Percentage of adolescents aged 11 to 18 years in the National Diet and Nutrition Survey with micronutrient intakes below LRNI by percentage of non-milk extrinsic sugars consumption of total energy ($n = 2587$) after the application of survey weights.

Table 4. Proportion of adolescents aged 11 to 18 years in the National Diet and Nutrition Survey with micronutrient intakes below LRNI by percentage of non-milk extrinsic sugars consumption of total energy (n = 2587) after the application of survey weights, expressed as percentage (99% CI).

Variables	Total	Quantiles of Non-Milk Extrinsic Sugars Consumption (% of Total Energy/Day)					p-Value
		≤5	>5–10	>10–15	>15–20	>20	
No. of participants, n	2587 (100%)	112 (4%)	470 (17%)	795 (34%)	699 (27%)	511 (18%)	
Micronutrients							
Vitamin A, µg/day	16 (13, 18)	21 (12, 35)	16 (11, 24)	12 (9, 17)	18 (13, 23)	17 (12, 25)	0.09
Riboflavin, mg/day	16 (13, 18)	39 (23, 56)	20 (15, 27)	13 (9, 17)	13 (9, 17)	16 (11, 22)	<0.01
Vitamin B12, µg/day	2 (1, 3)	5 (2, 13)	1 (1, 3)	1 (0, 4)	1 (0, 3)	2 (1, 6)	0.31
Folate, µg/day	7 (5, 9)	12 (5, 26)	6 (3, 11)	5 (3, 8)	6 (4, 10)	12 (7, 18)	0.03
Vitamin C, mg/day	1 (1, 2)	4 (1, 19)	2 (1, 6)	0 (0, 2)	1 (0, 5)	2 (1, 5)	0.11
Iron, mg/day	28 (25, 31)	44 (29, 61)	30 (23, 37)	25 (20, 30)	25 (20, 31)	33 (26, 41)	0.01
Calcium, mg/day	15 (13, 17)	31 (18, 49)	18 (13, 25)	10 (7, 14)	13 (10, 18)	18 (13, 25)	<0.01
Magnesium, mg/day	39 (36, 42)	51 (35, 67)	45 (37, 52)	33 (28, 38)	37 (31, 43)	44 (37, 52)	<0.01
Potassium, mg/day	25 (22, 28)	37 (23, 55)	30 (23, 38)	22 (17, 27)	21 (17, 27)	29 (22, 36)	0.01
Zinc, mg/day	19 (16, 21)	27 (15, 44)	19 (13, 26)	13 (10, 17)	19 (14, 25)	27 (21, 35)	<0.01
Iodine, mg/day	18 (16, 21)	37 (22, 54)	21 (15, 28)	14 (10, 18)	16 (12, 21)	22 (16, 28)	<0.01

4. Discussion

The intakes of NMES in UK adolescents within this nationally representative UK survey were 14.9%TE (75 g/day), with only 4% meeting the current UK or WHO [2] recommendations currently set at ≤5%TE. Twenty-one percent consumed less than 10%TE from NMES, and were therefore adherent to the previous UK recommendations set by the Department of Health in 1991 [8]. The low-sugars consumers consumed less sugar sweetened drinks, fruit juice, biscuits, cakes, sugar and sweet spreads, confectionery, yoghurts and ice-cream. Furthermore, low-sugars consumers ate more vegetables, pasta and rice, wholemeal and brown bread, and fish. In terms of nutrients, the NMES intake category with the lowest proportion of adolescents that were deficient (intakes below LRNI) was the 10–15% NMES category.

Our findings for average NMES intake among adolescents are similar to the NHANES (National Health and Nutrition Examination Survey) in the US (both surveys report approximately 14%TE for all age groups) [19]. Adolescents who meet the ≤5% energy from NMES recommendation were similar in numbers to those observed in other European countries, and consistent with observations elsewhere of higher consumption levels in adolescents than in adults [20]. In a recent analysis of the Dutch National Food Consumption Survey 2007–2010 [21], adherence to the ≤ 5% recommendation was even lower, at < 1% of the sample, suggesting that an NMES intake ≤5% TE might be too low to achieve within the general UK population and other countries. Interestingly, adolescents who consume 10–15% NMES were the least likely to be deficient in many micronutrients, and thus, arguably, consumed the most nutritionally balanced diets. It is likely that adolescents with extremely low NMES intakes are consuming diets atypical to the general population due to restrictions in intake, including dieting, as they also had much lower energy intakes than the remaining categories. As such, substantial changes in dietary patterns are needed to adhere to the new recommendations, not simply removing high-sugar foods from the diet.

Given this potential major shift in nutritional intake for the majority of the UK population, in order to achieve compliance, it is therefore important to have confidence that there is no evidence of detriment in terms of dietary micronutrient adequacy. However, our findings suggest a U-shaped relationship between odds of micronutrient inadequacy and NMES intake by %TE for several micronutrients, where adolescents with the lowest %TE from NMES appeared to have the highest likelihood of micronutrient inadequacy. This is broadly consistent with a systematic review of 30 cross-sectional and prospective studies investigating associations between added sugar and nutrient intakes, where 21 found a negative association between added sugar and micronutrient intakes [22]. Our finding that micronutrient inadequacy increased with higher NMES consumption was consistent with the systematic review. However, it is unclear whether the observed effects from the systematic review are clinically meaningful, as the differences were reported to be small to moderate. None of the previous studies in the review reported a positive association with lower diet quality at lower sugar intakes, as we saw here. This may be because none of the studies in the review specifically compared categories of sugars at 5% or below with higher intake categories; 10% of sugars intake or below was the lowest category reported by any of the included studies. No mention was made of excluding dieters in the review but dieters or participants restricting their diet in other ways could be dominating this low-sugars group. However, we did not see any major differences in dietary patterns or nutrient adequacy in the low-sugars consumers when dieters were excluded.

Among food categories, drinks consumption, especially high-calorie soft drinks, is perhaps the strongest driver of added sugars intake, followed by confectionery, cakes and biscuits. These food groups were strongly associated with the odds of a 10-fold increase in NMES intake (13 g vs. 122 g) between the lowest and highest sugars consumers. This is consistent with earlier findings by a repeated cross-sectional study of 1991 English school children aged 11–12 years that reported substantial increases in the percentage of added sugars from drinks and breakfast cereals since 1980 [23], and that sugar sweetened drinks are the highest source of added sugars in most age groups [14]. In contrast, we did not find significantly higher intakes of breakfast cereals, either whole-fibre or other cereals in high-sugars consumers in comparison to the repeated cross-sectional English study [23], perhaps because sugars from breakfast cereals contribute a relatively small amount to the overall intake of NMES despite increased breakfast cereal consumption in the last two decades.

We also found a clear relationship between %TE from NMES and total energy intakes, with participants in the highest NMES intake category reporting intakes that provided 35% more energy than the lowest consumers. This supports contentions that higher intakes of added sugars drive up energy intake [9]. However, the reported differences may be overestimated since the lowest NMES consumption group may largely have be under-reporting, and also contained a higher proportion of individuals who were 'dieting' compared with other NMES categories. In terms of nutrient quality, a minimum amount of energy and foods may be necessary to reduce risk of deficiency.

Intakes in foods low in sugar, such as vegetables, wholemeal bread, pasta, rice, high-fibre breakfast cereal and fish, were higher in the lower-sugars consumers. Whilst it is clearly feasible to reduce NMES consumption to 5% of energy or less and still adhere to other dietary guidelines [24], it is clear that dietary choices between high and low NMES consumers are notably different, and this would involve a substantial shift in current eating habits. Changes may include consuming more protein-rich foods with fresh vegetables and high-fibre carbohydrates, including more plant foods such as beans and pulses [25], which may mean less snacking and more cooking with concomitant time and cost implications. However, in practical terms, these changes are highly challenging, and we do not have the evidence that the general public are able to do this without individual assistance.

The British Nutrition Foundation published a seven-day meal plan with suggested meals and snacks that meet the recommendations for a range of nutrients, including NMES, but this is very different from a typical diet in the UK [13]. In order for the British population to meet the new recommendations for added sugars, significant reductions in the consumption of sugar sweetened drinks, including fruit juice, beer and cider, confectionery, cakes and biscuits, would be necessary. For example, sweetened drinks could ideally be replaced with water but could also be replaced with milk or unhealthier sweetened milk-based drinks such as flavoured milk. Additional replacements for foods with both high sugar and fat, such as confectionery, cakes and biscuits, with higher-fat content foods need to be considered and avoided.

The national survey NHANES in the US found that most of the added sugars are consumed through food bought in shops such as supermarkets rather than in restaurants, so improvements in the retail sector may potentially have more impact [19], but a holistic approach is needed to target the out-of-home sector as well as supermarkets and other retailers. Diet quality in NHANES is also reduced with higher intakes of sweetened drinks and higher intakes of energy-dense foods [6]. Whether nutrient dilution effects of added sugars are counteracted by micronutrient fortification of foods is controversial.

An analysis of German children and adolescents suggested that food fortification improvements to nutrient density outweighed the nutrient dilution impact of added sugars [26]. However, food fortification alone is unlikely to adequately improve diet quality at very high sugar and energy intakes.

A previous cross-sectional analysis of NDNS data reported that large portion sizes of soft drinks, were associated with higher BMI in adolescents [27]. Certainly, the evidence on the associations between specific sources of added sugars and health are strongest for sugar sweetened drinks, with recent systematic reviews of trials or cohorts in adults reporting increased weight gain [28] and increased risk of type 2 diabetes [29,30] for higher intakes of sweetened drinks. The evidence from individual food sources of added sugars is scarce, with a lack of reviews on sugar-rich foods such as confectionery, cakes and biscuits. Epidemiological evidence on different sugar substrates, such as glucose and fructose, are also scarce. A systematic review of trials on the effect of total sugar consumption on weight gain reported that higher total added sugars consumption increased the risk of weight gain [7]. However, the impact of sugars from foods was not separated from the impact from drinks [7]. Furthermore, most included trials had a short duration. There may be biological reasons why sugars in drinks are more obesogenic than other sources of sugars in foods, related to lack of satiety in energy-containing drinks [31] and glycaemic factors [32]. One suggested biological pathway is de novo lipogenesis (DNL), whereby refined carbohydrates and sugars are converted to fatty acids endogenously in the liver. Rates of DNL and fatty acid production (which leads to obesity and NAFLD) were largely increased with increased consumption of carbohydrates and sugars in parallel with decreasing levels of fat [33]. Similar findings were reported in an RCT with adolescent boys with hepatic steatosis [34].

Policies to reduce added sugars intakes were introduced by Public Health England, including a levy on sweetened drinks, reducing portion sizes of energy-dense foods and drinks, reducing promotions and marketing and encouraging reformulation [35]. Sustained behaviour change is difficult, and any one policy is unlikely to have the level of impact on dietary behaviour needed to improve population health outcomes. Contentious policies can take many years to be implemented, as seen in US attempts to reduce the sizes of drinks sold in fast food restaurants [36]. Although reductions in preference for salty foods were reported within adults [37–39], there is less evidence for a reduction in the preferred sweetness levels following the adoption of 'low-sugar' diets [40], suggesting that dietary patterns incorporating sugars-sweetened foods may potentially be more resistant to change than those incorporating salty foods. Sugar reduction policies may also need to involve programmes to change cooking practices at home in order to reduce snack foods and increase meals containing pasta, rice, and vegetables and increase the availability of healthy meals and snacks in restaurants and fast food outlets. It is also necessary to be mindful of the other equally important recommendations made to increase dietary fibre intakes, moderate total and saturated fat intakes, and select foods providing adequate amounts of vitamins and minerals.

Strengths and Limitations

There were notable strengths and limitations in this analysis. The recommendations concerned free sugars but our current study investigated NMES, as there was limited data on free sugars from the NDNS when this study was designed. However, differences in these intakes are minor in the British diet, and many organisations, including Public Health England, have tended to present NMES and free sugars intakes interchangeably to date [41]. Information in the NDNS summary for years 7 to 8 reported that free sugars was between 15.9 and 14.1% TE for each pair of survey years, very similar to our mean NMES value of 14.9% TE [42]. Furthermore, different countries use different definitions and regions where the definition of added sugars does not include fruit juice report different results. However, our findings for foods and drinks other than fruit juice are likely to be similar. A limitation was that the NDNS data is prone to under-reporting, despite the best efforts to use data collection methods to reduce this, and is estimated to be in the region of 30% for food diaries of over 16 year-olds [14] using the Oxford and Goldberg equations. Furthermore, under-reporting may also be more common in certain groups of the population (i.e., female, or being overweight/obese) and for energy-dense foods and drinks [43,44], which had an impact on the validity of the results. We did not exclude under-reporters from the current analysis. The particularly high proportion of low-sugars consumers who reported 'dieting' (9%) and with implausible energy intakes suggests that this group of individuals may be dominated by individuals actively attempting to lose weight by dietary restriction, perhaps via elimination of sugar-rich foods and increased intake of protein-rich foods. Equally, it may be that this low-sugars group was dominated by individuals who were particularly poor food diary record-keepers, with both general and/or selective under-reporting of particularly sugary foods. These contributing factors made the interpretation of the results more difficult, as there were very few participants who were low-sugars consumers and reported valid energy intakes. However, reporting NMES as %TE may have negated some of the effects from under-reporters. Furthermore, the NDNS is comprised of repeated cross-sectional data. Although the NDNS is broadly representative of the dietary behaviour of the population, it is not possible to identify any causal factors. The results showing that lower sugar consumers tended to have a higher BMI were likely because these adolescents were more likely to be restricting their intakes due to excess weight. The strengths of the study were the robust methodology used to analyse the data and the use of logistic regression to generate odds ratios while adjusting for known confounders. A further strength was use of national data, which used validated dietary assessment methods.

5. Conclusions

The typical British adolescent diet is currently very different from the levels of free sugars recommended by the Department of Health. Low-sugars consumers have lower intakes of many sweet foods and drinks, including sugar sweetened drinks (not low calorie), fruit juice, confectionery, sugars and sweet spreads and cakes and biscuits. In addition, low-sugars consumers eat a healthier diet in terms of more vegetables and fish, and more low-fat starchy foods such as rice, pasta, and wholemeal bread. However, micronutrient intake was lower in this group than for adolescents consuming 10–15% free sugars. These findings are useful for public health nutrition policy makers in planning priorities for future action to improve the diet quality of adolescents.

Supplementary Materials: The following are available online at http://www.mdpi.com/2072-6643/11/7/1621/s1, Table S1: Categories of food group, respective portion sizes and foods included, Table S2: The age and gender-adjusted odds (99% confidence interval, *p*-value) of being a low NMES consumer (≤5% total energy) in all adolescents aged 11 to 18 years with increasing food intake by typical portions (g/day), and after excluding participants who reported being a diet or on a special diet (*n* = 152) in the NDNS with increasing consumption of various foods by portion (g/day), Table S3: Percentage (99% CI) of adolescents aged 11 to 18 years in the National Diet and Nutrition Survey with micronutrient intakes below LRNI by percentage of non-milk extrinsic sugars consumption of total energy excluding dieters (*n* = 2434) after the application of survey weights, Figure S1: Percentage of adolescents aged 11 to 18 years excluding dieters in the National Diet and Nutrition Survey with micronutrient intakes below LRNI by percentage of non-milk extrinsic sugars consumption of total energy (*n* = 2434) after the application of survey weights.

Author Contributions: C.E.L.E. planned the analysis. J.H. and H.T.L. undertook the statistical analysis. C.E.L.E. wrote the first drafts of the papers. All authors were involved in subsequent and final drafts.

Funding: V.B. and C.E.L.E. received funding from Sugar Nutrition UK who commissioned the study in 2015 to analyse NDNS years 1–4. Updated analysis from years 1–8 was funded by the University of Leeds.

Acknowledgments: We are indebted to the UK National Diet and Nutrition Survey for providing the data. We are grateful for the contributions made by Victoria Burley (V.B.), the principal investigator of the original research who was involved in planning the original analysis and writing the first draft.

Conflicts of Interest: The study was partly funded by Sugar Nutrition UK. Sugar Nutrition UK was not involved in the design or analysis of the study or the later versions of the manuscript with the analysis from years 1–8.

References

1. Public Health England. PHE Obesity. Available online: https://www.gov.uk/guidance/phe-data-and-analysis-tools#obesity-diet-and-physical-activity (accessed on 14 July 2019).
2. World Health Organization. *Guideline: Sugars Intake for Adults and Children, Obesity and Overweight: Fact Sheet No 311*; WHO: Geneva, Switzerland, 2015.
3. Simmonds, M.; Llewellyn, A.; Owen, C.G.; Woolacott, N. Predicting adult obesity from childhood obesity: A systematic review and meta-analysis. *Obes. Rev.* **2016**, *17*, 95–107. [CrossRef] [PubMed]
4. Swan, G.E.; Powell, N.A.; Knowles, B.L.; Bush, M.T.; Levy, L.B. A definition of free sugars for the UK. *Public Health Nutr.* **2018**, *21*, 1636–1638. [CrossRef] [PubMed]
5. Kant, A.K. Reported consumption of low-nutrient-density foods by American children and adolescents: Nutritional and health correlates, NHANES III, 1988 to 1994. *Arch. Pediatr. Adolesc. Med.* **2003**, *157*, 789–796. [CrossRef] [PubMed]
6. Kant, A.K. Consumption of energy-dense, nutrient-poor foods by adult Americans: Nutritional and health implications. The third National Health and Nutrition Examination Survey, 1988–1994. *Am. J. Clin. Nutr.* **2000**, *72*, 929–936. [CrossRef] [PubMed]
7. Te-Morenga, L.; Mallard, S.; Mann, J. Dietary sugars and body weight: Systematic review and meta-analyses of randomised controlled trials and cohort studies. *BMJ* **2013**, *346*. [CrossRef] [PubMed]
8. Department of Health. *Committee on Medical Aspects of Food Policy. Panel on Dietary Reference Values. Dietary Reference Values For Food Energy And Nutrients For the United Kingdom*; HMSO: London, UK, 1991; p. xxv.
9. Scientific Advisory Committee on Nutrition. *SACN Carbohydrates and Health Report*; TSO: London, UK, 2015.
10. Gibson, S.A. Dietary sugars intake and micronutrient adequacy: A systematic review of the evidence. *Nutr. Res. Rev.* **2007**, *20*, 121–131. [CrossRef]
11. Rennie, K.L.; Livingstone, M.B.E. Associations between dietary added sugar intake and micronutrient intake: A systematic review. *Br. J. Nutr.* **2007**, *97*, 832–841. [CrossRef]
12. Gibson, S.A. Do diets high in sugars compromise micronutrient intakes? Micronutrient intakes in the Dietary and Nutritional Survey of British Adults according to dietary concentration of 'added', 'non-milk extrinsic' or 'total' sugars. *J. Hum. Nutr. Diet.* **1997**, *10*, 125–133. [CrossRef]
13. British Nutrition Foundation. New Recommendations for Free Sugars and Fibre-the Scale of the Challenge. Available online: https://www.nutrition.org.uk/nutritioninthenews/headlines/newrecommendationsfibresugars.html (accessed on 14 July 2019).
14. National Diet and Nutrition Survey Results from Years 1, 2, 3 and 4 (combined) of the Rolling Programme (2008/2009–2011/2012). Available online: https://www.gov.uk/government/statistics/national-diet-and-nutrition-survey-results-from-years-1-to-4-combined-of-the-rolling-programme-for-2008-and-2009-to-2011-and-2012 (accessed on 14 July 2019).
15. Whitton, C.; Nicholson, S.K.; Roberts, C.; Prynne, C.J.; Pot, G.K.; Olson, A.; Fitt, E.; Cole, D.; Teucher, B.; Bates, B.; et al. National Diet and Nutrition Survey: UK food consumption and nutrient intakes from the first year of the rolling programme and comparisons with previous surveys. *Br. J. Nutr.* **2011**, *106*, 1899–1914. [CrossRef]
16. MRC Elsie Widdowson Laboratory. *MRC Elsie Widdowson Laboratory, National Diet and Nutrition Survey Years 1–8, 2008/09–2015/16. [Data Collection]*, 11th ed.; UK Data Service: London, UK, 2018.
17. Henry, C. Basal metabolic rate studies in humans: Measurement and development of new equations. *Public Health Nutr.* **2005**, *8*, 1133–1152. [CrossRef]
18. Goldberg, G.R.; Black, A.E.; Jebb, S.A.; Cole, T.J.; Murgatroyd, P.R.; Coward, W.A.; Prentice, A.M. Critical evaluation of energy intake data using fundamental principles of energy physiology: 1. Derivation of cut-off limits to identify under-recording. *Eur. J. Clin. Nutr.* **1991**, *45*, 569–581. [PubMed]
19. Drewnowski, A.; Rehm, C.D. Consumption of added sugars among US children and adults by food purchase location and food source. *Am. J. Clin. Nutr.* **2014**, *100*, 901–907. [CrossRef] [PubMed]
20. Newens, K.; Walton, J. A review of sugar consumption from nationally representative dietary surveys across the world. *J. Hum. Nutr. Diet.* **2015**, *29*, 225–240. [CrossRef] [PubMed]
21. Sluik, D.; van Lee, L.; Engelen, A.I.; Feskens, E.J.M. Total, Free, and Added Sugar Consumption and Adherence to Guidelines: The Dutch National Food Consumption Survey 2007–2010. *Nutrients* **2016**, *8*, 70. [CrossRef] [PubMed]

22. Louie, J.C.; Tapsell, L.C. Association between intake of total vs added sugar on diet quality: A systematic review. *Nutr. Rev.* **2015**, *73*, 837–857. [CrossRef]
23. Rugg-Gunn, A.J.; Fletcher, E.S.; Matthews, J.N.; Hackett, A.F.; Moynihan, P.J.; Kelly, S.; Adams, J.; Mathers, J.C.; Adamson, A. Changes in consumption of sugars by English adolescents over 20 years 1. *Public Health Nutr.* **2007**, *10*, 354–363. [CrossRef]
24. British Nutrition Foundation. Let's Take Another Look at Sugar. Available online: https://www.nutrition.org.uk/nutritioninthenews/headlines/letstakeanotherlookatsugar.html (accessed on 4 March 2015).
25. Public Health England. Eatwell Plate. Available online: https://assets.publishing.service.gov.uk/government/uploads/system/uploads/attachment_data/file/528193/Eatwell_guide_colour.pdf (accessed on 28 June 2019).
26. Alexy, U.; Sichert-Hellert, W.; Kersting, M. Fortification masks nutrient dilution due to added sugars in the diet of children and adolescents. *J. Nutr.* **2002**, *132*, 2785–2791. [CrossRef]
27. Albar, S.A.; Alwan, N.A.; Evans, C.E.; Cade, J.E. Is there an association between food portion size and BMI among British adolescents? *Br. J. Nutr.* **2014**, *112*, 841–851. [CrossRef]
28. Malik, V.S.; Pan, A.; Willett, W.C.; Hu, F.B. Sugar-sweetened beverages and weight gain in children and adults: A systematic review and meta-analysis. *Am. J. Clin. Nutr.* **2013**, *98*, 1084–1102. [CrossRef]
29. Greenwood, D.C.; Threapleton, D.E.; Evans, C.E.; Cleghorn, C.L.; Nykjaer, C.; Woodhead, C.; Burley, V.J. Association between sugar-sweetened and artificially sweetened soft drinks and type 2 diabetes: Systematic review and dose-response meta-analysis of prospective studies. *Br. J. Nutr.* **2014**, *112*, 725–734. [CrossRef]
30. Imamura, F.; O'Connor, L.; Ye, Z.; Mursu, J.; Hayashino, Y.; Bhupathiraju, S.N.; Forouhi, N.G. Consumption of sugar sweetened beverages, artificially sweetened beverages, and fruit juice and incidence of type 2 diabetes: Systematic review, meta-analysis, and estimation of population attributable fraction. *BMJ* **2015**, *351*, 3576. [CrossRef] [PubMed]
31. Maersk, M.; Belza, A.; Holst, J.J.; Fenger-Gron, M.; Pedersen, S.B.; Astrup, A.; Richelsen, B. Satiety scores and satiety hormone response after sucrose-sweetened soft drink compared with isocaloric semi-skimmed milk and with non-caloric soft drink: A controlled trial. *Eur. J. Clin. Nutr.* **2012**, *66*, 523–529. [CrossRef] [PubMed]
32. Schwingshackl, L.; Hoffmann, G. Long-term effects of low glycemic index/load vs. high glycemic index/load diets on parameters of obesity and obesity-associated risks: A systematic review and meta-analysis. *Nutr. Metab. Cardiovasc. Dis.* **2013**, *23*, 699–706. [CrossRef] [PubMed]
33. Volk, B.M.; Kunces, L.J.; Freidenreich, D.J.; Kupchak, B.R.; Saenz, C.; Artistizabal, J.C.; Fernandez, M.L.; Bruno, R.S.; Maresh, C.M.; Kraemer, W.J.; et al. Effects of step-wise increases in dietary carbohydrate on circulating saturated Fatty acids and palmitoleic Acid in adults with metabolic syndrome. *PLoS ONE* **2014**, *9*, 113605. [CrossRef]
34. Schwimmer, J.B.; Ugalde-Nicalo, P.; Welsh, J.A.; Angeles, J.E.; Cordero, M.; Harlow, K.E.; Alazraki, A.; Durelle, J.; Knight-Scott, J.; Newton, K.P.; et al. Effect of a Low Free Sugar Diet vs Usual Diet on Nonalcoholic Fatty Liver Disease in Adolescent Boys: A Randomized Clinical Trial. *JAMA* **2019**, *321*, 256–265. [CrossRef]
35. Public Health England. Sugar Reduction and Wider Reformulation. Available online: https://www.gov.uk/government/collections/sugar-reduction (accessed on 5 June 2019).
36. Wang, Y.C.; Vine, S.M. Caloric effect of a 16-ounce (473-mL) portion-size cap on sugar-sweetened beverages served in restaurants. *Am. J. Clin. Nutr.* **2013**, *98*, 430–435. [CrossRef]
37. Bertino, M.; Beauchamp, G.K.; Engelman, K. Long-term reduction in dietary sodium alters the taste of salt. *Am. J. Clin. Nutr.* **1982**, *36*, 1134–1144. [CrossRef]
38. Beauchamp, G.K.; Bertino, M.; Engelman, K. Modification of salt taste. *Ann. Intern. Med.* **1983**, *98*, 763–769. [CrossRef]
39. Mattes, R.D. The taste for salt in humans. *Am. J. Clin. Nutr.* **1997**, *65*, 692S–697S. [CrossRef]
40. Wise, P.M.; Nattress, L.; Flammer, L.J.; Beauchamp, G.K. Reduced dietary intake of simple sugars alters perceived sweet taste intensity but not perceived pleasantness. *Am. J. Clin. Nutr.* **2016**, *103*, 50–60. [CrossRef]
41. Public Health England. Sugar Reduction: The Evidence for Action. 2015 14 July. Available online: https://www.gov.uk/government/publications/sugar-reduction-from-evidence-into-action (accessed on 14 July 2019).
42. Public Health England. NDNS: Results from Years 7 and 8 (Combined). Available online: https://www.gov.uk/government/statistics/ndns-results-from-years-7-and-8-combined (accessed on 5 July 2019).

43. Macdiarmid, J.; Blundell, J. Assessing dietary intake: Who, what and why of under-reporting. *Nutr. Res. Rev.* **1998**, *11*, 231–253. [CrossRef] [PubMed]
44. Poppitt, S.D.; Swann, D.; Black, A.E.; Prentice, A.M. Assessment of selective under-reporting of food intake by both obese and non-obese women in a metabolic facility. *Int. J. Obes.* **1998**, *22*, 303–311. [CrossRef]

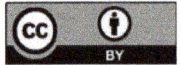

© 2019 by the authors. Licensee MDPI, Basel, Switzerland. This article is an open access article distributed under the terms and conditions of the Creative Commons Attribution (CC BY) license (http://creativecommons.org/licenses/by/4.0/).

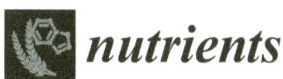

Article

Using Food Models to Enhance Sugar Literacy among Older Adolescents: Evaluation of a Brief Experiential Nutrition Education Intervention

María Isabel Santaló *, Sandra Gibbons and Patti-Jean Naylor *

School of Exercise Science, Physical and Health Education, Faculty of Education, University of Victoria, Victoria, BC V8P 5C2, Canada
* Correspondence: marisantalo@hotmail.com (M.I.S.); pjnaylor@uvic.ca (P.-J.N.); Tel.: +1-250-900-6725 (M.I.S.); +1-250-721-7844 (P.-J.N.)

Received: 28 June 2019; Accepted: 26 July 2019; Published: 31 July 2019

Abstract: Adolescent diets high in sugar are a public health concern. Sugar literacy interventions have changed intake but focused more on children, adults, and early adolescents and on sugar sweetened beverages rather than total sugar consumption. Food models are an efficacious experiential learning strategy with children. This study assessed the impact of two 45 min nutrition lessons using food models on adolescents' sugar literacy. Classes ($n = 16$) were randomized to intervention or control with knowledge, label reading skills, intentions to limit sugar consumption measured at baseline and follow-up. Two hundred and three students aged 14 to 19 from six schools on Vancouver Island, BC, Canada participated in the study. Adolescents' knowledge of added sugar in foods and beverages and servings per food group in a healthy diet was limited at baseline but improved significantly in the intervention condition ($F(1, 201) = 104.84$, $p < 0.001$) compared to controls. Intention to consume less added sugar increased significantly after intervention ($F(1, 201) = 4.93$, $p = 0.03$) as did label reading confidence ($F(1, 200) = 14.94$, $p < 0.001$). A brief experiential learning intervention using food models was efficacious for changing student's knowledge about sugar guidelines and sugar in food, label reading confidence, and intention to change sugar consumption.

Keywords: sugar; knowledge; education intervention; food models; adolescent

---

1. Introduction

Sugar in the diet is present naturally or as an added ingredient which has been related to both tooth decay and excess weight gain [1]. Overweight and obesity in populations has been rising worldwide, and is a significant public health concern as they are associated with health problems such as diabetes and cardiovascular disease [2]. Canadian adolescent overweight and obesity rates have mirrored this pattern; with 30% of children age 5 to 17 overweight or obese in 2018 [3].

It is well accepted that a major cause of overweight and obesity in the last three decades has been sedentary lifestyles and changes in the diet including consumption of less fruits and vegetables and more energy dense foods and beverages in the diet [4]. One World Health Organization (WHO) recommendation for addressing the overweight and obesity epidemic is limiting intake from total fats and free sugar, the sugar added to food and beverages, and sugars naturally present in honey, syrups, and fruit juices [5].

Although there is not yet an international consensus around the maximum amount of sugar that should be present in a healthy diet, recommendations from the WHO are widely used. These state that less than 10% of the calories in the diet should come from free sugar [5]. In Canada, adolescents are consuming 14.1% of their calories from added sugar [6] (sugars that are incorporated into foods and beverages and sugars naturally present in honey, syrups, and undiluted juices concentrates [7]).

Added sugar is consumed by adolescents in sugar-sweetened beverages (SSBs) but in solid foods as well [8]. Adolescent sugar consumption is a concern since this is an age where eating habits are formed and diet quality deteriorates [9]. Strategies and interventions to change this public health trend are needed. One approach has been to address food literacy, which is not only about knowledge and awareness, but also concerns the skills/capacity to act [10].

Brooks and Begley [11] reviewed literature focused on adolescent food literacy and found there was a lack of food literacy interventions for older adolescents (i.e., high school students). Additionally, based on their review of effective interventions, they suggested using innovative teaching aids, including opportunities for experiential or "hands-on" learning. Experiential learning is designed to develop personal understanding, knowledge, skills, and attitudes through active engagement and reflection on certain activities [12]. Atkins and Michie [13] suggest that it is important to include one or more behavioral change techniques to influence capacity building, motivation or opportunity to change behavior (COM-B model). Finally Brooks and Begley suggested schools, community centers or sporting clubs as possible delivery settings for food literacy intervention.

Schools represent an ideal setting to facilitate dietary behavior change since youth regularly attend for prolonged periods across a year and as they age [14] and they are responsible for the delivery of health curricula. Therefore, the school presents an opportunity to provide nutrition-related education interventions that incorporate evidence-based intervention techniques to increase health literacy levels.

In British Columbia, Canada, the Physical and Health Education (PHE) curriculum for secondary students includes teaching students about the role of nutrition in health and performance in order to help them develop the ability to choose to eat healthy foods [15,16]. The Ministry of Education encourages flexibility in finding different ways to bring this learning to students. Including sugar literacy education sessions as part of physical and health education could be a way to help adolescents make healthy food choices.

Nutrition education addressing sugar literacy for adolescents has mostly targeted SSB consumption [17,18]. Sugar-sweetened beverages are the single category of food/beverages through which adolescents consume the most added sugar; although the highest amount of added sugar they consume comes from across all other food groups together [6]. Therefore, interventions that consider not only knowledge, awareness, and skills related to sugar in SSBs but also in other foods are vital to reducing total added sugar in the diet. There appears to be no published literature related to broader sugar literacy interventions targeting older adolescents although a recent study intervened with 10 to 12 year old children in the United Kingdom [19]. The researchers provided two 45 min educational sessions across 2 days that also incorporated experiential activities using a teaching aid (heaped teaspoons of sugar to illustrate the amount of sugar in a variety of foods). At baseline, children had limited knowledge of sugar in foods and beverages. The educational intervention improved their knowledge significantly at follow-up ($p < 0.001$). This is not surprising, as visual teaching aids have been shown to make learning more effective. Shabiralyani et al. [20] suggest that 83% of what is learned is gained from the sense of sight, 11% from what we hear, and the remaining from the senses of smell, touch, and taste.

Life-sized food models are visual aids that have been used in nutrition education. The literature shows that two- or three-dimensional food models have been used to assess the amount of food consumed [21–25], to examine and teach nutrition knowledge in early childhood [26–28] and for nutrition education with families [29]. However, to date, there appears to be little evidence about the use of life-sized food models for nutrition education with adolescents. Two-dimensional food models may be a more feasible option for use in schools because of their lower cost, weight, and size but their efficacy needs to be tested.

The purpose of this study was to explore the impact of two 45 min nutrition lessons using life-sized two-dimensional food models on adolescents' sugar literacy. Specifically, the study objectives were to determine the effect of this experiential learning strategy on the knowledge and awareness of sugar content in foods and beverages and the recommendations for limits on sugar consumption as well as the impact on skills and intention to consume less added sugar.

2. Materials and Methods

The research design included a randomized controlled trial with baseline and follow-up measures (see Figure 1), with randomization by class to either a regular Physical and Health Education class condition (control group) with delayed nutrition education sessions or two nutrition education sessions using food models during physical and health education (intervention group).

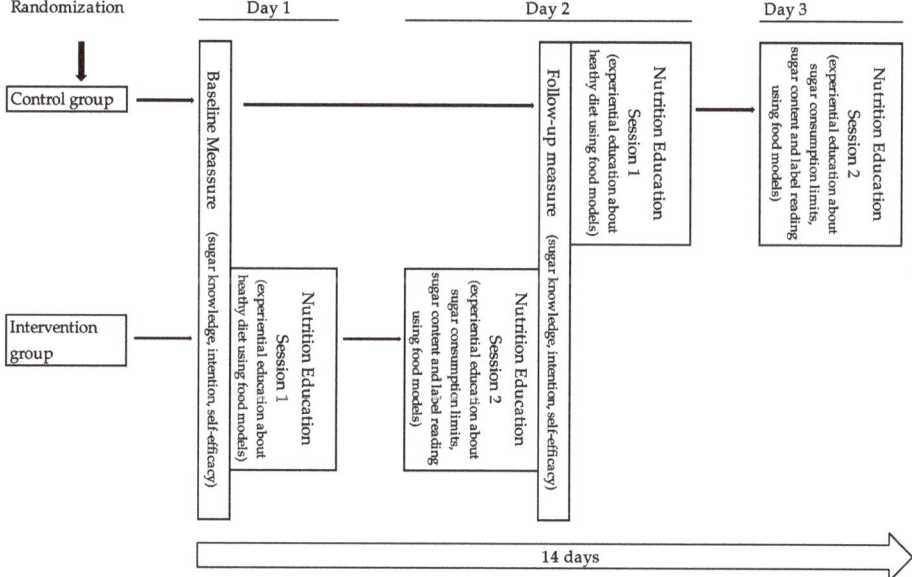

Figure 1. Research design diagram and timeline.

The sample size was calculated using G*Power analysis program [30] with the power set at 0.9, significance at $p < 0.05$, and an effect size d = 0.8 (large effect). A minimum of forty-nine participants was needed in each condition to be able to detect a difference between groups.

A 5 min recruitment presentation explaining the project was shared at a Physical and Health Education teachers meeting (representing 5 different school districts on Vancouver Island). Teachers were asked to contact the researcher if they were interested.

Eleven teachers from six schools in six communities indicated interest in participating in the project. An information letter and a consent to participate form were sent to the principals of the six schools. After University Human Research Ethics approval (#17-477), principal consent, and school district approval were received, a presentation about the study (i.e., objectives, participation dates, and evaluation guidelines) was conducted with the participating teachers' PHE classes, and an information package including consent forms asking for their and their parents' consent to participate in the research component (measurement) was handed out to each student. The schedule for nutrition education sessions was coordinated directly with each teacher.

Sixteen classes with a total of 334 students received the two 45 min nutrition education sessions. Each school participated with either 2 or 4 classes taking part. Half of the classes in each school were randomly assigned to the usual practice control condition (n = 8) and half to intervention conditions (n = 8). The consort study flow diagram (see Figure 2) shows that 214 students consented, 110 were in the intervention condition and 104 in the control group. All students that were present received the nutrition education as part of their physical education curriculum; however, only questionnaire data from the students that consented and participated in the baseline measure were analyzed. All control class students received the intervention after measurement was completed.

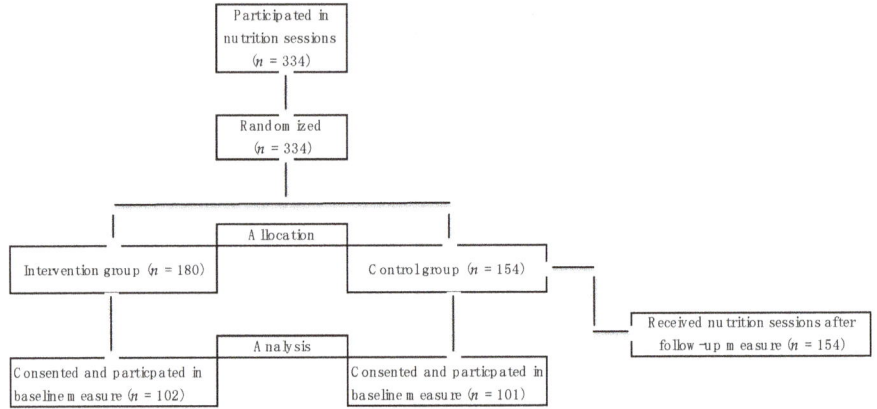

Figure 2. Flow of participants throughout the study.

The primary purpose of the nutrition education sessions was to enhance sugar literacy (knowledge, awareness, skills and intention to change) among youth. The sessions included an experiential learning component according to Michie's behavior change model (COM-B; [31]) to increase knowledge and understanding around sugar content in food and beverages and the daily amount of added sugar in a healthy diet placed into the context of Canada's Food Guidelines to promote healthy eating and lower consumption of added sugar. The sessions also included a component to help students develop the necessary skills to interpret nutrition fact labels in packaged products and design healthy eating patterns.

Each nutrition education session took place during PHE class time (45–65 min depending on the school schedule) and was held either in a room with large tables or on the gym floor so students could have enough space to work with the food models. Participants were provided with 2 didactic lectures plus experiential learning activities. For the experiential learning activities, participants were teamed in groups of 3 or 4, and each team was given a kit with more than 150 life-sized food and beverage models, 100 models of sugar teaspoons, and colored copies of seven nutrition fact labels of commercial foods and beverage packages. NutriKitUSA and Sip Smart BC life-sized two-dimensional food and beverage models with nutrition information including added sugar on the back were used (see the example in Appendix A). The food models in the kit included servings of fruits, vegetables, grain products, milk products, protein-rich foods, and beverages. For understanding added sugar content in packaged foods and beverages, seven additional nutrition fact labels of sugar-containing foods and beverages were analyzed.

The schedule and intervention curriculum content are described in detail in the following section.

Session 1:

Lecture: A brief educational lecture focused on overall diet and diet quality, which includes:

- Canada's Food Guide and the number of recommended daily servings from each food group for the age of participants;
- Limiting consumption of added sugar as part of a healthy lifestyle;
- The use of two-dimensional food models.

Experiential learning activities: food models were used to:

- Visualizing an everyday personal diet (students used the models to represent their previous day's diet);
- Designing a daily menu according to Canada's Food Guide Servings (students were asked to use the food models to create a healthy daily diet according to food guide servings)
- Setting goals on how to modify the personal diet to consume the number of servings suggested by Canada's Food Guide

Session 2:

Lecture: A brief educational lecture focused solely on sugar content in food and beverages, including the following:

- World Health Organization recommendations/guidelines for consumption of sugars;
- How to read and interpret ingredients lists on packaged foods and beverages, specifically, the added sugar content in Nutrition Fact tables.

Experiential learning activities: use of two-dimensional food models (including models of teaspoons of sugar) to help students (see Figure 3):

- Visualizing the amount of added sugar in food and beverages by expressing the content of sugar in teaspoons of sugar;
- Identifying added sugar information in packaged food (real food labels were provided) and converting added sugar content to teaspoons of sugar;
- Analyzing an example of an adolescent diet (supplied by the researcher) and determining the teaspoons of added sugar included in that diet. Make recommendations on how to reduce total added sugar and incorporate the right amount of servings from each Food Group for that particular diet.

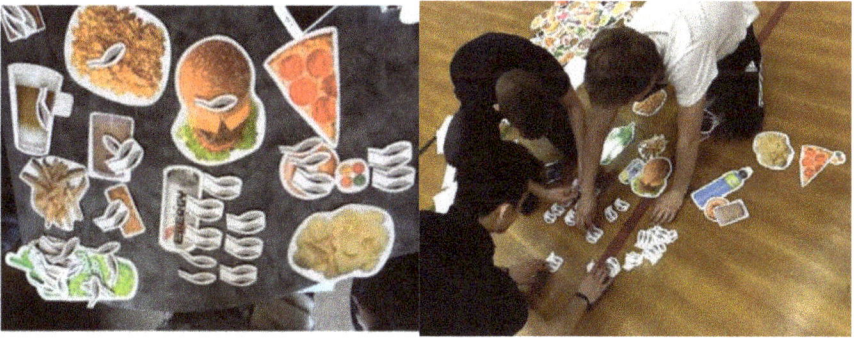

Figure 3. Pictures of interactive activity with two-dimensional food models.

The following section describes research procedures, measurement instruments and data analysis.

2.1. Procedures

After randomization, visits to each class were scheduled. All students had the benefit of the nutrition education lessons; however, intervention groups had the lessons between baseline and follow-up measures and the control group received them after the follow-up measure (see Figure 2). Measures and nutrition education lessons took place April–May 2018. Due to the pragmatic constraints, baseline measures were implemented just prior to the first education session and follow-up measures immediately after session 2. Control condition students completed the baseline measure on the same day as the intervention students but did not receive the two sessions. They received the first session immediately after the follow-up measure, and then a second session was scheduled.

2.2. Measurement Instrument

The 20 item survey instrument (completed at both baseline and follow-up) was composed of modified questions extracted purposively from two validated questionnaires: the Canadian Behavior, Attitude, and Nutrition Knowledge Survey [32] and the Intentions to Eat Low-Glycemic Index Foods questionnaire [33] and is described following (see the instrument in Appendix B):

Demographics: The age, gender, and grade of the participants were asked. Each participant was assigned a code to protect the confidentiality of their data.

2.3. Experimental Variables

Knowledge of daily portions: the questions were open-ended and asked the student to approximate the number of daily food group servings according to Canada's Food Guide for their particular age and gender.

Knowledge of the maximum amount of added sugar consumption: this item was open-ended and asked the maximum number of teaspoons of added sugar that an average person (14 years and up) could eat each day to maintain a healthy diet.

Knowledge of added sugar content in food and beverages: four questions for sugar content in different foods and two for different beverages were included.

Self-efficacy: Five items with a 7 point Likert scale were included. Scale reliability analysis showed the self-efficacy measure was internally consistent (Cronbach's Alpha = 0.74). The five questions were summed together to produce an overall score ranging from 5 to 35 representing their belief in their ability to eat/drink fewer foods and beverages with added sugar.

Intention to eat/drink foods and beverages with less added sugar: Three items that had a 7 point Likert scale with the response format "Strongly disagree to Strongly agree" were included. Cronbach's alpha for this subscale was 0.839. Items were summed together to produce an overall score. A higher score represented a higher intention to eat/drink fewer foods and beverages with added sugar in the following two weeks.

The frequency of limiting foods high in sugar: a 7 point Likert scale question (from rarely to always) about how often foods high in sugar were limited when making food choices was used.

Nutrition fact label reading confidence. Two 7 point Likert scale questions were used. In the first question, students were asked if, when reading nutrition facts labels, they would look for information about sugar and on the second question, if they were confident that they could interpret that information.

2.4. Data Analysis

Data analysis was conducted using SPSS (IBM Corp. Released 2016, Version 24, Armonk, NY, USA). Data were screened for completeness, missing data, and normality. One outlier was eliminated, four outliers in the knowledge variables for the control group were not removed because they were possible values. Twenty-four participants in the control group and 13 in the intervention group completed the baseline measure but were not present for the second measure. Intention-to-treat protocols for missing and absent data were used and the baseline value carried forward. Descriptive statistics (means, SD) were calculated and one-way analysis of variance (ANOVA) was used to determine if there were differences between groups at baseline. A regression analysis determined if there was a relationship between baseline demographic variables, including age and sex and the dependent variables. A repeated measures ANOVA determined if the groups differed over time and by condition. An apriori statistical cut-off point based on an alpha level of 0.05 was used for significance.

3. Results

3.1. Baseline

Participant characteristics are displayed in detail in Table 1. As noted in Table 1, almost three-quarters of the participants were female. The majority of students in the control group were grade 9 or 10, and for the intervention group, grade 10 or 11 and, thus, the average age of students in the control group was approximately 1 year younger than those in the intervention.

One-way ANOVA scores showed that there was a significant difference in age, sex, and grade by group at baseline. Regression analysis showed, however, that there was no correlation between age (grade) and sex, with the dependent variables at baseline and after the intervention. The percent of variance (R squared) explained in the dependent variables by age (grade) and sex was always below 30% ($R^2 < 0.3$). See Appendix C for regression analysis results.

Table 1. Characteristics of participants at baseline.

Characteristic	Total ($n = 203$)		Control ($n = 101$)		Intervention ($n = 102$)		F (df)	p
	Mean (SD)	%	Mean (SD)	%	Mean (SD)	%		
Age (years)	15.9 (1)		15.4 (0.7)		16.4 (1.0)		70.34 (201)	0.00
Gender							16.29 (201)	0.00
Female		74.3		62.5		86.3		
Male		25.7		37.5		13.7		
Grade	10.0 (0.9)		9.5 (0.6)	0.6	10.4 (0.9)		72.72 (201)	0.00
9		31.1		51.0		10.8		
10		49.0		47.1		51.0		
11		12.1				24.5		
12		7.8		1.9		13.7		
Knowledge (correct answers)								
Daily portions of Food Groups				18.3		23.0		
Suggested maximum amount of added sugar				11.0		2.0		
Added sugar content in food and beverage				14.8		18.5		
Total Knowledge				15.7		18.6	2.92 (201)	0.09
Self-efficacy (5—35 [a])	23.9 (5.8)		23.17 (5.1)		24.7 (6.3)		2.58 (201)	0.11
Intention to consume less added sugar (3—21 [b])	14.4 (4.4)		13.9 (4.6)		14.9 (4.1)		3.70 (201)	0.06
Ability to interpret sugar content in food labels (1—7 [c])	4.8 (1.5)		4.9 (1.6)		4.6 (1.4)		1.81 (201)	0.18
Frequency of limiting foods high in added sugar (1—7 [c])	4.1 (1.5)		4.1 (1.6)		4.1 (1.4)		0.02 (201)	0.89
Frequency of added sugar being read in food labels (1—7 [c])	4.5 (1.9)		4.6 (1.9)		4.5 (1.8)		0.13 (201)	0.72

Note. SD = Standard deviation; F = F value; df = degrees of freedom; p = probability value. [a] Sum of five 7 point Likert scale questions. [b] Sum of three 7 point Likert scale question. [c] 7 point Likert scale

Baseline means and standard deviations for the dependent variables are also shown in Table 1. This table shows that knowledge was low and that this did not differ by group. No difference was found between groups at baseline for self-efficacy, intention to consume less added sugar, ability to interpret sugar content in food labels, frequency of limiting foods high in added sugar, and frequency of added sugar being read in food labels.

3.2. Follow-Up

Means and main effect for time by condition are reported in Table 2 and summarized in the following section. An intervention effect was found for all knowledge variables across time. The intervention condition had a significantly higher score in their knowledge about daily food group portions, the maximum daily recommended amount of added sugar that should be consumed, and the added sugar content in foods and beverages at follow-up compared to controls. Eighty percent of the intervention group correctly answered the maximum recommended amount of added sugar that can be present in a healthy diet compared to 10% of the control group. The intervention group correctly answered 60% of the daily food group portion questions compared to 20% of correct answers for the control group at follow-up. Knowledge about sugar content in foods and beverages increased from 18% to 48% correct answers for the intervention group and was significantly different than the correct responses in the follow-up measure for control group. Effect sizes ranged were large in all knowledge dependent variables.

Intention to consume less food and beverages with added sugar and the ability to interpret sugar content in food labels differed significantly over time as well, with intentions to consume less added sugar increasing in the intervention condition. Effect sizes were respectively small and intermediate

($\eta^2 = 0.02$, $\eta^2 = 0.07$) however. There were no significant differences among groups over time in student's beliefs in their ability to limit added sugar (self-efficacy) nor in the frequency with which they reported limiting food that contained sugar or read the added sugar on food labels.

Table 2. Means and repeated measures ANOVA for change pre–post intervention in knowledge, self-efficacy, intentions, ability to read and interpret food labels, and frequency of limiting food with added sugar.

Dependent Variable	Control (n = 101)		Intervention. (n = 102)		F (df)	p	η2
	Mean (SD)	% (SD)	Mean (SD)	% (SD)			
Knowledge (correct answers)							
Daily portions of Food Groups							
Baseline		18.3 (20.0)		23.0 (22.2)	59.84 (201)	0.00	0.23
Follow-up		21.0 (19.3)		59.3 (32.6)			
Suggested maximum amount of added sugar							
Baseline		11.0 (31.3)		2.0 (13.9)	138.14 (201)	0.00	0.41
Follow-up		14.0 (34.7)		75.0 (43.2)			
Added sugar content in food and beverage							
Baseline		14.8 (14.3)		18.5 (16.4)	64.68 (201)	0.00	0.24
Follow-up		17.7 (18.2)		47.7 (26.2)			
Total knowledge							
Baseline		15.7 (11.4)		18.6 (11.7)	104.84 (201)	0.00	0.34
Follow-up		20.1 (18.3)		54.5 (22.4)			
Self-efficacy (5—35 [a])							
Baseline	23.2 (5.1)		24.7 (6.3)		0.49 (201)	0.49	0.00
Follow-up	23.8 (5.8)		25.5 (6.0)				
Intention to consume less added sugar (3—21 [b])							
Baseline	13.9 (4.6)		14.9 (4.1)		4.93 (201)	0.03	0.02
Follow-up	13.3 (4.6)		15.3 (4.1)				
Ability to interpret sugar content in food labels (1—7 [c])							
Baseline	4.9 (1.6)		4.6 (1.4)		14.94 (200)	0.00	0.07
Follow-up	4.6 (1.7)		5.3 (1.8)				
Frequency of limiting foods high in added sugar (1—7 [c])							
Baseline	4.1 (1.6)		4.1 (1.4)		0.19 (201)	0.67	0.00
Follow-up	4.3 (1.7)		4.3 (1.6)				
Frequency of added sugar being read in food labels (1—7 [c])							
Baseline	4.6 (1.9)		4.5 (1.8)		3.42 (201)	0.07	0.02
Follow-up	4.5 (1.9)		4.8 (1.6)				

Note. SD = Standard deviation; F = F value; df = degrees of freedom; p = probability value; η2 = partial eta squared; [a] Sum of five 7 point Likert scale questions. [b] Sum of three 7 point Likert scale question. [c] 7 point Likert scale question.

4. Discussion

With the importance of preventing obesity and enhancing dietary quality during adolescence highlighted in the literature, addressing the adolescent consumption of added sugars is critical. This study addressed a gap in the evidence-based literature by targeting adolescents rather than children and addressing sugar literacy across the spectrum of foods consumed rather than just through sugary drinks. Additionally, it tested a brief nutrition intervention delivered in high school Physical and Health Education classes using food models to provide an experiential learning component. Finally, it incorporated two-dimensional food models which are potentially more feasible to adopt in school-based health promotion efforts.

This study showed that a two 45 min brief nutrition education intervention using food models significantly improved adolescents' food and sugar literacy. Specifically, the intervention enhanced knowledge of added sugar content in foods and beverages, the maximum amount of added sugar in a healthy diet, food group servings in a healthy diet, and it also increased the ability of adolescents to interpret sugar content in food labels and increased their intention to reduce the consumption of added sugar. Not surprisingly given the post measurement was conducted immediately after the second lesson, the reported frequency of limiting foods with added sugar and reading labels was not significant. These results are discussed in the context of the following literature.

Knowledge has been recognized as an essential component in behavioral change theories of health promotion [34]. Adolescents' knowledge about added sugar content in food and about recommendations related to the maximum amount of sugar in a healthy diet was low at baseline for all participants, but it increased significantly following the intervention. This is consistent with a previous study that showed that two interactive classroom sessions about sugar given to 10–12 year-old children significantly improved their knowledge of sugar in food and beverages [19]. Further research is needed to evaluate if this knowledge was sustained over time.

This study also examined if adolescents knew the number of servings of each of the food groups that should be present in a healthy diet at their age and if that knowledge changed with the intervention. Even though the study focused on sugar literacy, education about food guidelines was included to ensure students understood healthy eating patterns, how to analyze their own diet, and could place sugar consumption within the context of the overall picture of healthy eating. Adolescents had poor knowledge about servings at baseline, but that knowledge significantly increased with the education sessions; although remaining less than ideal. They used this knowledge to create and visualize a healthy diet utilizing the food models and compared it to their everyday diet. The instrument, however, tested only their knowledge and not their actual ability to use that knowledge to implement a healthy diet. Further studies using eating behavior measurement tools like Food Frequency Questionnaires should test if this type of experiential learning intervention has a short- or long-term impact on the diet.

Having the skills or ability to act is an essential component of food literacy, in this case, sugar literacy. The intervention helped adolescents interpret sugar content in food labels. Nutrition courses including label reading have been given to college students with similar results [35]. Tallant's [35] study also reported that being able to understand food labels influenced students' decisions to include healthier foods in their diet. Once again, further studies are needed to evaluate whether or not over time the ability to interpret labels is sustained and if less added sugar is consumed.

This study evaluated if the nutrition education lessons had an effect on intentions to reduce the consumption of added sugar. The intervention group had a higher intention to reduce the amount of added sugar consumed after intervention, but the effect size was minimal. It may be that a brief intervention is less effective for shifting intentions.

Self-efficacy, as the confidence in one's personal ability to eat/drink less added sugar, was tested but did not change after the intervention. No change was expected after intervention since the follow-up measure was completed immediately after the second nutrition education session. Success is a key component of self-efficacy [36] and they had no opportunity to "apply'" their skills in real-life. Further studies that examine self-efficacy over time are needed.

As suggested by Michie [13], incorporating educational and training techniques did affect knowledge about sugar and increased the skills to interpret sugar content in food, beverages, and food labels. This theoretically influences the capacity (capability) of the students to engage in changing sugar eating behaviors by reducing the amount of added or free sugar consumed. In keeping with the concept of opportunity in Michie's model, these changes in adolescent sugar consumption could be enhanced by implementing policies to reduce the consumption of foods and beverages high in sugar [37]. Examples of policies suggested by the American Academy of Pediatrics to reduce consumption of SSBs, but that might also be able to be applied to other foods high in sugar as well, are taxes to increase the price of these products and the use of part of the tax revenues to reduce health and socioeconomic disparities, and decreasing marketing to adolescents about products high in added sugar and making healthy low added sugar beverages and foods the default in vending machines, parks, and restaurants [37].

Based on the experience gained in this study, a brief intervention had an impact on important food and sugar literacy variables. Given that session 1 addressed broader food education, an even briefer intervention of one sugar literacy lesson using food models and their impact on awareness of sugar content and sugar consumption in adolescents should be tested. This is consistent with the conclusions of a systematic review on brief nutrition interventions conducted in 2018 that proved that brief interventions can be sufficient to improve short-term dietary behavior [38].

Limitations

The results of the study should be viewed in the context of the limitations. Validated questionnaire items were adapted and not re-validated. We did re-establish scale reliabilities where more than one item contributed to a sub-scale. We randomized by class not individual student and did not adjust for class as a cluster. We accommodated for school as a cluster by having both an intervention and control class in the same school. This opened the study up to the potential for contamination and a manipulation check question was not included. Finally, due to the pragmatic constraints, actual behavior was not measured. The follow-up measurement was administered immediately after the second nutrition education session, which did not give the participants an opportunity to implement what they learned.

5. Conclusions

A brief sugar nutrition education intervention delivered in school Physical and Health Education classes appeared efficacious for increasing sugar literacy among adolescents. Knowledge around the number of portions and sugar content in food and beverages as well as the maximum amount of added sugar in a healthy diet was low in adolescents but increased significantly after just two 45 min nutrition sessions, as did their label reading confidence and intention to consume less added sugar. Increasing sugar literacy in adolescents is important in the context of escalating obesity rates and health issues related to poor diet and evidence that eating behaviors track across the lifespan and are influenced by nutrition knowledge and food literacy.

Two-dimensional food models appear to have potential as a teaching tool for nutrition education in the school environment as they offer visual and simulated hands-on experiences with food. They also have an advantage in terms of cost, weight, and size (storability and variety of foods) when compared to three-dimensional models but may be less durable.

Future work needs to look at the relationship between measures of sugar literacy and label reading behaviors and actual sugar consumption. Also, studies on brief nutrition education interventions using food models should involve a longer-term follow-up and more sensitive measurement tools.

Author Contributions: M.I.S., S.G., and P.-J.N. contributed to the conceptualization of the study and methodology; data collection, investigation, and formal analysis was conducted by M.I.S. and supervised by P.-J.N.; the original draft was prepared by M.I.S.; review and editing was conducted by M.I.S., S.G., and P.-J.N.; project administration, M.I.S.; and funding acquisition, P.-J.N.

Funding: This research received no external funding.

Acknowledgments: The authors would like to gratefully acknowledge and thank the School Districts and Administrators that gave permission to conduct the study and the teachers and students that agreed to participate in the study; without them it would have been impossible to explore this intervention. In addition, we would like to acknowledge the contribution of John Walsh who consulted with M.I.S. on the statistical analysis.

Conflicts of Interest: The first author declares a conflict of interest in that she owns a company that designs and produces two-dimensional food models called NutritKit educational materials.

Appendix A Examples of Food Models Used

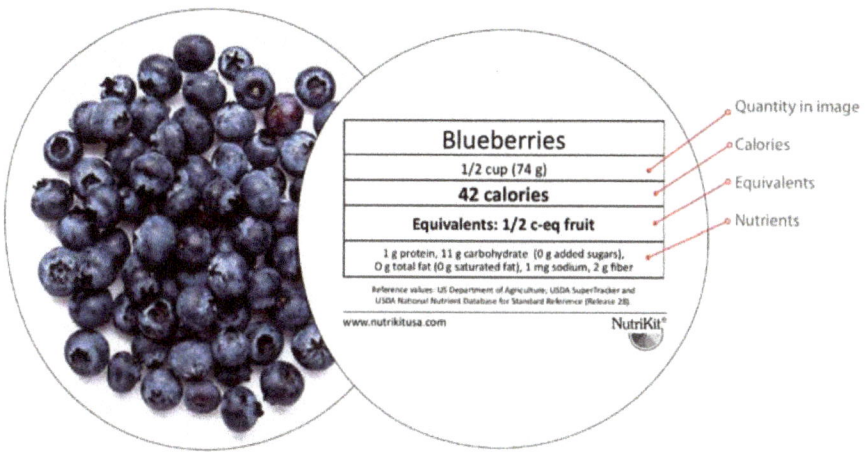

Figure A1. NutriKitUSA.

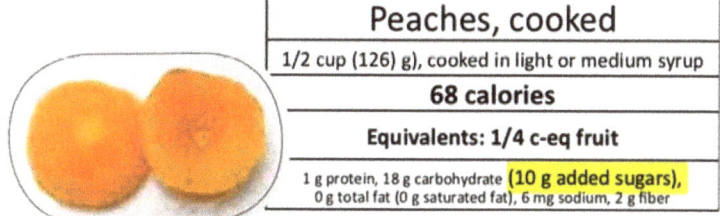

Figure A2. NutriKitUSA.

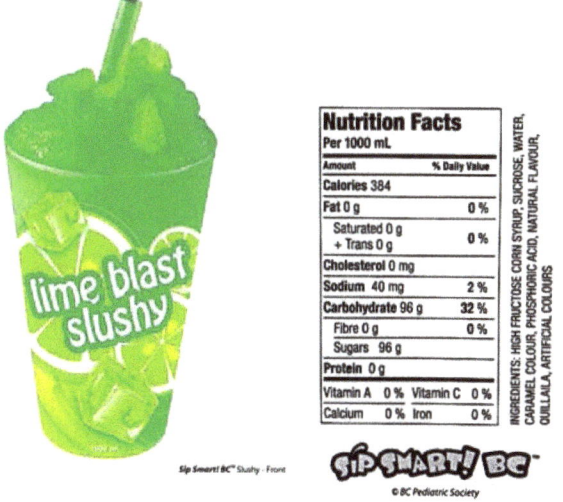

Figure A3. Sip Smart BC image.

Appendix B Questionnaire.

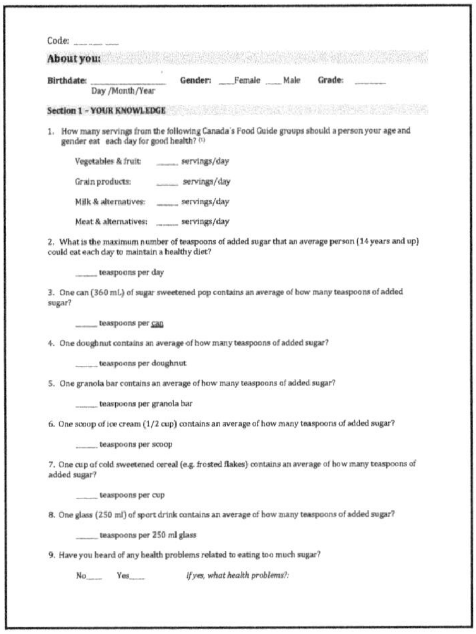

Code: ___ ___ ___

About you:

Birthdate: ______________ **Gender:** ___Female ___ Male **Grade:** ______
Day /Month/Year

Section 1 – YOUR KNOWLEDGE

1. How many servings from the following Canada's Food Guide groups should a person your age and gender eat each day for good health? (1)

   Vegetables & fruit: _____ servings/day

   Grain products: _____ servings/day

   Milk & alternatives: _____ servings/day

   Meat & alternatives: _____ servings/day

2. What is the maximum number of teaspoons of added sugar that an average person (14 years and up) could eat each day to maintain a healthy diet?

   _____ teaspoons per day

3. One can (360 mL) of sugar sweetened pop contains an average of how many teaspoons of added sugar?

   _____ teaspoons per can

4. One doughnut contains an average of how many teaspoons of added sugar?

   _____ teaspoons per doughnut

5. One granola bar contains an average of how many teaspoons of added sugar?

   _____ teaspoons per granola bar

6. One scoop of ice cream (1/2 cup) contains an average of how many teaspoons of added sugar?

   _____ teaspoons per scoop

7. One cup of cold sweetened cereal (e.g. frosted flakes) contains an average of how many teaspoons of added sugar?

   _____ teaspoons per cup

8. One glass (250 ml) of sport drink contains an average of how many teaspoons of added sugar?

   _____ teaspoons per 250 ml glass

9. Have you heard of any health problems related to eating too much sugar?

   No____ Yes____ *If yes, what health problems?:*

Figure A4. Page 1 Questionnaire.

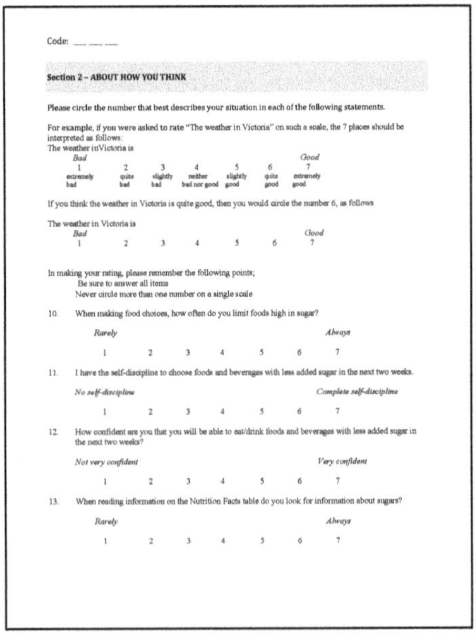

Code: ___ ___ ___

Section 2 – ABOUT HOW YOU THINK

Please circle the number that best describes your situation in each of the following statements.

For example, if you were asked to rate "The weather in Victoria" on such a scale, the 7 places should be interpreted as follows:
The weather inVictoria is

Bad						*Good*
1	2	3	4	5	6	7
extremely bad	quite bad	slightly bad	neither bad nor good	slightly good	quite good	extremely good

If you think the weather in Victoria is quite good, then you would circle the number 6, as follows

The weather in Victoria is

Bad						*Good*
1	2	3	4	5	6	7

In making your rating, please remember the following points;
Be sure to answer all items
Never circle more than one number on a single scale

10. When making food choices, how often do you limit foods high in sugar?

    Rarely *Always*

    1 2 3 4 5 6 7

11. I have the self-discipline to choose foods and beverages with less added sugar in the next two weeks.

    No self-discipline *Complete self-discipline*

    1 2 3 4 5 6 7

12. How confident are you that you will be able to eat/drink foods and beverages with less added sugar in the next two weeks?

    Not very confident *Very confident*

    1 2 3 4 5 6 7

13. When reading information on the Nutrition Facts table do you look for information about sugars?

    Rarely *Always*

    1 2 3 4 5 6 7

Figure A5. Page 2 Questionnaire.

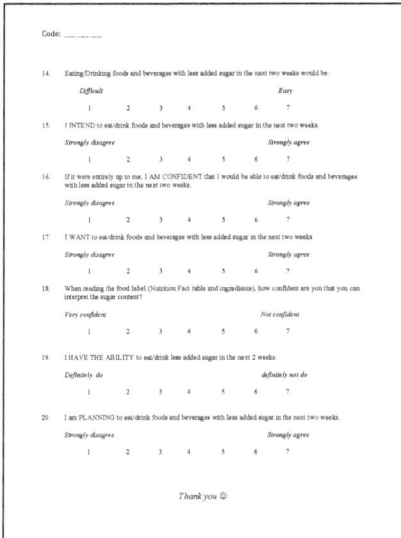

Figure A6. Page 3 Questionnaire.

Appendix C Regression Analysis Outcomes

Table A1. Correlation between age (grade) and sex, with the dependent variables at baseline and after the intervention.

Dependent Variable	Age			Sex		
	F	p	R^2	F	p	R^2
Total knowledge						
Baseline	0.74	0.39	0.004	0.81	0.37	0.004
Follow-up	0.21	0.65	0.002	0.00	0.99	0.000
Self efficacy						
Baseline	3.01	0.08	0.015	0.54	0.46	0.003
Follow-up	0.08	0.78	0.001	2.93	0.09	0.028
Intention to consume less added sugar						
Baseline	2.19	0.14	0.011	9.65	0.00	0.041
Follow-up	3.08	0.08	0.030	0.70	0.40	0.007
Ability to interpret sugar content in food labels						
Baseline	0.09	0.77	0.000	0.01	0.93	0.000
Follow-up	0.35	0.55	0.004	0.17	0.68	0.002
Frequency of limiting foods high in added sugar						
Baseline	0.04	0.85	0.000	1.70	0.19	0.008
Follow-up	0.51	0.48	0.005	0.04	0.84	0.000
Frequency of added sugar being read in food labels						
Baseline	0.13	0.72	0.001	5.27	0.02	0.021
Follow-up	0.59	0.44	0.006	1.52	0.22	0.015

References

1. Newens, K.J.; Walton, J. A review of sugar consumption from nationally representative dietary surveys across the world. *J. Hum. Nutr. Diet.* **2016**, *29*, 225–240. [CrossRef] [PubMed]
2. Hammond, R.A.; Levine, R. The economic impact of obesity in the United States. *Diabetes Metab. Syndr. Obes.* **2010**, *3*, 285–295. [CrossRef] [PubMed]
3. Pulmonary Hypertension Assn of Canada. Tackling obesity in Canada: Childhood Obesity and Excess Weight Rates in Canada, Aem. 2018. Available online: https://www.canada.ca/en/public-health/services/publications/healthy-living/obesity-excess-weight-rates-canadian-children.html (accessed on 28 April 2019).

4. Manger, W.M.; Manger, L.S.; Minno, A.M.; Killmeyer, M.; Holzman, R.S.; Schullinger, J.N.; Roccella, E.J. Obesity prevention in young schoolchildren: Results of a pilot study. *J. Sch. Health* **2012**, *82*, 462–468. [CrossRef] [PubMed]
5. World Health Organization. *Guideline: Sugars Intake for Adults and Children, WHO UK Distributor*; Stationery Office: Geneva, Switzerland, 2015.
6. Brisbois, T.D.; Marsden, S.L.; Anderson, G.H.; Sievenpiper, L.J. Estimated intakes and sources of total and added sugars in the canadian diet. *Nutrients* **2014**, *6*, 1899–1912. [CrossRef] [PubMed]
7. Bowman, S.A. Added sugars: Definition and estimation in the USDA food patterns equivalents databases. *J. Food Compos. Anal.* **2017**, *64*, 64–67. [CrossRef]
8. Reedy, J.; Krebs-Smith, S.M. Dietary Sources of Energy, Solid Fats, and Added Sugars Among Children and Adolescents in the United States. *J. Am. Diet. Assoc.* **2010**, *110*, 1477–1484. [CrossRef] [PubMed]
9. Delisle, H.; World Health Organization. *Nutrition in Adolescence: Issues and Challenges for the Health Sector: Issues in Adolescent Health and Development*; World Health Organization: Geneva, Switzerland, 2015.
10. Krause, C.; Sommerhalder, K.; Beer-Borst, S.; Abel, T. Just a subtle difference? Findings from a systematic review on definitions of nutrition literacy and food literacy. *Health Promot. Int.* **2016**, *33*, 378–389. [CrossRef]
11. Brooks, N.; Begley, A. Adolescent food literacy programmes: A review of the literature. *Nutr. Diet.* **2014**, *71*, 158–171. [CrossRef]
12. What Is Experiential Learning? Experiential Learning. (n.d.). Available online: https://www.experientiallearning.org/about-mta/what-is-experiential-learning/ (accessed on 25 June 2019).
13. Atkins, L.; Michie, S. Changing eating behaviour: What can we learn from behavioural science? *Nutr. Bull.* **2013**, *38*, 30–35. [CrossRef]
14. Peralta, L.R.; Dudley, D.A.; Cotton, W.G. Teaching Healthy eating to elementary school students: A scoping review of nutrition education resources. *J. Sch. Health* **2016**, *86*, 334–345. [CrossRef]
15. Physical and Health Education 11|Building Student Success—BC's New Curriculum, (n.d.). Available online: https://curriculum.gov.bc.ca/curriculum/physical-health-education/11/courses (accessed on 10 December 2018).
16. Physical and Health Education 12|Building Student Success—BC's New Curriculum, (n.d.). Available online: https://curriculum.gov.bc.ca/curriculum/physical-health-education/12/courses (accessed on 10 December 2018).
17. Lane, H.; Porter, K.; Estabrooks, P.; Zoellner, J. A Systematic review to assess sugar-sweetened beverage interventions for children and adolescents across the socioecological model. *J. Acad. Nutr. Diet.* **2016**, *116*, 1295–1307. [CrossRef]
18. Lane, H.; Porter, K.J.; Hecht, E.; Harris, P.; Kraak, V.; Zoellner, J. Kids SIPsmartER: A feasibility study to reduce sugar-sweetened beverage consumption among middle school youth in central appalachia. *Am. J. Health Promot.* **2018**, *32*, 1386–1401. [CrossRef] [PubMed]
19. TGriffin, L.; Jackson, D.M.; McNeill, G.; Aucott, L.S.; Macdiarmid, J.I. A brief educational intervention increases knowledge of the sugar content of foods and drinks but does not decrease intakes in scottish children aged 10–12 years. *J. Nutr. Educ. Behav.* **2015**, *47*, 367–373. [CrossRef]
20. Shabiralyani, G.; Hasan, K.S.; Hamad, N.; Iqbal, N. Impact of visual aids in enhancing the learning process case research: District dera ghazi khan. *J. Educ. Pract.* **2015**, *6*, 226–233.
21. Luevano-Contreras, C.; Durkin, T.; Pauls, M.; Chapman-Novakofski, K. Development, relative validity, and reliability of a food frequency questionnaire for a case-control study on dietary advanced glycation end products and diabetes complications. *Int. J. Food Sci. Nutr.* **2013**, *64*, 1030–1035. [CrossRef] [PubMed]
22. Nieman, D.C.; Henson, D.A.; Sha, W. Ingestion of micronutrient fortified breakfast cereal has no influence on immune function in healthy children: A randomized controlled trial. *Nutr. J.* **2011**, *10*, 36. [CrossRef] [PubMed]
23. Sheehy, T.; Kolahdooz, F.; Mtshali, T.L.; Khamis, T.; Sharma, S. Development of a quantitative food frequency questionnaire for use among rural South Africans in KwaZulu-Natal. *J. Hum. Nutr. Diet.* **2014**, *27*, 443–449. [CrossRef]
24. Sheehy, T.; Roache, C.; Sharma, S. Eating habits of a population undergoing a rapid dietary transition: Portion sizes of traditional and non-traditional foods and beverages consumed by Inuit adults in Nunavut, Canada. *Nutr. J.* **2013**, *12*, 70. [CrossRef]

25. Zemel, M.B.; Donnelly, J.E.; Smith, B.K.; Sullivan, D.K.; Richards, J.; Morgan-Hanusa, D.; Mayo, M.S.; Sun, X.; Cook-Wiens, G.; Bailey, B.W.; et al. Effects of dairy intake on weight maintenance. *Nutr. Metabo.* **2008**, *5*, 28. [CrossRef]
26. Holub, S.C.; Musher-Eizenman, D.R. Examining preschoolers' nutrition knowledge using a meal creation and food group classification task: Age and gender differences. *Early Child Dev. Care* **2010**, *180*, 787–798. [CrossRef]
27. Reynolds, K.D.; Hinton, A.W.; Shewchuk, R.M.; Hickey, C.A. Social cognitive model of fruit and vegetable consumption in elementary school children. *J. Nutr. Educ.* **1999**, *31*, 23–30. [CrossRef]
28. Matheson, D.; Spranger, K.; Saxe, A. Preschool children's perceptions of food and their food experiences. *J. Nutr. Educ. Behav.* **2002**, *34*, 85–92. [CrossRef]
29. Park, O.-H.; Brown, R.; Murimi, M.; Hoover, L. Let's Cook, Eat, and Talk: Encouraging Healthy Eating Behaviors and Interactive Family Mealtime for an Underserved Neighborhood in Texas. *J. Nutr. Educ. Behav.* **2018**, *50*, 836–844. [CrossRef] [PubMed]
30. Faul, F.; Erdfelder, E.; Lang, A.-G.; Buchner, A. G*Power 3: A flexible statistical power analysis program for the social, behavioral, and biomedical sciences. *Behav. Res. Methods* **2007**, *39*, 175–191. [CrossRef] [PubMed]
31. Michie, S.; van Stralen, M.M.; West, R. The behaviour change wheel: A new method for characterising and designing behaviour change interventions. *Implement. Sci.* **2011**, *6*, 42. [CrossRef] [PubMed]
32. Lafave, L.M.Z.; Lafave, M.R.; Nordstrom, P. *Development of a Canadian Behaviour. Attitude and Nutrition Knowledge Survey (BANKS)*; CanadianCouncilonLearning: Ottawa, Ontario, Canada, 2008.
33. Watanabe, T.; Berry, T.R.; Willows, N.D.; Bell, R.C. Assessing intentions to eat low-glycemic index foods by adults with diabetes using a new questionnaire based on the theory of planned behaviour. *Can. J. Diabetes* **2015**, *39*, 94–100. [CrossRef] [PubMed]
34. Wardle, J.; Parmenter, K.; Waller, J. Nutrition knowledge and food intake. *Appetite* **2000**, *34*, 269–275. [CrossRef] [PubMed]
35. Tallant, A. First-year college students increase food label–reading behaviors and improve food choices in a personal nutrition seminar course. *Am. J. Health Educ.* **2017**, *48*, 331–337. [CrossRef]
36. Bandura, A. On the functional properties of perceived self-efficacy revisited. *J. Manag.* **2012**, *38*, 9–44. [CrossRef]
37. Muth, N.D.; Dietz, W.H.; Magge, S.N.; Johnson, R.K. American academy of pediatrics, section on obesity, committee on nutrition, american heart association, public policies to reduce sugary drink consumption in children and adolescents. *Pediatrics* **2019**, *143*, e20190282. [CrossRef]
38. Whatnall, M.C.; Patterson, A.J.; Ashton, L.M.; Hutcheson, M.J. Effectiveness of brief nutrition interventions on dietary behaviours in adults: A systematic review. *Appetite* **2018**, *120*, 335–347. [CrossRef] [PubMed]

© 2019 by the authors. Licensee MDPI, Basel, Switzerland. This article is an open access article distributed under the terms and conditions of the Creative Commons Attribution (CC BY) license (http://creativecommons.org/licenses/by/4.0/).

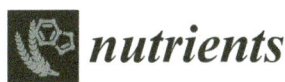

Article

Examining the Efficacy of a 'Feasible' Nudge Intervention to Increase the Purchase of Vegetables by First Year University Students (17–19 Years of Age) in British Columbia: A Pilot Study

Matheus Mistura [1], Nicole Fetterly [1], Ryan E. Rhodes [1,2], Dona Tomlin [1] and Patti-Jean Naylor [1,*]

1. Chronic Disease Prevention Research and Knowledge Exchange Unit, School of Exercise Science, Physical and Health Education, University of Victoria, Victoria, BC V8W 2P1, Canada
2. Behavioural Medicine Lab, School of Exercise Science, Physical and Health Education, University of Victoria, Victoria, BC V8W 2P1, Canada
* Correspondence: pjnaylor@uvic.ca; Tel.: +1-250-721-7844

Received: 29 June 2019; Accepted: 1 August 2019; Published: 2 August 2019

Abstract: In the transition from high school to university, vegetable consumption tends to deteriorate, potentially influencing immediate and longer-term health outcomes. Nudges, manipulation of the environment to influence choice, have emerged as important to behavior change goals. This quasi-experimental pilot study examined the impact of a contextually feasible evidence-informed nudge intervention on food purchasing behavior of older adolescents (1st year students) in a university residence cafeteria in British Columbia, Canada. A co-design process with students and staff identified a student relevant and operationally feasible nudge intervention; a placement nudge, fresh vegetables at the hot food table, combined with a sensory and cognitive nudge, signage encouraging vegetable purchase). Using a 12-week single-case A-B-A-B design, observations of the proportion of vegetables purchased were used to assess intervention efficacy. Data analysis included visual trend inspection, central tendency measures, data overlap, variability and latency. Visual trend inspection showed a positive trend when nudges were in place, which was more apparent with female purchases and during the first intervention (B) phase. However, further analysis showed lack of baseline stability, high variability across phases and overlapping data, limiting efficacy conclusions. Menu choices, staff encouragement, term timing and student finances are other potential influences. Further 'real world' nudge research is needed.

Keywords: nudge; choice architecture; vegetable; food; university; students; adolescents; cafeteria

1. Introduction

Vegetables are one of the most important foods we consume as humans due to their nutrient density and fiber, as well as their low energy contribution to the diet. Low consumption levels are linked to poorer health outcomes, including obesity and the development of diseases, such as cardiovascular disease, diabetes and some cancers [1]. The consumption of vegetables can also promote satiety and reduce the risk of obesity, which is a growing concern globally and specifically affects the target population of this study—older adolescents (17–19) in their first year of university, who have documented weight gain [2]. The consumption of vegetables is low in adolescence and tends to deteriorate even more during the transition from adolescence to young adulthood [3]. It has also been found that unhealthy eating habits and weight gain established in youth tend to be maintained during aging [4,5]. This worldwide scenario highlights the importance of developing strategies to increase vegetable consumption in this population and attempt to slow the global obesity epidemic.

Food decisions are made many times throughout the day and are shaped by many factors. The intention to eat well may be modulated by convenience, availability, taste or mood. Environmental interventions that influence these daily food decisions have gained importance as they have been shown to positively shape dietary behaviors [6]. Nudge theory or choice architecture has been gaining momentum in public health to subtly guide an individual's decisions without denying them autonomy of choice or significantly changing their economic incentives [7]. Nudges have been categorized and shown to be effective with a variety of populations through systematic review and meta-analyses [8–11]. However, there are not many studies targeting adolescents and evidence of their effectiveness in terms of vegetable intake in the school setting has been labelled as both weak and inconclusive [12].

One categorization scheme emerging from a recent meta-analysis identified three nudge classifications: cognitive/educational, hedonistic/sensory and placement/behavior and found that effect size increased from cognitive to placement/behavior nudges [9]. An example of a cognitive or educational nudge is the display of nutrition facts at point-of-sale or messaging about the importance of eating vegetables or drinking fewer sugary beverages. A recent Toronto, Canada study found that using physical activity caloric equivalents (PACE) was a more unique and eye-catching way to raise awareness about sugar content in beverages [13].

A sensory nudge might involve descriptive naming of dishes to make them more appealing, for example "farm to table bar" as compared to "salad bar". This has been tested with adolescents where a cross-country European study targeted adolescents using a sensory nudge (vegetable-forward entrée as the "dish of the day") and found that the "dish of the day" label did not have a significant effect on vegetable selection compared to the control groups (meat-forward or fish selection) [14,15]. Further, the Danish research group involved in the study did secondary analyses and found that self-reported social norms (e.g., friends and family that were high vegetable consumers) and attitudes had a positive association with choosing the vegetable-forward entrée. In addition, males were much less likely to choose the vegetable-forward dish than females [14].

Finally, a placement or behavior nudge might modify the listing of dishes on a menu to place healthier choices more prominently, or make the healthier choice the default (e.g., side salad not french fries). A placement study conducted with university-aged males in a laboratory setting placed vegetables at the beginning of a buffet versus the end and measured the quantity of vegetables on the plate; finding a significant increase in vegetable selection after exposure to the nudge [16].

Although there are many nudge interventions that show effectiveness, overall there is still a growing need for more real-life studies of scalable nudging strategies targeting adolescents and their food choices. In that context, this pilot study arose with the purpose of implementing a contextually feasible nudge intervention in the University of Victoria's residence cafeteria to evaluate its impact on vegetable purchases by first-year students (typically aged 17–19 years). A secondary aim was to explore whether this appeared to vary based on the sex of the participant. The hypothesis was that a placement, cognitive and sensory nudge intervention would increase the purchase of vegetables by this population of young adults and this may be more salient among females. UVIC Human Research Ethics Board approved the study (Protocol Number 15-445).

2. Materials and Methods

2.1. Formative Research and Co-Design Process

Prior to the intervention, along with a review of the literature, formative research was conducted that involved surveying students and conducting focus groups with food services staff to help inform which nudges to trial in this real-life setting with this target audience. This has been referred to in the literature as co-design, allowing for better translation of evidence to practice and resulting in a more successful implementation [17,18]. The web-based student survey asked about their demographics, their daily consumption of vegetables and fruit, and what affects their decision to purchase vegetables. Three hundred and forty adolescent (average age 18) undergraduate students responded to the survey.

On average, the adolescents reported consuming 4.6 servings of vegetables and fruit daily (excluding potatoes), approximately half of the recommended amount for their age group. The six reasons most commonly identified for choosing vegetables were (in order of most to least common) healthiness, freshness/appearance, taste/preference, cost, cooking method and convenience (see Table 1). These are similar to other studies with university students [19]. A variety of nudges from the literature that represented the study survey data were presented to food services staff in focus groups to determine which efficacious nudges were feasible for implementation within the operation, and yet addressed what was relevant to the adolescents as per the survey results. Each staff member had three votes to rank their top choices.

Table 1. Qualitative summary of the main drivers of vegetable purchase by adolescents.

Top Reasons	% of Students Citing the Reason as Important	Main Themes
Healthiness	36%	Healthy; vitamins; nutrients; feel good; good for you
Freshness	11%	Freshness; look fresh
Taste	10%	Taste; personal preference
Cost	9%	Cost; price
Cooking method	5%	Steamed vs fried; cooked; frozen; raw; added sauce
Convenience	4%	Quick; time; easy access

Table 2 shows the rankings given by staff on the feasibility of nudges. This data was presented back to the management team, including the dietitian. The co-design of the intervention was thus created jointly by the research team and food services, and the types of nudges were agreed upon by both groups.

Table 2. Ranking of nudge feasibility by the staff focus group (n = 8).

Nudge	Votes
Vegetables as default	8
Convenience 'to go'	7
Increased choice	6
Veg 1st on menu	3
Taste testing, fresh veg side	2
Enhance appearance	1
Color coded sign	0
Pathway	0

2.2. Research Design and Sampling

This pilot study utilized a quasi-experimental single case A-B-A-B comparison design. In order to measure the efficacy of the intervention, data was collected for two periods at baseline (A), the first one described the current level of vegetables purchased and the second described whether the behavior continued without the intervention or returned to baseline. The four phases were conducted during the fall term of 2016 over a 10-week period, eliminating both the first few weeks of term when students were adjusting, and the end of term, just prior to the exam period, when cafeteria use changes. Each baseline period lasted two weeks and each intervention phase was three weeks in length. See Table 3 for sample sizes.

Table 3. Number of data points and number of hot table purchases by sex and phase.

	Baseline 1	Intervention 1	Baseline 2	Intervention 2
Data points per phase	n = 10	n = 13	n = 12	n = 15
Hot Table Purchases	n	n	n	n
Females	2037	2566	2476	3063
Males	3061	3607	3278	4322
Overall	5098	6173	5754	7385

2.3. Setting

The study was conducted in the main residence cafeteria that serves mostly older adolescent students, on meal plans, who are either first-year or student staff (residence advisors). The cafeteria is not exclusive to this population, so adults that appeared visibly older than the target population of undergraduate students were excluded from the observations. The focus of the nudge was at the "hot table" or "steam line" at lunch and dinner where two choices of entrées are served along with 2–3 choices of side dishes, such as grains, other starches and hot vegetables. An example of an entrée would be lasagna or chicken breasts with mushroom sauce, grain or starches would be items, such as rice, potatoes or noodles depending on the main course, and side dish vegetables could be items such as steamed carrots, pea pods or broccoli. Students make their decisions a la carte and their purchases are charged to their student card in a declining balance.

2.4. Intervention

The nudges chosen were placement nudges that involved altering the properties of the vegetables to enhance freshness and appearance. This was implemented by adding an option of fresh, raw vegetables to the existing cooked vegetable option, in combination with an environmental cue (sensory and cognitive) in the form of a small poster displayed at eye level, which highlighted the addition of the fresh vegetable option with a colorful character and message about its health benefits (See Table 4 and Figure 1).

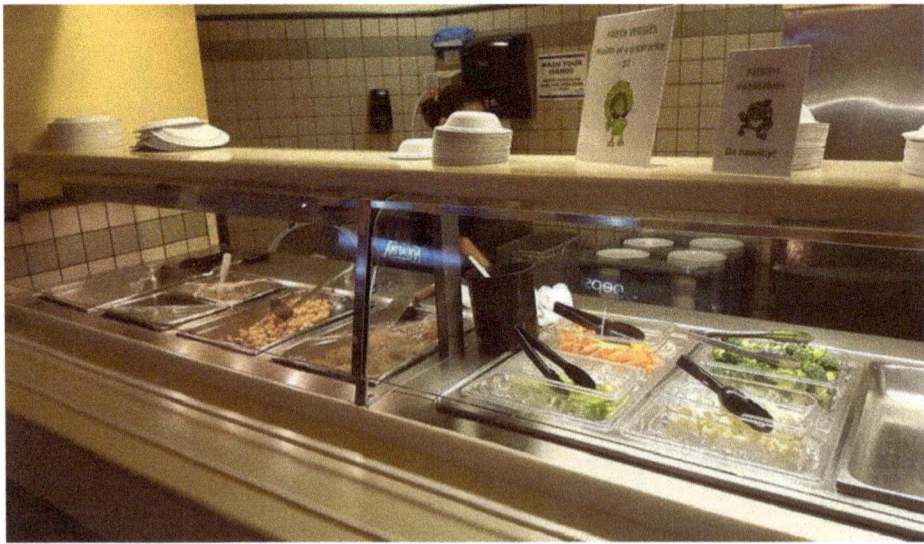

Figure 1. Display of sensory and cognitive nudges and hot table placement of fresh vegetables.

Table 4. Nudge interventions by category.

Nudge Categorizations	Study Interventions
Placement Nudge	Adding raw vegetables on the hot line, not just at the salad bar, making them easier to choose with an entrée.
Hedonistic/Sensory	Adding colourful, fresh vegetable option alongside cooked; colourful poster (see supplementary Figure S1).
Cognitive/Educational	Poster with messaging about vegetable benefits (see supplementary Tables S1–S3).

2.5. Data Collection

The primary measure was the count of students observed purchasing either one of the vegetable side options (raw or cooked) compared to the total count of students that purchased from the hot table. To address the secondary aim, the counts were recorded by sex (male or female). To provide context for the analysis, prior to each observation period the researcher also recorded all of the foods being served at the hot table and whether they were observing a lunch or dinner. The observations took place during both lunch and dinner for a period of 2 h each from a junction area of about 2.5 m distance with good visibility of the hot table and serving activities. The primary researcher recorded 80% of the observations, with trained assistants supporting the remaining observation periods. To avoid inconsistency, research assistants were provided with a 2-h orientation by the primary researcher on how to observe and track purchases.

2.6. Data Analysis

All visual and statistical analyses were made using IBM SPSS V.23® (IBM Corp, Armonk, NY, USA) and Microsoft Excel 2016® software (Redmond, WA, USA). To avoid overestimation of vegetable purchases based on cafeteria attendance, the proportion of vegetables purchased was calculated for each meal daily and then plotted in Excel, both for the overall sample and for females and males separately. Visual inspection is an accepted data analysis technique in single-case multiple baseline designs [20]. Steps in visual inspection as outlined in Kazdin [20] included: superimposing a line representing means for the phases on plots of the daily proportions and examining them visually; and calculating trend lines for each phase and superimposing them onto the data plots to allow for trend analysis where the researcher has looked for changes in the direction or slope of a trend in tandem with the change in study phase (e.g., from A to B).

Additional statistical analyses were conducted to examine mean differences between phases and trends, although, due to ascending and descending trends, these analyses had limitations. The Wilcoxon signed-ranks test was used to determine if the rank of proportions differed significantly across the phases. Descriptive statistics were also generated to allow assessment of variability (which can also be seen visually), latency and overlap between phases. Non-overlapping data refers to points during the baseline that do not reach some or any of the points during the intervention phase [20]. We used above 50%, and ideally >70%, non-overlap as the guideline for concluding efficacy [21].

3. Results

Visual inspection of the means used to assess the potential efficacy of the nudge interventions (B1, B2) showed neither intervention had an effect on the mean proportion of vegetables purchased between phases for the overall sample or for females or males analyzed separately. However, with ascending and descending trends, this was not unexpected. The results of the trend analysis are represented in Figures 2–4. During the first intervention (B1), there were visible changes in the direction of trend lines compared to baseline (A1) and withdrawal (A2) for both the overall sample and for females and males separately. During the second intervention (B2), the visible differences in trend direction and slope A-B phases were not substantive and control over the outcome variable was not fully demonstrated visually. Further analysis using the Wilcoxon signed-rank test showed that the interventions did not elicit a statistically significant change (see Table 5) in the ranking of the proportion of vegetables purchased from baseline to intervention to withdrawal in either the B1 or B2 phases, and effect sizes were small.

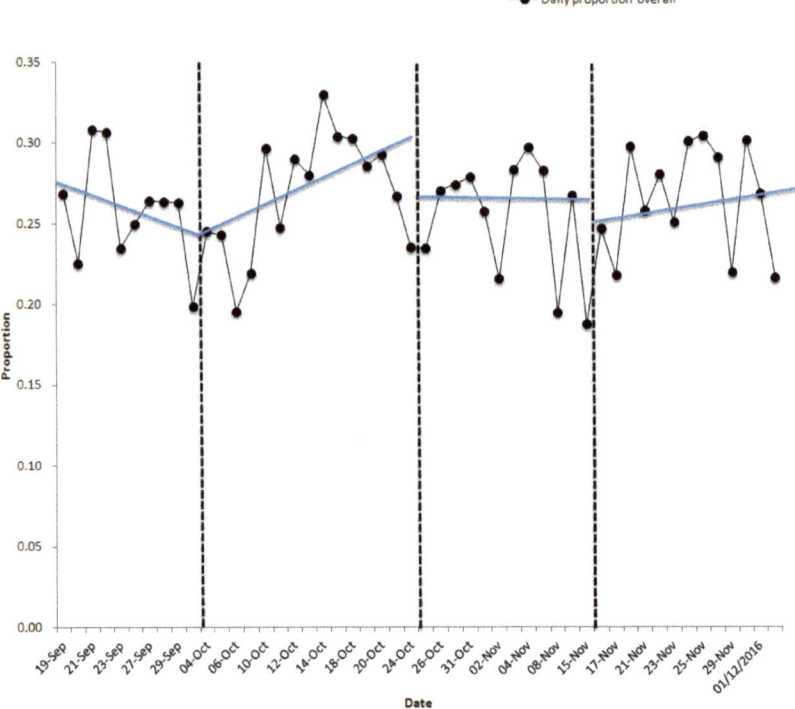

Figure 2. Proportion of vegetables purchased and trend lines across all periods for the overall sample in the university cafeteria.

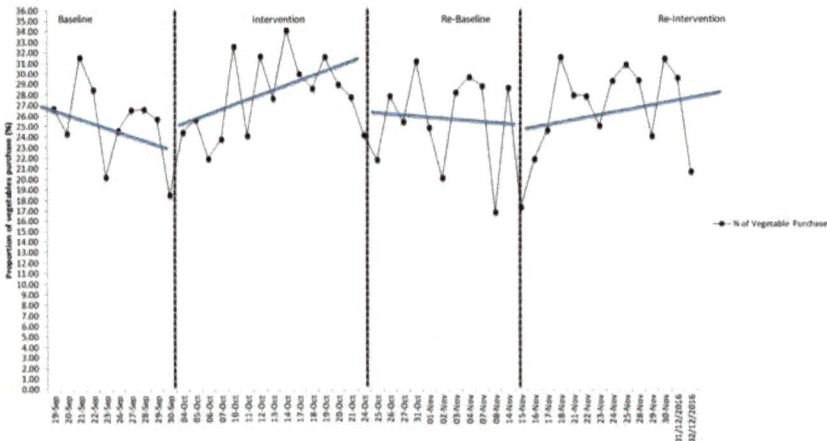

Figure 3. Proportion of vegetables purchased and trend lines across all periods for the female young adults in the university cafeteria.

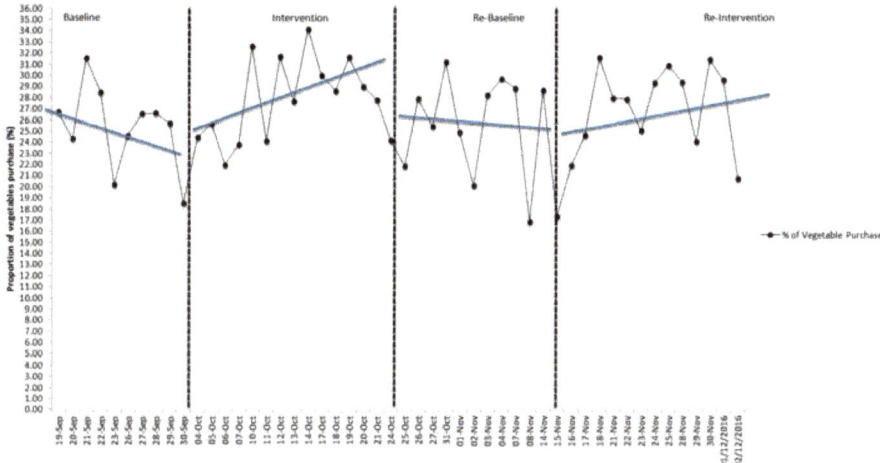

Figure 4. Proportion of vegetables purchased and trend lines across all periods for the male young adults in the university cafeteria.

Table 5. Analysis of the Wilcoxon signed-rank test across three phases with means.

Condition	A1–B1 Means (SD) Statistic, p Effect Size *	B1–A2 Means (SD) Statistic, p Effect Size *	A2–B2 Means (SD) Statistic, p Effect Size *
Overall	$\overline{X}^1 = 25.81\ (3.38)$ $\overline{X}^2 = 26.51\ (4.17)$ $Z = -0.459, p = 0.646$ $D = 0.192$	$\overline{X}^2 = 26.51\ (4.17)$ $\overline{X}^3 = 26.28\ (2.63)$ $Z = -0.561, p = 0.575$ $D = 0.226$	$\overline{X}^3 = 26.28\ (2.63)$ $\overline{X}^4 = 26.13\ (3.77)$ $Z = -0.051, p = 0.959$ $D = 0.02$
Female	$\overline{X}^1 = 25.30\ (3.78)$ $\overline{X}^2 = 28.05\ (3.70)$ $Z = -0.968, p = 0.333$ $D = 0.412$	$\overline{X}^2 = 28.05\ (3.70)$ $\overline{X}^3 = 25.33\ (4.4)$ $Z = -0.746, p = 0.445$ $D = 0.302$	$\overline{X}^3 = 25.33\ (4.4)$ $\overline{X}^4 = 26.65\ (4.25)$ $Z = -0.051, p = 0.959$ $D = 0.02$
Male	$\overline{X}^1 = 26.24\ (3.60)$ $\overline{X}^2 = 26.80\ (4.02)$ $Z = -0.255, p = 0.799$ $D = 0.106$	$\overline{X}^2 = 26.80\ (4.02)$ $\overline{X}^3 = 26.40\ (2.81)$ $Z = -0.153, p = 0.878$ $r = 0.060$	$\overline{X}^3 = 26.40\ (2.81)$ $\overline{X}^4 = 26.40\ (3.68)$ $Z = -0.051, p = 0.959$ $r = 0.010$

* Effect sizes estimated as Cohen's D using https://www.psychometrica.de/effect_size.html [22].

To be considered effective, the percentage of non-overlapping data (PND) must be >50, and ideally >70% [21], and that did not occur in this study. Overall, between the first baseline and intervention phase, the PND was 7.7%, 0% for the re-baseline, and 0% for the re-intervention (all data overlapped). For males only, the first baseline and intervention phase had 0% non-overlapping data. For both males and females, the period between re-baseline and re-intervention had 13.33% PND, and the most substantive amount of non-overlapping data was during the first baseline-intervention phase for females only; equaling 30% PND.

4. Discussion

We set out to test the efficacy of contextually relevant nudges targeting older adolescents in their first year of university by conducting a quasi-experiment A-B-A-B design trial in a natural setting: a university residence cafeteria. The evidence-based nudges were selected based on student needs and staff feasibility assessments and were thus potentially more scalable into a 'real world' setting if found efficacious. Currently, there is a need for evidence on the impact of nudge strategies on older adolescents, as well as those that have put been put into real world practice and evaluated.

Although visual inspection showed changes in the direction of trends with each presentation and with removal of the intervention, this pattern appeared to weaken over time. Visual inspection also showed high variability in the data, which was confirmed by descriptive measures of variability (standard deviation and range) and by an analysis of overlapping data challenging the strength of conclusions possible from the visual inspection. Although this was also supported by non-significant findings from the Wilcoxon signed-rank tests, the effect sizes were commensurate with the literature [9] and more substantive for females. Combining the multiple analyses conducted in this study failed to definitively support the presence of an intervention effect for the combined placement, cognitive and sensory nudges. These results, although counter to the hypothesis, may be the result of methodological (sample size) and practical limitations, but are also not out of step with other nudge studies, many of which have not shown efficacy [15,23–25]. The findings are discussed in the context of the literature below.

Despite student survey results showing that they chose vegetables for health reasons, we know that the university cafeteria and overall food environment decreases students' intention to make healthy food choices due to the plethora of less healthy foods they must navigate through at every meal opportunity [23]. A couple of research teams have surveyed students and found that health was reported as a primary consideration when choosing foods [19,23], but Bevet and colleagues found that a placement nudge intervention adding vegetable-rich entrées and a healthy snack bar could not steer students away from chicken nuggets [23].

Friis et al. (2017) tested the effects of three nudges, cognitive, placement and perceived nudges, on university-aged students in a lab setting buffet dinner. Only the 'healthy default' placement nudge (salad in 200 g jars versus the salad tray in the buffet) resulted in an increase in vegetable intake. The cognitive nudge (benefiting the environment) and perceived variety (different display of salad on the buffet) promoted a reduction in caloric intake but further examination showed that this was due to a lower intake of red meat with no increase in vegetable consumption [24].

A previous study that tested nudges with European adolescents showed that a salience nudge was not effective and highlighted the importance of other psychosocial factors, such as social norms, sex and attitudes [14]. A systematic review of interventions targeted at university-aged students showed a broader set of behavior change techniques that were effective, including nutrition education and enhanced self-regulation, as well as point-of-choice messaging (which can be classified as a cognitive or salience nudge) were effective options [26]. Sunstein (2017) discussed the reasons that nudges fail, one being strong antecedent preferences of the target [27].

A non-randomized intervention conducted by Broers and colleagues (2019) showed that cues increased selections from the hot vegetable buffet in a university cafeteria, but increasing the accessibility of pre-biotic vegetables and cues (tray liners promoting prebiotic vegetables) decreased the chances of students picking the target vegetable [28]. The variability in findings from previous nudge studies has been demonstrated in systematic reviews [9–11].

Novel attempts to educate consumers at the point of selection may be needed, rather than straight calorie labeling or cognitive messaging identifying foods as 'healthy'. Scourboutakos et al. (2017) stated that young people want more shocking educational messaging. They found an effect in their real-life university cafeteria study that used physical activity caloric equivalents (e.g., minutes exercising to burn the calories from the beverages) labeling to reduce sugary beverage purchases, despite it being an all-you-care-to-eat cafeteria where cost was not a factor in selection [13].

Strengths and Limitations

The study is one of the few nudge interventions applied in a real-world cafeteria setting and targeting adolescents. Identifying the feasibility and efficacy of scalable nudges is important for public health decision-making. The formative work to ensure the evidence-based nudges were contextually relevant to students and staff is a strength, as was the contextually relevant research design, notwithstanding the limitations described below. Additionally, numerous analytical approaches were adopted to ensure a transparent and fulsome analysis, and effect sizes commensurate with previous literature [9] were identified. Conversely, there were many limitations, which is a result of the real-life context and related research design. First, the single case A-B-A-B research design is a quasi-experimental design and relies on a return to baseline or change in the direction or slope of a trend after removal of the intervention, followed by a replication of the effect following re-presentation of the intervention to demonstrate 'control' over the effect [20]. The trend weakened over time, bringing into question whether there was an intervention effect. There appeared to be a replication of the effect, but the trend weakened over time, challenging the conclusion that there was experimental control. As discussed earlier there was high variability in the data (overlapping data was high) and data stability is also a pre-requisite to demonstrating an effect in single case designs [20].

The research design did not include a comparison group, nor were adjustments for confounding variables possible. The observation itself may have acted as a salience nudge. Furthermore, although data was collected for 4 h/day across lunch and dinner for a full university term, and a large number of meals were observed (>5000 meals per phase), it was a relatively small data set in the analysis with only one data point per day (the proportion of vegetable servings per hot table purchases).

The study would have had to have approximately 100 data points per phase to detect the effect sizes achieved between baseline and intervention phases if a parametric design was used. There were only 186 days in the university year, and implementation over the entire period was pragmatically impossible. The small to modest effect sizes between the first baseline and intervention and the second baseline were comparable to typical nudge effect sizes reported by Cadario and Chandon in 2017 [9], suggesting that a more robust sample size may have increased the likelihood of seeing a significant effect.

The intervention seemed to visibly lose efficacy over time, with minimal changes in trends in the second phase compared to the first phase. The nudges may have lost their impact due to students' familiarity with the addition of the fresh vegetables, lack of variety in the fresh vegetable offering (observed by the research assistant) and/or elements related to the signage and vegetable tray placement. For instance, the primary offering was raw carrot and celery sticks, which may be considered lower value or 'conventional' vegetables. Sunstein named five reasons why nudges may fail, and having a short-term effect was one of them, as well as strong antecedent preferences, perhaps including the preferred type of vegetables [27]. The choice of raw vegetables was out of the control of the research team and was determined by the affordability and ease of preparation by food service staff. In a future intervention, using other fresh vegetables, may increase the selection of vegetables by students [28,29].

The signage or cognitive messaging used was also limited by time and cost of designing and printing. Floor decals and large posters may have proved more effective and eye-catching. Naming the vegetables (a greater sensory nudge) and the variety and placement of the nudges may also have improved the effect [30].

Additionally, pragmatic considerations (e.g., distance from the steam unit) led cafeteria staff to place the raw vegetable trays at the end of the food offerings rather than the beginning. This may have influenced the results as previous research has shown that food positioning affects food choice [16,28]. Kongsbak et al. found that placement of vegetables in different bowls at the beginning of a buffet significantly increased selection as compared to the vegetables served altogether in one bowl and at the end of the buffet after the pasta and bread choices. This was conducted in a laboratory, not a real-world setting, and only once, so the results may have varied if issues like price and habituation were encountered, which likely occurred in this real-life study [16,27].

Other factors were elucidated by cafeteria staff anecdotally and included the financial situation of students over the term. Budgetary concerns may have resulted in the purchase of similarly priced highly satiating foods (e.g., fried potatoes, perogies) over less satiating vegetables [29]. Stressful events such as exams, projects, and the end of the term may have also influenced the students' choice for more 'comforting' foods [31]. Control over what else was available in the cafeteria (e.g., grill items, french fries) also belonged solely to the food service staff and not the researchers. That said, nudges are supposed to work without the limitation of choice to the consumer.

Another issue that developed in this setting was menu composition, which was out of the control of the research team. Specifically, the menu composition was two entrées, usually animal proteins, two starchy side dishes, one option of cooked vegetables, and during the intervention period, the raw vegetables (crudités). Often the color of the entrée was similar to the vegetable offering (observation by research staff). Also, each item was purchased a la carte at $6.95 for each entrée and $2 for each option of side dishes and vegetables. Purchasing each item separately has been shown to decrease the purchase of vegetables, while a combination of products with a fixed single price (such as an entrée plus vegetable) increases the purchase of vegetables [32–34]. Finally, the perceived value assigned to certain products may have been problematic. It is possible that students in this study perceived that $2 for a portion of vegetables was not good value and would rather spend their meal plan dollars on other, more calorically-dense items (e.g., entrées, fries, drinks, desserts) [29].

Overall, there are many more unintended nudges occurring in a cafeteria than the one being studied, for example the smell of fries, the colorful packaging of soda pop and the ordering and naming of items on a menu. Although the co-design methodology did result in staff buy-in and successful implementation, it did not prove successful in increasing adolescent student vegetable consumption despite the engagement of the target audience and their needs via the student survey. Sunstein (2017) cautioned that sometimes a "plausible (and abstractly correct) understanding about what drives human behavior turns out to be wrong in a certain context", p. 5 [27].

5. Conclusions

Co-design of interventions in real-life settings is related to better implementation, as interventions typically reflect and/or are relevant for the context [17,18]. The impact of this intervention on older adolescent vegetable purchasing remains in question but the effect sizes were promising. Thus future research should incorporate innovative research designs and achieve power in such real world contexts. Nudge researchers must also accommodate for other operational issues within the full cafeteria that may over-power the effect of small nudges in constrained areas. More research is needed in this field and specifically in this target population, where there is lower than recommended vegetable consumption and documented weight gain. Nudges in real-life settings, rather than laboratories, need to have more controls in place that also balance the operational needs of the food service establishment. They may also need to be strengthened or speak to the 'actual' issues of the target population using more salient cognitive messages, innovative use of social media and reflect current food trends. Interventions may need to be incentivized to mitigate decreases in consumption and establish healthy eating habits throughout the lifespan [26]. These findings will inform re-design and testing of future nudges. in real world settings.

Supplementary Materials: The following are available online at http://www.mdpi.com/2072-6643/11/8/1786/s1, Figure S1: Specific signage images used as cognitive educational nudge, Table S1. Breakdown in numbers and percentage of cooked and fresh vegetables for the overall sample by phase, Table S2. Breakdown numbers and percentage of cooked and fresh vegetables for the female sample by phase, Table S3. Breakdown numbers and percentage of cooked and fresh vegetables for the male sample by phase.

Author Contributions: M.M., D.T. and P.-J.N. designed and implemented the trial. M.M. collected the data. M.M., D.T. and P.-J.N. analysed data and prepared initial drafts of reports and a thesis that served as the basis of the manuscript. N.F. helped to implement the study, drafted the final manuscript integrating sections of the reports and thesis. All authors co-edited.

Funding: This research was supported by funding from the British Columbia Ministry of Health.

Acknowledgments: The authors acknowledge the support by University of Victoria Food Services staff and management as well as the graduate student research assistants, without whom this research would not have been possible.

Conflicts of Interest: The authors declare no conflict of interest.

References

1. Wang, X.; Ouyang, Y.; Liu, J.; Zhu, M.; Zhao, G.; Bao, W.; Hu, F.B. Fruit and vegetable consumption and mortality from all causes, cardiovascular disease, and cancer: Systematic review and dose-response meta-analysis of prospective cohort studies. *BMJ* **2014**, *349*, g4490. [CrossRef] [PubMed]
2. Leone, R.J.; Morgan, A.L.; Ludy, M.J. Patterns and Composition of Weight Change in College Freshmen. *Coll. Stud. J.* **2015**, *49*, 553–564. [CrossRef]
3. Larson, N.; Laska, M.; Story, M.; Neumark-Sztainer, D. Predictors of Fruit and Vegetable Intake in Young Adulthood. *J. Acad. Nutr. Diet.* **2012**, *112*, 1216–1222. [CrossRef] [PubMed]
4. Kelder, S.; Perry, C.; Klepp, K.; Lytle, L. Longitudinal tracking of adolescent smoking, physical activity, and food choice behaviors. *Am. J. Public Health* **1994**, *84*, 1121–1126. [CrossRef] [PubMed]
5. Pope, L.; Hansen, D.; Harvey, J. Examining the Weight Trajectory of College Students. *J. Nutr. Educ. Behav.* **2017**, *49*, 137–141. [CrossRef] [PubMed]
6. Olstad, D.; Vermeer, J.; McCargar, L.; Prowse, R.; Raine, K. Using traffic light labels to improve food selection in recreation and sport facility eating environments. *Appetite* **2015**, *91*, 329–335. [CrossRef] [PubMed]
7. Thaler, R.H.; Sunstein, C.R.; Balz, J.P. Choice Architecture. Available online: http://dx.doi.org/10.2139/ssrn.1583509 (accessed on 2 April 2010).
8. Blumenthal-Barby, J.; Burroughs, H. Seeking Better Health Care Outcomes: The Ethics of Using the "Nudge". *Am. J. Bioeth.* **2012**, *12*, 1–10. [CrossRef] [PubMed]
9. Cadario, R.; Chandon, P. Which Healthy Eating Nudges Work Best? A Meta-Analysis of Field Experiments. *SSRN Mark. Sci.* **2017**. [CrossRef]
10. Arno, A.; Thomas, S. The efficacy of nudge theory strategies in influencing adult dietary behaviour: A systematic review and meta-analysis. *BMC Public Health* **2016**, *16*, 676. [CrossRef]
11. Wilson, A.; Buckley, E.; Buckley, J.; Bogomolova, S. Nudging healthier food and beverage choices through salience and priming. Evidence from a systematic review. *Food Qual. Prefer.* **2016**, *51*, 47–64. [CrossRef]
12. Nørnberg, T.; Houlby, L.; Skov, L.; Peréz-Cueto, F. Choice architecture interventions for increased vegetable intake and behaviour change in a school setting: A systematic review. *Perspect. Public Health* **2016**, *136*, 132–142. [CrossRef] [PubMed]
13. Scourboutakos, M.J.; Mah, C.L.; Murphy, S.A.; Mazza, F.N.; Barrett, N.; McFadden, B.; L'Abbé, M.R. Testing a Beverage and Fruit/Vegetable Education Intervention in a University Dining Hall. *J. Nutr. Educ. Behav.* **2017**, *49*, 457–465. [CrossRef] [PubMed]
14. dos Santos, Q.; Federico, S.; Cueto, J.; Mello, V.; Rodrigues, K.; Giboreau, A.; Saulais, L.; Monteleone, E.; Dinnella, C.; Brugarolos, M.; et al. Impact of a nudging intervention and factors associated with vegetable dish choice among European adolescents. *Eur. J. Nutr.* **2019**. [CrossRef] [PubMed]
15. dos Santos, Q.; Vanessa, N.; Rodrigues, M.; Hartwell, H.; Giboro, A.; Monteleone, E.; Dinnella, C.; Perez-cueto, F. Nudging using the 'dish of the day' strategy does not work for plant-based meals in a Danish sample of adolescent and older adults. *Int. J. Consum. Stud.* **2018**, *42*, 327–334. [CrossRef]
16. Kongsbak, I.; Skov, L.R.; Nielsen, B.K.; Ahlmann, F.K.; Schaldemose, H.; Atkinson, L.; Pérez-Cueto, F.J.A. Increasing fruit and vegetable intake among male university students in an ad libitum buffet setting: A choice architectural nudge intervention. *Food Qual. Prefer.* **2016**, *49*, 183–188. [CrossRef]
17. Glasgow, R.E.; Lichtenstein, C.; Marcus, A.C. Why don't we see more translation of health promotion research to practice? Rethinking the efficacy-to-effectiveness transition. *Am. J. Public Health* **2003**, *93*, 1261–1267. [CrossRef] [PubMed]
18. Buckley, B.; Thijssen, D.; Murphy, R.; Graves, L.; Whyte, G.; Gillison, F.; Crone, D.; Wilson, P.; Hindley, D.; Watson, P. Preliminary effects and acceptability of a co-produced physical activity referral intervention. *Health Educ. J.* **2019**, 0017896919853322. [CrossRef]
19. Tam, R.; Yassa, B.; Parker, H.; O'Connor, H.; Allman-Farinelli, M. University students' on-campus food purchasing behaviors, preferences, and opinions on food availability. *Nutrition* **2017**, *37*, 7–13. [CrossRef] [PubMed]
20. Kazdin, A. *Single-Case Research Designs*; Oxford University Press: New York, NY, USA, 1982.
21. Scruggs, T.E.; Mastropieri, M.A. How to Summarize Single-Participant Research: Ideas and Applications. *Exceptionality* **2001**, *9*, 227–244. [CrossRef]

22. Lenhard, D. Computation of Different Effect Sizes Like d, f, r and Transformation of Different Effect Sizes: Psychometrica. 2019. Available online: https://www.psychometrica.de/effect_size.html (accessed on 18 July 2019).
23. Bevet, S.; Niles, M.; Pope, L. You can't "nudge" nuggets: An investigation of college late-night dining with behavioral economics interventions. *PloS ONE* **2018**, *13*, e0198162. [CrossRef]
24. Friis, R.; Skov, L.; Olsen, A.; Appleton, K.M.; Saulais, L.; Dinnella, C.; Hartwell, H.; Depezay, L.; Monteleone, E.; Giboreau, A.; et al. Comparison of three nudge interventions (priming, default option, and perceived variety) to promote vegetable consumption in a self-service buffet setting. *PLoS ONE* **2017**, *12*, e0176028. [CrossRef] [PubMed]
25. Steenhuis, I. The impact of educational and environmental interventions in Dutch worksite cafeterias. *Health Promot. Int.* **2004**, *19*, 335–343. [CrossRef] [PubMed]
26. Deliens, T.; Van Crombruggen, R.; Verbruggen, S.; De Bourdeaudhuij, I.; Deforche, B.; Clarys, P. Dietary interventions among university students: A systematic review. *Appetite* **2016**, *105*, 14–26. [CrossRef] [PubMed]
27. Sunstein, C.R. Nudges that fail. *Behav. Public Policy* **2017**, *1*, 4–25. [CrossRef]
28. Broers, V.; Van den Broucke, S.; Taverne, C.; Luminet, O. Investigating the conditions for the effectiveness of nudging: Cue-to-action nudging increases familiar vegetable choice. *Food Qual. Prefer.* **2019**, *71*, 366–374. [CrossRef]
29. Pollard, J.; Kirk, S.; Cade, J. Factors affecting food choice in relation to fruit and vegetable intake: A review. *Nutr. Res. Rev.* **2002**, *15*, 373. [CrossRef]
30. Turnwald, B.P.; Boles, D.Z.; Crum, A.J. Association Between Indulgent Descriptions and Vegetable Consumption: Twisted Carrots and Dynamite Beets. *JAMA Int. Med.* **2017**, *177*, 1216–1218. [CrossRef]
31. Sulkowski, M.; Dempsey, J.; Dempsey, A. Effects of stress and coping on binge eating in female college students. *Eat. Behav.* **2011**, *12*, 188–191. [CrossRef]
32. Bucher, T.; van der Horst, K.; Siegrist, M. Improvement of meal composition by vegetable variety. *Public Health Nutr.* **2011**, *14*, 1357–1363. [CrossRef]
33. Carroll, K.A.; Samek, A.S.; Zepeda, L. Product bundling as a behavioral nudge: Investigating consumer fruit and vegetable selection using Dual-Self Theory. In Proceedings of the Agricultural and Applied Economics Association, 2016 Annual Meeting, Boston, MA, USA, 31 July–2 August 2016.
34. Harris, J. Consumer Preference for Product Bundles: The Role of Reduced Search Costs. *J. Acad. Mark. Sci.* **2006**, *34*, 506–513. [CrossRef]

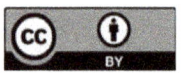

© 2019 by the authors. Licensee MDPI, Basel, Switzerland. This article is an open access article distributed under the terms and conditions of the Creative Commons Attribution (CC BY) license (http://creativecommons.org/licenses/by/4.0/).

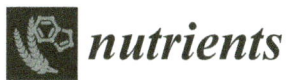

Article

Healthy Planet, Healthy Youth: A Food Systems Education and Promotion Intervention to Improve Adolescent Diet Quality and Reduce Food Waste

Melissa Pflugh Prescott [1,*], Xanna Burg [1], Jessica Jarick Metcalfe [1], Alexander E. Lipka [2], Cameron Herritt [3] and Leslie Cunningham-Sabo [3]

[1] Department of Food Science and Human Nutrition, University of Illinois at Urbana-Champaign, Champaign, IL 61820, USA
[2] Department of Crop Sciences, University of Illinois at Urbana-Champaign, Champaign, IL 61820, USA
[3] Department of Food Science and Human Nutrition, Colorado State University, Fort Collins, CO 80523, USA
* Correspondence: mpp22@illinois.edu; Tel.: +(217)-300-7489

Received: 28 June 2019; Accepted: 8 August 2019; Published: 11 August 2019

Abstract: Emerging evidence suggests a link between young people's interest in alternative food production practices and dietary quality. The primary purpose of this study was to examine the impact of a student-driven sustainable food systems education and promotion intervention on adolescent school lunch selection, consumption, and waste behaviors. Sixth grade science teachers at two middle schools (n = 268 students) implemented a standards-based curriculum on sustainable food systems, addressing the environmental impacts of food choices and food waste. The cumulating curriculum activity required the 6th grade students to share their food systems knowledge with their 7th and 8th grade counterparts (n = 426) through a cafeteria promotional campaign to discourage food waste. School-wide monthly plate waste assessments were used to evaluate changes in vegetable consumption and overall plate waste using a previously validated digital photography method. At baseline, the intervention students consumed significantly less vegetables relative to the control group (47.1% and 71.8% of vegetables selected, respectively (p = 0.006). This disparity was eliminated after the intervention with the intervention group consuming 69.4% and the control consuming 68.1% of selected vegetables (p = 0.848). At five months follow up, the intervention group wasted significantly less salad bar vegetables compared to the control group (24.2 g and 50.1 g respectively (p = 0.029). These findings suggest that food systems education can be used to promote improved dietary behaviors among adolescent youth.

Keywords: food systems; school nutrition; food waste; adolescents; implementation science

1. Introduction

School meal programs combat childhood hunger and inadequate nutrition by providing children with the nutrients needed for physical and educational development. These programs also present an important opportunity to simultaneously address child diet quality and food waste. About 95% of U.S. children aged 9–18 do not meet the federal dietary recommendations for vegetable intake [1–3], and childhood obesity continues to be a major public health problem [4]. U.S. Students who participate in both the National School Lunch Program (NSLP) and School Breakfast Program consume up to 47% of their daily energy intake from school meals [5], and school nutrition programs reduce household income disparities in adolescent fruit and vegetable intake [6]. Strengthened nutrition standards mandated under the Healthy, Hunger-Free Kids Act of 2010 (HHFKA) promote important improvements to school meal programs, such as increasing vegetable variety, offering only low- and non-fat milk, and establishing meal calorie minimums and maximums [7]. However, concerns about the amount of food selected but not consumed by students [8] threaten the viability of these standards [9,10]. Additionally, wasted food squanders the natural resources used to derive food and is a major contributor to climate change [11,12]. Traditional nutrition education interventions that target students' selection, consumption, and waste of fruits and vegetables during school meals are rarely effective past the short-term [13,14], suggesting that a novel approach is warranted.

Emerging evidence suggests a link between young people's interest in alternative food production practices, like locally grown foods and foods grown using sustainable agricultural techniques, and dietary quality [15,16]. Yet, the limited available evidence suggests adolescents may not be aware of the impact that their eating behaviors have on the environment [17]. Researchers in the United Kingdom [18], Canada [19], and Australia [20] have demonstrated the intersection between food systems and health in the public school setting, and in the United States, food systems education is considered a form of farm-to-school programs [21,22]. A recent systematic literature review of farm-to-school programs questioned the feasibility of incorporating these interventions into classroom curricula and identified the failure to quantify intervention fidelity as one of the major limitations of existing research on these programs [23]. Schools have educational priorities that may compete with health priorities [24], and the constrained budget, time, and staff of school systems [25,26] can make it difficult to sustain school-based health interventions in the short and long term. This makes schools an ideal setting for implementation science research, which examines the effective dissemination and implementation of evidence-based interventions in the real world, with a focus on evaluating program feasibility, acceptability, and fidelity [27].

Middle schools are an ideal setting for our student intervention since lessons on food systems concepts are well aligned with the academic learning standards required for middle school (grades 6–8) [28]. Also, compared to younger children, adolescent students are making more of their own food choices and may be better able to connect their food choice and waste actions to health and environmental consequences. Yet, there is little information on the impact of food systems education in this age group. The primary purpose of this study was to examine the impact of a student-driven sustainable food systems education and promotion intervention on adolescents' food selection, consumption, and waste behaviors, particularly for fruits and vegetables, during school lunch. In addition, we aimed to understand the influence of the intervention on students' knowledge and attitudes towards the food system and to estimate the intervention acceptability and fidelity.

2. Materials and Methods

2.1. Study Design and Setting

The Healthy Planet, Healthy Youth (HPHY) study used an experimental embedded mixed methods design [29], in which the qualitative data were embedded within and generally played a supportive role in the non-randomized controlled trial which was primarily based on quantitative data. Figure 1 details the sequence of study events with qualitative data indicated by yellow boxes and quantitative date in blue boxes. In addition, a community-based participatory research approach was used [30], which promotes the value of community members as equal partners throughout the research process. The HPHY Advisory Committee met quarterly the year prior to the intervention and semi-annually during the intervention year. The HPHY Advisory Committee included school nutrition staff from three local school districts, staff from the state office of school nutrition, and university faculty with a variety of expertise, including science education, food safety, nutrition, and agricultural economics. HPHY was implemented in two Colorado middle schools within the same school district. The school nutrition programs at both middle schools had salad bars, scheduled lunch periods lasting 30–32 min, and offer vs. serve provisions which allowed students to decline some of the foods offered. The Blinded for Review Institutional Review Board approved this project.

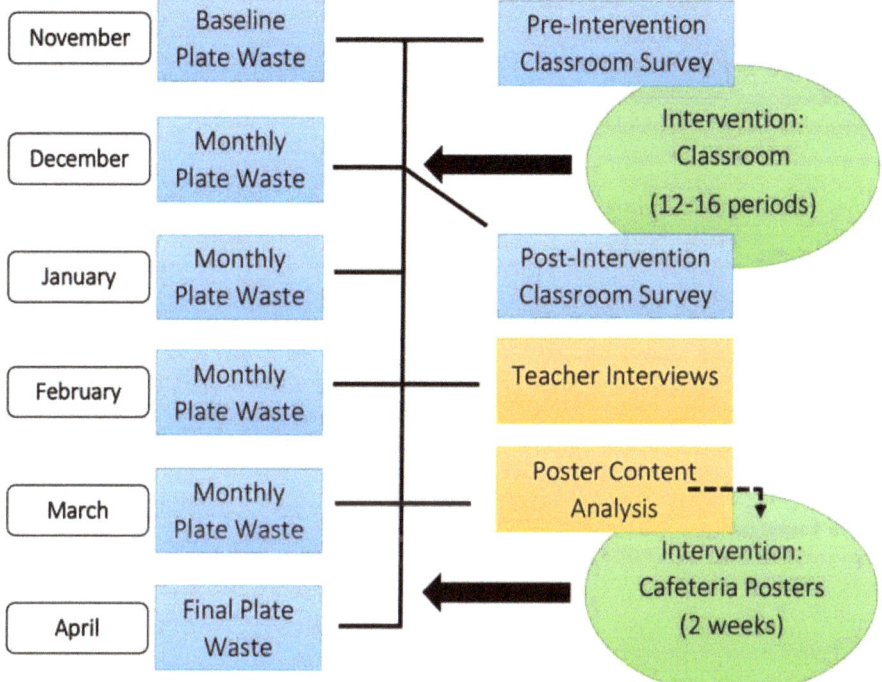

Figure 1. Overview of the Healthy Planet, Healthy Youth experimental embedded mixed methods design, including timeline of intervention and data collection. Rectangular elements illustrate data collection, where blue signifies quantitative data and yellow signifies qualitative data. Oval elements illustrate intervention points and duration of intervention. The dotted line indicates that the poster content analysis results were used to develop the cafeteria poster intervention.

2.2. Participant Selection and Recruitment

The local school district's science education coordinator circulated recruiting advertisements to 6th grade science teachers via email. The district school nutrition program was actively involved in the HPHY Advisory Committee, facilitating engagement with the kitchen managers at the recruited middle schools. Participating teachers were provided a $250 cash incentive for their time, a copy of the curriculum, curriculum supplies, a one-hour in person training, and a curriculum outline that provided suggestions for how to amend the original curriculum so that it could be delivered in a shorter time frame.

All sixth-grade students enrolled in the science classes taught by the recruited teachers received the food system education intervention implemented as a unit during their science class. No parental consent, nor student assent, was required to receive the intervention, but written parental consent and electronic student assent were provided for all students participating in the classroom pre- and post-surveys. Verbal student assent was provided for all 6th–8th grade students participating in the monthly plate waste assessments and voting on food systems promotion posters; these two activities qualified for a waiver of parental consent.

2.3. Intervention and Theoretical Underpinnings

HPHY draws upon the Self-Determination Theory (SDT) [31], which underscores the importance of motivation quality, ranging from intrinsic to amotivation. In addition, SDT theorizes that people are more likely to achieve intrinsic motivation when their basic needs for autonomy, competence, and relatedness are met. In particular, the current study aimed to satisfy the participants' need for relatedness by incorporating curriculum activities that facilitated student interactions, such as group projects and voting for food systems posters. Through these interactions we hypothesized that the intervention would nurture shared values of environmental conservation among students and would increase their motivation to make healthy food choices and waste less food.

An abbreviated version of an existing curriculum, Farm to Table and Beyond (FTTB) [28], was used for this intervention. This curriculum was selected since it is aligned to the required 6th grade science academic standards. The principal investigator and a local retired science teacher reviewed the entire curriculum and selected five lessons from FTTB that were central to the research questions, appeared feasible to implement, and provided maximum academic benefit to science teachers. These units included: Introduction to the Food System, Environmental Impacts of Food, Food Changes as it Moves through the Food System, Food Waste, and School Cafeteria Waste. Teachers were also encouraged to implement a supplementary lesson on Transporting Food. As a part of the School Cafeteria Waste lesson, students were tasked with estimating their personal lunch food waste over the course of one week. Teachers helped the students aggregate and graph the data as a part of a class project. For the culminating intervention project, students were asked to create a poster to teach the 7th–8th grade students in their school the most important thing they learned in the food systems unit.

For the promotion part of the intervention, researchers conducted a content analysis of the posters and used the findings to create professional-quality posters to promote waste reduction during school meals. At each school, the 6th–8th grade students voted on which poster they liked best using bingo chips, and the two posters with the most votes were hung in each school's cafeteria during the final month of the intervention.

2.4. Measures and Data Collection

2.4.1. Qualitative Measures and Data Collection

The qualitative data consisted of student posters and teacher interviews. Students at one school created individual posters, and the other created posters in groups; all were digitally photographed. Student names were removed or obstructed during photography. Teacher interviews were conducted using a structured interview protocol, audiotaped, and transcribed verbatim. Protocol questions included inquiries on overall feedback and adaptations used for each lesson, facilitators, and barriers to implementing the intervention, and the sustainability of the intervention. Transcriptions were assessed for quality. Written informed consent was acquired for each interview participant.

2.4.2. Classroom Survey Measures and Data Collection

We adapted an existing 46-item, unpublished survey targeting 5th to 6th graders to evaluate FTTB [28]. The original FTTB survey focused on the nature and human relationship, student interest in science, and their attitudes towards healthy foods. We used a three-step process to ensure the validity and reliability of our adapted survey. First, we assessed survey constructs for our project by holding two 60-min focus groups (1 for boys, 1 for girls) with 8th grade students and revised survey items accordingly. Second, individual 30-min cognitive interviews were completed in July–August 2017 with rising middle school students at a school district summer program to establish face validity of the revised survey questions. The survey was updated to improve participant comprehension and promote increased congruence between researcher and participant understanding of key terms used in the survey [32,33]. Third, an online survey repeated twice within a 10–21 day timeframe assessed test-retest reliability. Participants ($n = 65$) were recruited through a direct mailing list of local families with children aged 11–13. Unreliable survey questions were not used in further analyses. Reliable survey questions were grouped according to pre-identified themes based upon the self-determination theory and curriculum units: relatedness, regulatory style, stewardship, food processing, local food, natural resources, packaging, food waste, climate change, food systems, and transport. Themes with at least two items showing acceptable internal consistency (Cronbach's alpha greater than 0.7) were used in analysis. Final classroom survey scales included: relatedness (6 items), regulatory style (7 items), natural resources (2 items), and food packaging (3 items). Three food waste items that were reliable but did not fit into a scale score were also included.

2.4.3. School Meal Component Selection, Consumption, and Waste Data Collection

Plate waste data collection was conducted one day per month for six months (November 2017–April 2018; Figure 1) at each school using a previously validated digital photography method [34–36]. Monthly plate waste assessments for each school typically occurred within seven calendar days of each other. Plate waste dates were chosen after consulting with the school principal to work around school events and field trips and according to the availability of research staff. Students had no advance knowledge of when data would be collected and were not told that the plate waste measures were related to the classroom curricular intervention. The baseline plate waste collection occurred prior to the start of the classroom lessons. Students went through the lunch serving line using the normal school procedures. Trained researchers met students at the cashier, obtained verbal assent, and completed tray tags to indicate the sex, grade, and selected food items for each student. Tray tags were pre-printed with the day's menu options. Researchers circled the selected entrees, hot vegetables, whole fruit, beverages, and a la carte items on the tray tag, and documented selected salad bar items and the corresponding visual estimates of served portions. After students were finished eating lunch, their tray was brought to the research station located near the garbage cans. Researchers labeled trays with a unique tray number, measured beverage waste to the nearest 0.5 ounce using a liquid measuring cup, and then photographed the remaining food on the tray against a reference board with the camera 26 inches above at a 45-degree angle. Three to five reference foods of each item served that day were collected and photographed prior to the start of lunch. Reference foods were taken back to the lab and weighed to the nearest 0.5 g. An average weight for each reference food was calculated from the three to five reference food samples.

Photographs were independently, visually assessed for the percent of each food item wasted by two, trained researchers. A third researcher, experienced in the digital photography plate waste method, compared the two assessments. Estimates for percent wasted were confirmed identical or were averaged if the two estimates were within 20%. The third researcher reconciled any percent wasted estimates that differed more than 20%. Standardized weights and standardized percent wasted amounts were used when possible, such as items that could be broken down by food component (i.e., bread and bun estimates for sandwiches). Reference food weights were merged with portion/amount taken and percent wasted estimates to calculate the weight of each food item wasted.

2.4.4. Research Staff Data Trainings

Researchers attended a 1.5-h data collector training which consisted of an overview of the study purpose and rationale, review of the data collection protocol and data collection sheets, hands-on practice assessing menu items selection and estimation of salad bar portion size selection, and expectations for professional conduct. The 1-h data analysis training consisted of an overview of the study purpose and rationale, orientation to reference photographs and standardized percent wasted amounts, and practice assessing the percent wasted of actual participant lunch trays.

2.5. Data Analyses

2.5.1. Qualitative Analyses

Teacher interview transcripts were analyzed using ATLAS.ti (Version 8.0.4; Berlin, Germany, 2017). We used a single researcher, two-pass hybrid deductive–inductive qualitative approach, where the implementation science research questions informed the initial codebook and additional unique themes emerged during the coding process [37].

Digital photographs of student posters were also analyzed using ATLAS.ti (Version 8.0.4; Berlin, Germany, 2017). Seven food systems themes were identified a priori based upon the curriculum content and feedback interviews with classroom teachers: food waste prevention, food recovery, prevention of other related waste (packaging, food implements), recycling, reasons to reduce waste, natural resources, and growing your own food. A two-pass deductive content analysis coding method [38] was used by a single researcher to classify student messages written and drawn on the posters utilizing these a priori themes, and descriptive statistics were used to explore differences in theme frequencies across schools.

2.5.2. Classroom Survey Pre and Post Data Analyses

Classroom survey analyses were completed using R 3.4.1 and the following packages: dplyr, ggplot2, lme4, lmerTest, and emmeans. Statistical significance was set at $\alpha = 0.05$. The overall mean for each outcome measure was calculated for pre and post and compared using a paired t-test or paired Wilcoxon signed-rank test (for non-normal data). The mean difference between pre and post (post score − pre score) was calculated for each outcome measure by school and schools were compared using a Wilcoxon signed-rank test. Linear mixed models were used to assess change in outcome measures over time. All models included an individual random effect for unique subject ID to account for repeated measures (pre and post). Demographic factors (school, sex, race, ethnicity, how a student eats lunch, farm experience, garden experience, and cooking frequency) were included as fixed effects in all models to assess whether demographic groups differed in the outcome measure. For the demographic factors that had different pre to post trends, interaction terms were added individually to the mixed model to assess differences by demographic groups. Farm experience and garden experience were continuous variables calculated from a multiple answer question, where zero represented no experience and each additional experience (total of four for farming and three for gardening) added one. Cooking frequency was also a continuous variable from zero to seven and represented the average number of days per week a student helped make breakfast, lunch, dinner, and snacks. For each outcome measure, the model with the lowest Akaike information criterion was considered the final model for interpretation. Model assumptions were checked using the residuals versus fitted plots and Q-Q plots. Model results for fixed effects were investigated using a Type 3 ANOVA table, and estimated marginal means were used to investigate contrasts between time points and demographic factors.

2.5.3. Plate Waste Data Analyses

Plate waste data analyses were completed using SPSS software (Version 24; Armonk, NY, USA, 2016). Statistical significance was set at $\alpha = 0.05$. Descriptive statistics (overall means or frequencies for each outcome variable) were calculated for the intervention (6th graders) and control groups (7th–8th graders) at each of the six time points (pre-intervention through five month follow-up).

Food selection outcomes were binary (1 = student selected item from food group, 0 = student did not select item from food group) and were presented as the percent of participants who selected items from each food group (vegetables, fruit, entrée, and milk). Food consumption outcomes were continuous and expressed as the percent of each food group (vegetables, fruit, entrée, and milk) that each participant consumed. Food waste outcomes were continuous and expressed as the weight (in grams for solid food items, in fluid ounces for milk) of the food that was wasted or thrown away at the end of lunch. The vegetable selection and waste variables included both hot vegetables and vegetables from the salad bar, and the fruit selection and waste variables included both whole fruits and fruit from the salad bar. Logistic regression analyses controlling for participants' gender and school were used to assess differences between the intervention and control group in food selection outcomes (vegetables, fruit, entrée, and milk) at key time points (pre-intervention, post-intervention, and five month follow-up). Two-way ANCOVAs were used to analyze the effect of condition (intervention vs. control group) and time point on food consumption and waste outcomes (vegetables, fruit, entrée, and milk). These analyses controlled for participants' gender, the school that they attended, and the percent of entrée consumed. Estimated marginal means (adjusted to account for the influence of control variables) were used to compare outcomes between the intervention and control group. Post-hoc analyses (with Tukey corrections) were used to determine whether there were significant differences between the intervention and control group in consumption and waste at key time points (pre-intervention, post-intervention, and five month follow-up). These logistic regression and ANCOVA analyses were also repeated with school A and school B individually to investigate differences in outcomes by school.

3. Results

The HPHY education and promotion intervention was delivered to approximately 268 6th grade students between the two schools, and an additional 650 students in 7th–8th grade were exposed to the promotional food systems posters in the cafeteria (Table 1). There were four total 6th grade science teachers between the two schools, and all of them agreed to deliver the classroom intervention. The results section provides findings for the intervention fidelity and feasibility, poster content analyses, classroom survey, and plate waste outcomes.

Table 1. Demographic characteristics of intervention schools ($n = 2$) and sample demographics of students participating in the classroom survey.

	School A	School B
School Enrollment [1]		
Total	568	129
Sex, n (%)		
Male	297 (52%)	64 (50%)
Female	271 (48%)	65 (50%)
Race, n (%) [2]		
White	254 (45%)	106 (82%)
Hispanic	274 (48%)	10 (8%)
Non-White or Non-Hispanic	40 (7%)	13 (10%)
Classroom Survey Sample		
Total	56	41
Sex, n (%)		
Male	23 (41%)	20 (49%)
Female	31 (55%)	19 (46%)
Not reported	2 (4%)	2 (5%)
Age, mean (SD)	11.31 (0.47)	11.32 (0.52)
Race, n (%) [3]		
White	40 (71%)	32 (78%)
Non-White	6 (11%)	3 (7%)
Unsure or not reported	10 (18%)	6 (15%)
Ethnicity, n (%)		
Hispanic/Latino	12 (21%)	5 (12%)
Not Hispanic/Latino	34 (61%)	29 (71%)
Not sure or not reported	10 (18%)	7 (17%)
How students eat lunch on school days, n (%)		
School lunch	25 (45%)	14 (34%)
Bring lunch from home	11 (20%)	15 (37%)
Combination of school lunch and food from home	11 (20%)	6 (15%)
Choose not to eat lunch	4 (7%)	5 (12%)
Not reported	5 (9%)	1 (2%)

Table 1. *Cont.*

	School A	School B
Farm Experience [4], n (%)		
Live on a farm	2 (4%)	3 (7%)
Worked on a farm before	14 (25%)	10 (24%)
Family member works on a farm	8 (14%)	6 (15%)
Visited a farm before	29 (52%)	23 (56%)
No farm experience	4 (7%)	4 (10%)
Not reported	14 (25%)	3 (7%)
Garden Experience [4], n (%)		
Garden at home	23 (41%)	23 (56%)
Help with school/community garden	6 (11%)	4 (10%)
Gardened in the past	19 (34%)	15 (37%)
Do not garden	2 (4%)	5 (12%)
Not reported	14 (25%)	3 (7%)
Cooking frequency [5] (overall), mean (SD)	3.85 (1.84)	3.35 (1.91)
Breakfast	4.17 (2.48)	3.02 (2.67)
Lunch	3.00 (2.27)	2.81 (2.20)
Dinner	3.41 (2.57)	3.08 (2.44)
Snacks	4.66 (2.48)	4.43 (2.65)

Notes: *SD*: standard deviation; [1] School enrollment is for grades 6 to 8 only and sourced from administrative data. [2] Non-White or Non-Hispanic races include Black, Asian, American Indian or Alaska Native, and 2+ Races; [3] Non-White races include Black, Asian, American Indian or Alaska Native, Native Hawaiian or Other Pacific Islander, 2+ Races, and Other; [4] Student could choose multiple responses, so percentages do not sum to 100%; [5] Cooking frequency was reported as average days per week each student helped prepare the specified meal; results are average days per week; overall is the average of all meal categories.

3.1. Intervention Fidelity

Table 2 summarizes the student activities for each lesson. Few lessons were implemented as suggested in the curriculum outline. One universal adaption was incorporating suggested homework activities into classroom learning since neither school typically assigned science homework. For school A, one lesson was omitted and substituted with a video due to standardized testing-related changes to the daily school schedule that made it difficult to implement an interactive learning activity across all class periods. In School B, one class period was omitted due to overlap in the previous month's science unit on climate change. In addition, the teacher at School B thought that her school was already progressively handling the food waste issue since they donate all cafeteria food scraps to a local pig farmer and omitted the Cafeteria Waste Inventory unit.

3.2. Teacher Feedback on Implementation: Feasibility, Acceptability, and Fidelity

Three of the four intervention teachers participated in individual interviews. Thematic analyses yielded six themes: age-appropriate content, student engagement, barriers and facilitators, teacher engagement, and building on related science topics. Definitions for each theme and example quotes are provided in Table 3. Taken together, the interview data underscore the importance of engaging teachers, as well as students. Teachers were overwhelmed with classroom time constraints and juggling the wide span of abilities among their students but reported that the freedom to tailor the curriculum to the needs of their students, amend lessons based on prior curricular topics, and adjust lessons due to school schedule changes were paramount to successfully implementing the intervention. In-person training, support from researchers, and an outline of strategies to amend the curriculum were also universally viewed as key facilitators.

Table 2. Intervention implementation summary by school.

	Summary of Class Activities Implemented	
Curriculum Unit: Aim	School A	School B
Introduction to the Food System: To assess what we already know about the food system and how it affects the environment	Students selected a food item of their choice and drew a diagram of all the steps that the food goes through from farm to table.	Students drew diagrams of the steps that apples and applesauce go through from farm to table.
Transporting Food: To gain an understanding of the role transportation systems play in food systems. (This was an optional supplementary lesson.)	Lesson omitted.	Students were each assigned information summaries to review about one of the following: food transport via airplane, railroads, inland waterways, ocean freighter, or truck. Later, students were put into groups with students who had been assigned different transport options from themselves. Each student had to teach their group about the advantages and disadvantages of their assigned method of food transport.
Environmental Impacts: To construct knowledge about the importance and use of natural resources, including fossil fuels	Students did a Point of View activity where they were each assigned different roles to play at a town meeting, such as Soil Scientist or Food-Packaging Manufacturer. The purpose of the town meeting was to decide whether or not to allow people to cut down unlimited trees on the nearby mountain to use in manufacturing or to place strict limits on the number of trees that can be cut down. Students had to build their argument, write their argument, review other students' written arguments, and vote to determine the outcome.	Lesson omitted.
Food Changes as it Moves through the Food System: To construct knowledge about the environmental effects of food processing	The lesson was replaced with a video about the impact of human consumption of food, everyday products, and fuel on the planet.	Students reviewed how trends in food packaging and garbage disposal have changed over time. Students were asked to create their own snack company that is profitable, yet minimizes the impact on the environment. Students mapped out the farm to table process of all ingredients in their company's food product, including food and packaging waste and fuel sources used to power their company's factories.
Food Waste: To analyze the amount of waste individuals generate and to develop a method for surveying school-cafeteria waste	The lesson was omitted, and students were assigned to read and answer questions on a magazine article on food waste. They were also challenged to track their weekend food waste at home. Findings were aggregated by the teachers and reviewed with students.	Lesson replaced with teacher-facilitated discussion on single-use products vs. reusable products, with an emphasis on cups and silverware.

Table 2. *Cont.*

Curriculum Unit: Aim	Summary of Class Activities Implemented	
	School A	School B
Cafeteria Waste Inventory: To collect, analyze and utilize data about food-related waste in the school cafeteria.	Students were given an index card to document how much food they threw away at lunch and why over the course of one week. They graphed the results as a class.	Lesson omitted
Share Most Important Message: To share the most important thing they learned in the unit with other students	Students created posters to share their messages, either individually or in groups.	Students created posters, individually, to share their messages.
Total classroom days devoted to the unit:	16 days	12 days

Table 3. Middle School Teacher Interview Theme Results ($n = 3$).

Theme	Illustrative Quote(s)
Adolescent development	I would suggest for other middle school students to use [the curriculum]. I think it's an appropriate time [for it]. [Middle school students] have enough of a world perspective to know that there is stuff outside the grocery store and outside their own kitchen. But I think we kind of take for granted that people notice things and unless we teach it, they won't [notice] because it's not part of everyday experience. I think [this topic] is perfectly appropriate for middle school.
	I think it's really relevant because [my students should] be more aware of the world around them, to be aware of some of the hardships that their families face. So, it's like, "Oh! That did cost mom and dad money when they threw this thing away." So, I think it's a very timely thing for them to be aware of.
	I think [this topic] is valuable. Sixth, seventh and eighth grade is when they start making food choices of their own. They might be like out with friends and buy a soda. So, I think the packaging piece was valuable for them to think like, okay, where this is going to go once it leaves me?
Student engagement with the material and each other	This was probably the best quality work of the two posters we had to make and the writing piece [from this unit]. That's the best quality work I've seen almost all semester. Because it was meaningful to them, it was impacting them.
	I think it was cool for them to be like, "Hey, that's my index card, that's my data, this isn't just some story problem out of a textbook. This is like my lunch last week." I think that was good, and they took some ownership of [the cafeteria waste assignment] that way.
	I think just because it was more engaging, they were more willing to take a risk and work with somebody that they hadn't worked with before. So, that's not content specific, but I think it speaks to the content and how engaging it is because it was cool to see kids specifically like between ethnic groups [work together].
Barrier: Time constraints	Unfortunately, the thing I would do differently would be I would back away, from winter break a tiny bit. Just because I think we could have a more meaningful discussion about, 'did you have change over the week,' 'did you have your mom pack your lunch differently' or 'did you ask for different things when you went through the line.' I would love to have had like an extra day, to have done some sort of post discussion or debriefing or survey or something like that, it just was like we never had time to do that.
	Yeah, I liked it a lot I guess I would like more time with it. I think I did it in 2 weeks or 3 weeks and it still felt like I needed more time.

Table 3. Cont.

Theme	Illustrative Quote(s)
Barrier: Wide span of student reading-levels and abilities	I have some sixth graders that read on like a fourth-fifth grade level. Some sixth graders read on like an eighth-grade, ninth grade level. So, it might be cool if [in the future] there were reading exerts that were tailored to that.
	We have a huge span of students' experiences, capabilities and language capabilities ... I think we have some students who probably could have developed their own research questions and probably could have made their own graph without any, or very little support. I have some students who, just a handful, but probably never understood why we were asking them to keep track [of their food waste]. So, a huge range. To try to close that gap [teacher name] and I [assigned the questions of] how many things are you throwing away and why [for each] day [during school lunch]. We felt like that was something that was approachable for almost all of our students, that they could do quickly, and that they wouldn't blow off so that they didn't lose their basketball time [at recess].
Facilitator: Academic standards	[Any new curriculum must] support stuff we are already doing because we don't have time as teachers, or days in the classroom to add in something that's totally new that we have never tried before that we don't know if it's going to work or support our curriculum. If it supports our curriculum and it's a fresher more engaging way to do it, then absolutely, but if it's going to be a ton of work and we are not sure if it's going to support what we are doing I would say, I would be reluctant to do it.
	So, we used this as a culminating piece of our ecology unit. So, we'd already been discussing like populations, niche ecosystems that kind of thing. So, it was taking the application of what they'd already learned about an ecosystem and kind of giving it a real-world application for them.
	The lessons are good. I think [the curriculum] takes things that we have to teach as [required academic] standards but puts them in an application that is often overlooked.
Facilitator: Curriculum outline	I think if you just gave a teacher this textbook, they'd never open it, as beautiful as it is. I think once a week somebody gives me a book and is like, "Oh, it's great, just read it. I just found this. I had it 10 years ago; it's all about this new thing about teaching Math." I'm like great, you love your resources, but [teaching resources] need to be accessible and that's what this [points to curriculum outline] is like. [The curriculum outline] made [the curriculum] accessible.
	I feel like you guys picked the lessons that were feasible, if not easy, to connect to one another. So, that is good, that's a huge amount of work just to go through that book and pull out meaningful lessons because we can't do them all.
Facilitator: support from researchers	I really appreciated the meeting with [Researcher Name] at the beginning with all of the teachers. We could all give our feedback and just how open she was with, "Call me if you have any questions, here is my e-mail and we can send a grad student." I felt very well supported by her. I appreciated the outline. I appreciated the textbook ... This is way more than I've ever gotten from anybody else. Like I said, a lot of people would be like, "Here's a unit that you can do but you have to find the resources. Here are the resources, but how do you structure it and sequence it?" and I got both. It was like a gift.
	You guys did a great job, you were available and prompt, but you weren't like staring over our shoulder or second-guessing the choices we made. It was great.
	That was awesome- you coming in and sitting down and going over [the curriculum outline]. Because you weren't going to give somebody a [curriculum] book like this and they were going to be like, "Yeah, no, I'm not doing this." So, you coming in and making it like, "Okay, here's the bare bones of what we want you to do," and just like running us through it really quick. So, then we could sit down as a team and go, okay, how do we modify this so it fits the needs for our students and they get something out of it?

Table 3. *Cont.*

Theme	Illustrative Quote(s)
Facilitator: teacher freedom to adapt the curriculum	Yeah, I don't want somebody to tell me how to teach it because they might be a great teacher, but they don't know my students the way I do.
	I really appreciated how open [Researcher Name] was to [us adapting the curriculum]. That made it really easy as a teacher because I think if she hadn't said that and she had said 'follow this piece by piece,' I would've been overwhelmed and not done it. Because you have to adapt it for what your kids already know. This kid needs an extension; this kid needs support. So, if I were unable to make changes to it like I did, I don't think I would have done it. So, that helped a lot.

Equally important, the teachers also agreed that adolescence was an ideal developmental period to teach food systems, particularly from a student-driven approach. One teacher said, "Honestly, [the best part of this unit was] the kids' excitement and just their knowledge that they could impact something and that they had control over something at this age. I think they feel like so much of what they're asked to do is from somebody else's direction. So, the ability to be like, 'I can make a choice in how much food I take' appeals to them." This view is supported by the high levels of reported student engagement in the topic. Yet, despite the developmental appropriateness of the topic, food systems was not an existing part of the science curriculum at either school. Both schools covered niche ecosystems in their ecology units, and School B had just finished a unit on climate change prior to starting the food systems education intervention. Teachers at both schools agreed that the intervention unit on food systems was an ideal complement to their existing science curriculum, particularly since it allowed them to cover the state-required scientific inquiry standards in a new way.

3.3. Content Analyses of Student Work and Student Voting Results

There were a total of 54 posters and 326 coded poster messages across the two schools. Figure 2 provides the frequency of the a priori poster message themes by school. Food waste prevention was the most common poster message overall, with school A featuring twice as many food waste prevention messages compared to school B. The most common poster message at school B was the prevention of packaging waste/disposable food implements, but this message was rarely included in posters at school A. Common stylistic factors of student posters included the incorporation of food into the letters of poster titles and statements to peers in the form of questions.

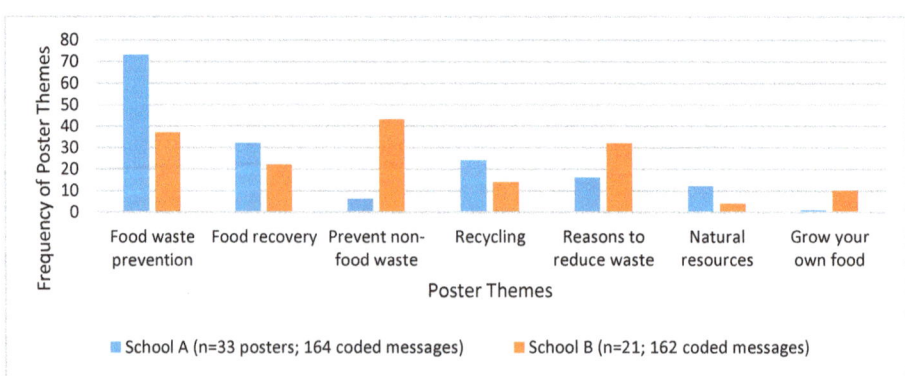

Figure 2. Student poster content analyses results, by school. A total of 54 posters were completed across both schools featuring 326 food systems themes. (Posters were completed in groups or individually, depending on teacher preference.) Food recovery are actions to avoid landfill disposal of wasted food, such as composting.

Figure 3 shows the posters receiving the most votes. These posters were displayed in the cafeterias during the final month of the intervention. Approximately 61.1% (*n* = 347) of the middle school students in School A and 55.1% (*n* = 66) in School B participated in the student poster voting.

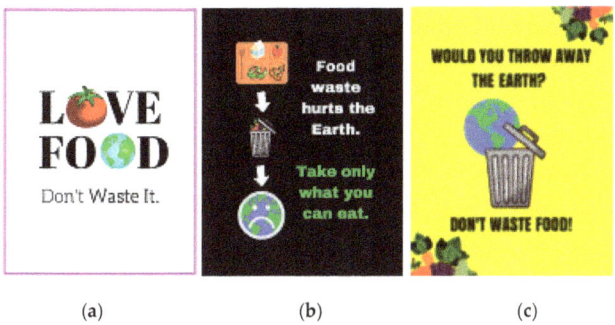

(a)   (b)   (c)

Figure 3. Food waste reduction poster winners, as voted on by school A (*n* = 347) and school B (*n* = 66) that were posted in school cafeteria during the final month of the intervention: (**a**) Top-voted poster at both schools (**b**) Second place poster at school A. (**c**) Second place poster at school B.

3.4. Classroom Survey Results

A total of 268 students were enrolled in a 6th grade science class at the two schools and eligible for the study. About half of the students eligible (*n* = 130, 50.4%) had parental consent and 97 students completed the classroom survey (36.2% of eligible students, 74.6% of consented students). Due to a technical error with the online survey platform, some students were unable to finish their classroom survey. Table 1 provides the demographic characteristics of students participating in the classroom survey, and Table 4 provides outcome results from the classroom survey measures.

Table 4. Comparison of changes in classroom survey measures pre to post.

	Overall Mean (SD)		*p*-Value [1]	Mean Difference (SD) Pre to Post [2]		*p*-Value [3]
	Pre	Post		School A	School B	
Relatedness [4]	3.44 (0.78)	3.39 (0.73)	0.703	−0.10 (0.65)	0.04 (0.51)	0.258
Regulatory style [5]	2.94 (0.82)	3.00 (0.84)	0.656	−0.01 (0.78)	0.18 (0.77)	0.079
Natural resource scale [4]	3.26 (0.92)	3.31 (0.98)	0.784	0.17 (0.89)	−0.18 (0.80)	0.037
Food packaging scale [4]	2.37 (1.09)	2.47 (1.06)	0.515	0.11 (0.83)	0.15 (0.72)	0.976
Food waste: *I try to limit how much food I throw away* [4]	3.56 (1.07)	3.69 (1.04)	0.321	0.20 (1.04)	0.13 (1.07)	0.974
Food waste: *When I am eating, I think about where my food came from* [4]	2.56 (1.19)	2.64 (1.11)	0.603	0.11 (1.25)	0.08 (1.01)	0.702
Food waste: *I feel that one person's food waste is bad for the environment* [4]	3.54 (0.86)	3.80 (0.78)	0.044	0.26 (0.98)	0.25 (0.77)	0.833

Notes: SD: standard deviation; [1] Paired t-test (for normal data) or paired Wilcoxon signed-rank test (for non-normal data); H_0: mean difference = 0; [2] Mean difference: Post score-Pre score; [3] Wilcoxon signed-rank test; H_0: mean difference = 0; [4] Responses were a 5-point Likert scale; [5] Mean from seven questions with the same five response categories that classified respondents into a spectrum of regulatory style: amotivation (1), external motivation (2), introjected motivation (3), identified motivation (4), intrinsic motivation (5).

3.4.1. Self-Determination Theory

Overall, *relatedness* and *regulatory style* did not differ pre to post. However, change in *relatedness* was different depending on ethnicity group (time by ethnicity interaction: F = 5.33, *p*-value = 0.007) with Hispanic students significantly increasing in mean *relatedness* from 2.82 (standard error [SE] = 0.28) at pre to 3.21 (SE = 0.28) at post (Figure 4). Non-Hispanic students and those students who were not sure of their ethnicity did not differ in mean *relatedness* from pre to post. Change in *relatedness* did not differ among other available demographic characteristics and change in *regulatory style* was not different among any demographic groups.

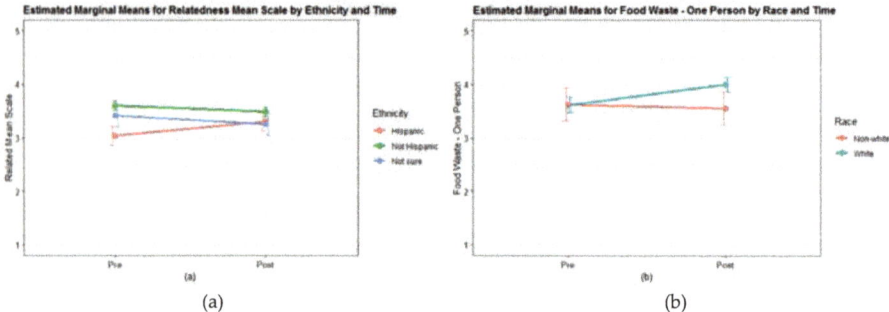

Figure 4. Interaction plots for (**a**) relatedness by time and ethnic group (*n* = 78; averaged over levels of school, sex, race, how a student eats lunch, farm experience, garden experience, and cooking frequency) and (**b**) food waste question ("I feel that one person's food waste is bad for the environment") by time and race group (*n* = 78; averaged over levels of school, sex, ethnicity, how a student eats lunch, farm experience, garden experience, and cooking frequency).

3.4.2. Food Systems and Food Waste Knowledge and Attitudes

Overall, only one of the food waste knowledge and attitudes measures was significantly different pre to post: "I feel that one person's food waste is bad for the environment." In addition to increasing overall, the change in response to this question differed by student race with white students increasing from 3.62 (SE = 0.14) at pre to 4.00 (SE = 0.14) at post (contrast *p*-value < 0.001; Figure 4). Students in non-white race categories were combined due to sample size and did not differ in response from pre to post. *Natural resource knowledge* was not significantly different pre to post overall or within each school group. However, while both schools had similar *natural resource knowledge* at pre, the two schools were significantly different at post (contrast *p*-value = 0.028). School A increased in *natural resource knowledge* from 3.51 (SE = 0.26) at pre to 3.71 (SE = 0.26) at post, where School B decreased from 3.33 (SE = 0.27) at pre to 3.18 (SE = 0.27) at post. *Food packaging knowledge* and the two remaining food waste knowledge and attitude measures did not change significantly pre to post overall or by any of the available demographic characteristics.

3.5. Plate Waste

A total of 1596 plate waste observations occurred across the six data collection dates between the baseline (pre-intervention) time point and the five month follow-up. Frequencies for selection and estimated marginal means for consumption in the intervention and control groups at each of the six time points are provided in Figure 5. Analyses focused specifically on the differences between intervention and control groups at pre-intervention (*n* = 256), immediately post-intervention (*n* = 236), and the five month follow-up (*n* = 286). Across the six time points, participants were 43% female and 57% male. Approximately 37% of participants were in sixth grade (intervention group), 36% were in seventh grade (control group), and 27% were in eighth grade (control group).

Logistic regression results are provided in Table 5. At baseline, the odds of students selecting vegetables was significantly higher in the control group (35.9% selection) compared to the intervention group (22.5% selection). Immediately post-intervention, the intervention group increased their vegetable selection by 29.3 percentage points and differences between groups were no longer significant.

Two-way ANCOVA results for food consumption and food waste at baseline, post-intervention, and five month follow-up are provided in Table 6. While two-way interactions between condition and time point were not significant (across all six time points) for any food consumption or food waste variables, some differences between experimental groups were observed at specific time points. The estimated marginal means for the average consumption of vegetables was significantly lower in the intervention group (47.1%) compared to the control group (71.8%) at baseline. The estimated marginal means for the average consumption of fruit were significantly higher in the control group (57.9%) compared to the intervention group (44.0%) at baseline.

The estimated marginal means for the average hot vegetable waste were significantly higher in the intervention group (26.4 g) compared to the control group (6.1 g) at baseline. There were no significant differences in salad bar vegetable waste between conditions at pre- and post-intervention time points, but at five month follow-up, the control group (on average) wasted significantly more vegetables from the salad bar. There were no significant differences in salad bar fruit waste between conditions at pre- and post-intervention time points, but at five month follow-up the control group (on average) wasted significantly more fruit from the salad bar.

For School B, there were no significant differences in vegetable consumption between the control and intervention groups at baseline, the first post intervention assessment, nor the five month follow up assessment. On the other hand, School A had a significant difference in vegetable consumption at baseline between the intervention and control group, had no differences at the first post intervention assessment, and no differences at the five month follow-up assessment. (Stratified analyses by school not shown in tables or figures.)

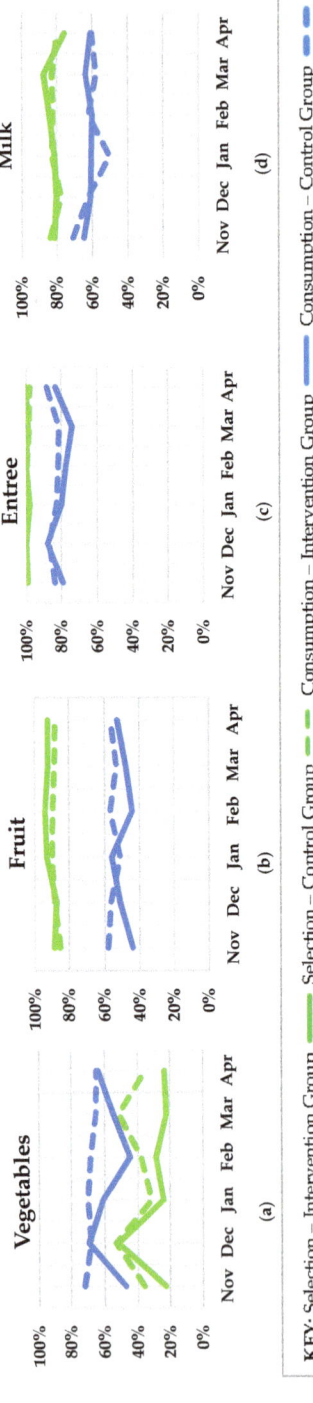

Figure 5. Selection (percent of students who selected food) and consumption (average percent of food consumed) outcomes at each of the six time points for the following food groups: (**a**) Vegetables (includes both hot vegetables and vegetables from the salad bar), (**b**) Fruit (includes both whole fruit and fruit from the salad bar), (**c**) Entrée, and (**d**) Milk. Sample size ranged from 85 to 112 for the intervention group and 145–187 for the control group across the six time points. Estimated marginal means are displayed for consumption variables while original frequencies are displayed for selection variables.

Table 5. Influence of Condition (Intervention vs. Control Group) on Food Selection at Pre-Intervention, Post-Intervention, and Five Month Follow-Up.

	Pre-Intervention (n = 256)			Post-Intervention (n = 236)			Five Month Follow-Up (n = 286)		
	Intervention % Selected	Control % Selected	p	Intervention % Selected	Control % Selected	p	Intervention % Selected	Control % Selected	p
Food Selection (% of students)									
Vegetables	22.5%	35.9%	0.021	51.8%	53.0%	0.880	23.2%	35.3%	0.054
Fruit	88.2%	84.8%	0.500	87.1%	88.1%	0.750	91.9%	87.7%	0.380
Entrée	99.1%	99.3%	0.875	100%	100%	-	100%	97.9%	0.996
Milk	81.1%	83.4%	0.438	80.0%	77.5%	0.859	75.7%	79.7%	0.121

Note: The p-values presented are for the influence of condition (intervention vs. control) on food selection outcomes at each time point.

Table 6. Differences in Food Consumption and Waste between Intervention and Control Groups at Pre-Intervention, Post-Intervention, and Five Month Follow-Up.

	Pre-Intervention			Post-Intervention			Five Month Follow-Up		
	Intervention Mean	Control Mean	p	Intervention Mean	Control Mean	p	Intervention Mean	Control Mean	p
Food Consumption (% consumed)									
Vegetables	47.1%	71.8%	0.006	69.4%	68.1%	0.848	63.8%	64.8%	0.905
Fruit	44.0%	57.9%	0.009	51.1%	56.3%	0.365	52.5%	56.4%	0.454
Entrée *	79.1%	83.5%	0.207	87.7%	86.8%	0.821	83.1%	88.1%	0.143
Milk	64.9%	71.0%	0.265	61.0%	62.4%	0.815	61.0%	60.3%	0.891
Food Waste (grams wasted)									
Hot Vegetable	26.4	6.1	0.015	15.4	19.2	0.384	9.5	9.8	0.965
Salad Bar Vegetable	26.6	19.0	0.466	15.1	18.5	0.756	24.2	50.1	0.029
Whole Fruit	79.9	68.9	0.241	61.2	52.4	0.384	62.0	67.1	0.577
Salad Bar Fruit	51.6	55.7	0.737	49.1	69.9	0.110	46.1	70.8	0.036
Entrée *	38.8	28.4	0.088	19.6	20.6	0.876	33.8	25.0	0.142
A La Carte	0.8	0.2	0.648	2.2	0.2	0.091	0.0	0.1	0.918
Milk †	2.9	2.3	0.219	3.3	3.1	0.782	3.2	3.2	0.940

Note. Estimated marginal means (controlling for gender, school, and entrée consumption) are displayed. The p-values presented are for differences between conditions (intervention vs. control) on food consumption and waste outcomes at each time point. The mean difference is the population mean difference is zero. Consumption means for vegetables and fruit include vegetables and fruit from the salad bar. Hot vegetable, salad bar vegetable, whole fruit, and salad bar fruit food waste outcomes are mutually exclusive. Consumption (n = 76–250) and waste (n = 52–245) depending upon time point and reimbursable meal component. * Entrée analyses did not control for entrée consumption. Entrées include combined protein and grain meal components. † Milk waste is displayed in fluid ounces.

4. Discussion

In this experimental embedded mixed methods study, adolescents who received a food systems education and promotion intervention increased their vegetable and fruit consumption relative to baseline, while the control group decreased their vegetable and fruit consumption. Although the percentage of intervention students selecting a vegetable was less than controls at the five-month follow-up, intervention students wasted less of the vegetables and fruit that they selected. These differences in wasted produce were primarily driven by reductions in salad bar fruit and vegetable waste, likely stemming from the autonomy students have in determining the portion size of salad bar items. Taken together, these findings suggest that food systems education can positively influence dietary behaviors among adolescent youth. However, the plate waste outcomes were not consistent over time with vegetable consumption rates approaching baseline levels three months after the intervention and then increasing back to the levels achieved at 1-month post intervention once the food systems cafeteria promotions were implemented. This may signify the waning influence of the classroom intervention over time, that was later bolstered by the food systems promotions at the end of the year. These changes over time suggest the need to find ways to reinforce the classroom curriculum messages throughout the school year.

The current study findings complement previous literature exploring the relationship between young people's interests in sustainable food systems and diet quality and extends this connection to younger adolescents. Robinson-O'Brien et al. reported that people aged 15–23 years who valued at least 2 alternative agriculture practices, such as locally grown, non-processed, or organic foods, were more likely than their peers to have a dietary pattern consistent with the Healthy People 2010 objectives [15]. Similarly, Pelletier et al. concluded that young adults (mean age 21.9 years) who place a higher importance on alternative food practices consumed 1.3 more servings of fruits and vegetables, more dietary fiber, fewer added sugars and sugar sweetened beverages, and less fat relative to their peers who placed low importance on these practices [16]. The findings from the current study illustrates that a sustainable foods intervention can promote improved diet quality and reduced food waste among a younger population and used an objective dietary assessment method.

The present study findings contrast with the findings of Goldberg et al.'s study on a communications campaign intervention that focused on the overlap between healthy eating and eco-friendly behaviors aiming to improve the quality of foods brought from in packed lunches among 3rd and 4th graders [39]. The authors found no significant changes in the quality of lunch food brought from home and were unable to conclude that classrooms were an effective tool to facilitate changing the school meal related behaviors [39], whereas the present study was able to leverage classroom experiences in the school cafeteria. It is likely that the relationship between healthy eating and environmental sustainability was too complex to be effectively transmitted from classroom teachers to children to parents, and it is also possible that the adolescents in the present study may be a more developmentally appropriate audience to understand this complex relationship than elementary school students.

Traditionally adolescent behavioral nutrition interventions have utilized health or nutrition education to change dietary behavior, but have shown little effectiveness in this age group [40]. The current study used food systems education, using an approach informed by the self-determination theory [41], to influence adolescent behavior. The intervention provided opportunities for students to engage in conversations and activities with their peers to discuss issues related to planetary health, taught students that individual's food decisions have important consequences, and reminded them that they have the power to change their own behaviors. These food systems concepts complement the underlying tenets of the self-determination theory: relatedness, competence, and autonomy. These concepts may also appeal to the increased concern for social justice that is often experienced during adolescence [42,43], further fostering intrinsic motivation to improve dietary behaviors. The teachers in the present study supported these constructs, universally viewing the food system lens as a developmentally appropriate strategy to influence adolescent eating and wasting habits.

In addition, students successfully created a variety of relevant messages after being exposed to food systems education, also demonstrating their level of understanding of this important topic and that 6th grade is an appropriate age for food systems interventions.

The relationship between healthy eating habits and food waste reduction is complicated, as messages to reduce waste could potentially have unintended negative consequences, such as increasing portion sizes and ignoring satiety cues. In the present study, the measured food environment exclusively consisted of food served through the National School Lunch Program, which meet strict nutrition standards. Thus, increases in consumption of these foods may be viewed favorably. Additionally, selection and consumption were measured as a percentage and do not necessarily indicate that an increased amount of food was selected or consumed, particularly since portions of salad bar items were self-selected. In the present study, significantly more control students a vegetable, while intervention students wasted significantly less vegetables and fruit from the salad bar at the five-month follow-up. These findings suggest that the differences in dietary behaviors are unlikely to be explained by overeating behaviors and are more likely attributed to intervention students being more selective about what and how much food they put on their trays. Taken together, this study underscores the importance of reporting the amount of food wasted, not just selection or consumption percentages.

The feasibility of classroom-based farm-to-school programs has previously been questioned [23]. Yet, the teachers in the current study reported that the intervention was feasible and acceptable, as evidenced by their continuation of the intervention without researcher involvement the following year. Teachers viewed the freedom to adapt the lesson to their classroom as essential to feasibility and acceptability. However, these adaptations resulted in important differences in how the curriculum was implemented between schools, and these differences impacted student intervention experiences. The school-level differences in poster themes across schools and differences in the natural resources' knowledge scores mirror the variation in intervention implementation. The lack of significant differences in vegetable consumption between the intervention and control groups at School B also suggest that the desirable changes in vegetable consumption and waste for the overall sample were primarily driven by School A, which also corresponds to the implementation differences on the cafeteria waste unit. These findings demonstrate the importance of incorporating intervention fidelity measures and other implementation metrics in school-based nutrition research.

This study also has important limitations to consider. First, the plate waste data uses controls that are 1–2 years older than the intervention participants. This age difference is consequential due to the likelihood of the older students experiencing increased growth velocity that occurs during puberty. Subsequently, we believe our consumption and waste estimates are conservative given that older children are likely to eat more and waste less relative to younger children. Second, we were unable to conduct plate waste on the same menu days throughout the year. While this does not impact comparisons between comparison and control groups, it makes it difficult to assess trends over time. Third, our implementation assessment only included qualitative measures. Quantitative measures would have allowed us to compare implementation indices relative to other published literature. Fourth, some of the classroom survey scales had poor internal consistency and were not included in our analyses. This may be a consequence of the interrelated nature of food systems concepts, making it difficult to differentiate sub-sections from one another. Fifth, the classroom survey, in particular, had low sample size. This limitation may have contributed to the inconsistencies in the survey findings, such as only 1 of the 3 food waste questions showing significant change. Finally, we did not include any academic outcome measures. Little is known about how nutrition and food systems education impact academic outcomes [44,45]. In order for more schools to incorporate these topics into their curricula, more evidence is needed to link to educational outcomes [23,45]. The teachers in our study were motivated by the high quality writing and group activity assignments submitted by their students during the intervention; this perceived impact on student academic performance likely influenced the teachers' desire to continue the program without researcher support. Quantitative evidence on the impact to academic outcomes may facilitate widespread adoption of a food systems curriculum in middle schools.

5. Conclusions

Adolescence is an ideal developmental period for food systems education. Our study demonstrated that food systems education implemented by science teachers can be used to improve fruit and vegetable consumption and wasting behaviors during school meals. Further, teacher freedom to adapt the lessons was viewed as essential for intervention feasibility and acceptability, but the adaptations hindered implementation fidelity. Additional research is needed to understand the impact of food systems education, particularly food waste reduction messages, on food served outside of the National School Lunch Program, such as desserts and other energy-dense foods. Future studies should also examine academic outcomes to aid widespread incorporation of food systems concepts into school curricula and investigate strategies to reinforce food systems concepts after the classroom instructions end to promote long-term dietary change.

Author Contributions: Conceptualization, M.P.P. and L.C.-S.; methodology, M.P.P. and L.C.-S.; formal analysis, X.B., C.H., J.J.M., A.E.L., and M.P.P.; resources, M.P.P. and L.C.-S.; data curation, X.B.; writing—original draft preparation, M.P.P., X.B., and J.J.M.; writing—review and editing, L.C.-S., C.H., and A.E.L.; funding acquisition, M.P.P.

Funding: This material is based upon work supported by the National Institute of Food and Agriculture, U.S. Department of Agriculture, under award number 2017-67012-28197. Any opinions, findings, or recommendations in this publication are those of the authors and do not necessarily reflect the view of the U.S. Department of Agriculture. Additional funding for this research was provided by the Colorado School of Public Health.

Acknowledgments: This research would not have been possible without the expertise and efforts of the science teachers and nutrition services staff at the intervention schools. We also acknowledge the diligent efforts of the graduate and undergraduate researchers involved in data collection and digital photography analyses. We also appreciate the support and recruitment assistance from Meena Balgopal and the assistance from Pam Koch and Betty Wayman during the survey development process. In addition, we are indebted to Lynn Gilbert for her insight and feedback on how to tailor the curriculum to Northern Colorado middle schools. Finally, we also appreciate the late Stephanie Smith for sharing her validated digital photography plate waste methodology and data collection tools with us. While she may no longer be with us, her scientific contributions and our warm memories of her courageous, positive attitude and infectious laughter will live on indefinitely.

Conflicts of Interest: The authors declare no conflict of interest.

References

1. Kimmons, J.; Gillespie, C.; Seymour, J.; Serdula, M.; Blanck, H.M. Fruit and vegetable intake among adolescents and adults in the United States: Percentage meeting individualized recommendations. *Medscape J. Med.* **2009**, *11*, 26. [PubMed]
2. Krebs-Smith, S.M.; Guenther, P.M.; Subar, A.F.; Kirkpatrick, S.I.; Dodd, K.W. Americans Do Not Meet Federal Dietary Recommendations. *J. Nutr.* **2010**, *140*, 1832–1838. [CrossRef] [PubMed]
3. U.S. Department of Health and Human Services; Office of Disease Prevention and Health Promotion. Scientific Report of the 2015 Dietary Guidelines Advisory Committee, Part D. Chapter 1: Food and Nutrient Intakes, and Health: Current Status and Trend-Continued. Available online: http://health.gov/dietaryguidelines/2015-scientific-report/06-chapter-1/d1-2.asp (accessed on 16 February 2016).
4. Ogden, C.L.; Carroll, M.D.; Kit, B.K.; Flegal, K.M. Prevalence of childhood and adult obesity in the United States, 2011–2012. *JAMA* **2014**, *311*, 806–814. [CrossRef] [PubMed]
5. Briefel, R.R.; Crepinsek, M.K.; Cabili, C.; Wilson, A.; Gleason, P.M. School food environments and practices affect dietary behaviors of US public school children. *J. Am. Diet. Assoc.* **2009**, *109*, S91–S107. [CrossRef]
6. Longacre, M.R.; Drake, K.M.; Titus, L.J.; Peterson, K.E.; Beach, M.L.; Langeloh, G.; Hendricks, K.; Dalton, M.A. School food reduces household income disparities in adolescents' frequency of fruit and vegetable intake. *Prev. Med.* **2014**, *69*, 202–207. [CrossRef] [PubMed]
7. US Department of Agriculture. Final Rule: Nutrition Standards in the National School Lunch and School Breakfast Programs. *Fed. Regist.* **2012**, *77*, 4088–4167.

8. National School Boards Association. School officials worry about wasted food. *Am. Sch. Board J.* **2014**, *201*, 13.
9. United States Government Accountability Office. *School Lunch: Implementing Nutrition Changes Challenging and Clarification of Oversight Requirements is Needed*; U.S. Government Accountability Office: Washington, DC, USA, 2014.
10. U.S. Department of Agriculture. *Ag Secretary Perdue Moves to Make School Meals Great Again*, 17th ed.; Release No. 0032; U.S. Department of Agriculture: Washington, DC, USA, 2017.
11. Gunders, D. *Wasted: How America Is Losing Up to 40 Percent of Its Food from Farm to Fork to Landfill*; IP:12-06-B; Natural Resources Defense Council: New York, NY, USA, 2012.
12. Buzby, J.C.; Farah-Wells, H.; Hyman, J. The estimated amount, value, and calories of postharvest food losses at the retail and consumer levels in the United States. *USDA-ERS Econ. Inf. Bull.* **2014**, *121*, 1–29.
13. Martins, M.L.; Rodrigues, S.S.; Cunha, L.M.; Rocha, A. Strategies to reduce plate waste in primary schools–experimental evaluation. *Public Health Nutr.* **2015**, *19*, 1517–1525. [CrossRef]
14. Upton, D.; Upton, P.; Taylor, C. Increasing children's lunchtime consumption of fruit and vegetables: An evaluation of the Food Dudes programme. *Public Health Nutr.* **2013**, *16*, 1066–1072. [CrossRef] [PubMed]
15. Robinson-O'Brien, R.; Larson, N.; Neumark-Sztainer, D.; Hannan, P.; Story, M. Characteristics and Dietary Patterns of Adolescents Who Value Eating Locally Grown, Organic, Nongenetically Engineered, and Nonprocessed Food. *J. Nutr. Educ. Behav.* **2009**, *41*, 11–18. [CrossRef] [PubMed]
16. Pelletier, J.E.; Laska, M.N.; Neumark-Sztainer, D.; Story, M. Positive Attitudes toward Organic, Local, and Sustainable Foods Are Associated with Higher Dietary Quality among Young Adults. *J. Acad. Nutr. Diet.* **2013**, *113*, 127–132. [CrossRef] [PubMed]
17. Bissonnette, M.M.; Contento, I.R. Adolescents' Perspectives and Food Choice Behaviors in Terms of the Environmental Impacts of Food Production Practices: Application of a Psychosocial Model. *J. Nutr. Educ.* **2001**, *33*, 72–82. [CrossRef]
18. Jones, M.; Dailami, N.; Weitkamp, E.; Salmon, D.; Kimberlee, R.; Morley, A.; Orme, J. Food sustainability education as a route to healthier eating: Evaluation of a multi-component school programme in English primary schools. *Health Educ. Res.* **2012**, *27*, 448–458. [CrossRef] [PubMed]
19. Black, J.L.; Velazquez, C.E.; Ahmadi, N.; Chapman, G.E.; Carten, S.; Edward, J.; Shulhan, S.; Stephens, T.; Rojas, A. Sustainability and public health nutrition at school: Assessing the integration of healthy and environmentally sustainable food initiatives in Vancouver schools. *Public Health Nutr.* **2015**, *18*, 2379–2391. [CrossRef] [PubMed]
20. Elsden-Clifton, J.; Futter-Puati, D. Creating a Health and Sustainability Nexus in Food Education: Designing Third Spaces in Teacher Education. *Aust. J. Environ. Educ.* **2015**, *31*, 86–98. [CrossRef]
21. United States Department of Agriculture. The Farm to School Census. Available online: https://farmtoschoolcensus.fns.usda.gov/ (accessed on 11 September 2018).
22. Ralston, K.; Beaulieu, E.; Hyman, J.; Benson, M.; Smith, M. *Daily Access to Local Foods for School Meals: Key Drivers*; U.S. Department of Agriculture, Economic Research Service, U.S Government Printing office: Washington, DC, USA, 2017.
23. Prescott, M.P.C.R.; Bonanno, A.; Costanigro, M.; Jablonski, B.B.R.; Long, A.B. Farm to School Activities and Student Outcomes: A Systematic Review. *Adv. Nutr..* Submitted.
24. Anderson, P.M.; Butcher, K.F.; Schanzenbach, D.M. Adequate (or Adipose?) Yearly Progress: Assessing the Effect of "No Child Left Behind" on Children's Obesity. *NBER Work. Pap. Ser.* **2011**, *12*, 54–76.
25. Ladd, H.F. *How School Districts Respond to Fiscal Constraint*; NCES 98-217; National Center for Educational Statistics: Washington, DC, USA, 1997.
26. Leachman, M.; Masterson, K.; Figueroa, E. *A Punishing Decade for School Funding*; Center on Budget and Policy Priorities: Washington, DC, USA, 2017.
27. Swindle, T.; Curran, G.M.; Johnson, S.L. Implementation Science and Nutrition Education and Behavior: Opportunities for Integration. *J. Nutr. Educ. Behav.* **2019**, *51*, 763–774. [CrossRef] [PubMed]
28. Saunders, K. Farm to Table and Beyond. *J. Nutr. Educ. Behav.* **2009**, *41*, e305–e306. [CrossRef]
29. Zoellner, J.; Harris, J.E. Mixed-Methods Research in Nutrition and Dietetics. *J. Acad. Nutr. Diet.* **2017**, *117*, 683–697. [CrossRef]
30. Cornwall, A.; Jewkes, R. What is participatory research? *Soc. Sci. Med.* **1995**, *41*, 1667–1676. [CrossRef]

31. A Case for Sustainable Food Service & Nutrition Education—CONVAL School District (NH). *Curric. Rev.* **2008**, *47*, 14.
32. Saldaña, J. *The Coding Manual for Qualitative Researchers*, 2nd ed.; Sage: London, UK, 2013.
33. Wayman, E.; Cunningham-Sabo, L.; Lohse, B. Cognitive Interviews Define Fuel for Fun Physical Activity Survey Items as Face Valid with Rochester, NY Area Fourth Graders. *J. Nutr. Educ. Behav.* **2017**, *49*, S25–S26. [CrossRef]
34. Williamson, D.A.; Allen, H.R.; Martin, P.D.; Alfonso, A.J.; Gerald, B.; Hunt, A. Comparison of digital photography to weighed and visual estimation of portion sizes. *J. Am. Diet. Assoc.* **2003**, *103*, 1139–1145. [CrossRef]
35. Swanson, M. Digital Photography as a Tool to Measure School Cafeteria Consumption. *J. Sch. Health* **2008**, *78*, 432–437. [CrossRef] [PubMed]
36. Smith, S.L.; Cunningham-Sabo, L. Food choice, plate waste and nutrient intake of elementary- and middle-school students participating in the US National School Lunch Program. *Public Health Nutr.* **2014**, *17*, 1255–1263. [CrossRef] [PubMed]
37. Swain, J. A Hybrid Approach to Thematic Analysis in Qualitative Research: Using a Practical Example. In *SAGE Research Methods Cases*; SAGE: London, UK, 2018. [CrossRef]
38. Schreier, M. *Qualitative Content Analysis in Practice*; SAGE Publications: Thousand Oaks, CA, USA, 2012.
39. Goldberg, J.P.; Folta, S.C.; Eliasziw, M.; Koch-Weser, S.; Economos, C.D.; Hubbard, K.L.; Tanskey, L.A.; Wright, C.M.; Must, A. Great Taste, Less Waste: A cluster-randomized trial using a communications campaign to improve the quality of foods brought from home to school by elementary school children. *Prev. Med.* **2015**, *74*, 103–110. [CrossRef]
40. Stice, E.; Shaw, H.; Marti, C.N. A meta-analytic review of obesity prevention programs for children and adolescents: The skinny on interventions that work. *Psychol. Bull.* **2006**, *132*, 667–691. [CrossRef]
41. Ryan, R.M.; Deci, E.L. Self-determination theory and the facilitation of intrinsic motivation, social development, and well-being. *Am. Psychol.* **2000**, *55*, 68. [CrossRef]
42. Yeager, D.S.; Henderson, M.D.; Paunesku, D.; Walton, G.M.; D'Mello, S.; Spitzer, B.J.; Duckworth, A.L. Boring but important: A self-transcendent purpose for learning fosters academic self-regulation. *J. Pers. Soc. Psychol.* **2014**, *107*, 559–580. [CrossRef]
43. Fuligni, A.J. The Need to Contribute During Adolescence. *Perspect. Psychol. Sci.* **2018**, *14*, 331–343. [CrossRef] [PubMed]
44. Joshi, A.; Azuma, A.M.; Feenstra, G. Do Farm-to-School Programs Make a Difference? Findings and Future Research Needs. *J. Hunger Environ. Nutr.* **2008**, *3*, 229–246. [CrossRef]
45. Langford, R.; Bonell, C.; Jones, H.; Pouliou, T.; Murphy, S.; Waters, E.; Komro, K.; Gibbs, L.; Magnus, D.; Campbell, R. The World Health Organization's Health Promoting Schools framework: A Cochrane systematic review and meta-analysis. *BMC Public Health* **2015**, *15*, 130. [CrossRef] [PubMed]

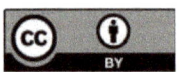

© 2019 by the authors. Licensee MDPI, Basel, Switzerland. This article is an open access article distributed under the terms and conditions of the Creative Commons Attribution (CC BY) license (http://creativecommons.org/licenses/by/4.0/).

MDPI
St. Alban-Anlage 66
4052 Basel
Switzerland
Tel. +41 61 683 77 34
Fax +41 61 302 89 18
www.mdpi.com

Nutrients Editorial Office
E-mail: nutrients@mdpi.com
www.mdpi.com/journal/nutrients

www.ingramcontent.com/pod-product-compliance
Lightning Source LLC
LaVergne TN
LVHW071948080526
838202LV00064B/6707